Pediatric and Adolescent Sports Traumatology

This book is affectionately dedicated to my daughter, Valentina, who, through her vigorous participation in volleyball, skiing and swimming kept alive in me a passion for sport; to Rossella, who waited with infinite patience and understanding during this project; and to my parents who allowed me a place to design, write and edit the chapters of the book in the peace and quiet of my country home.

Foreword

Organized orthopaedic sports medicine's emergence began in earnest in the US in the 1970s. At that time, emphasis was placed on information presented by team physicians for elite collegiate and/or professional teams, especially American football. Societies were formed, courses developed, and journals initiated to accommodate the burgeoning interest in this newly organized field. Non-orthopaedic disciplines such as exercise physiology, sports psychology, nutrition, athletic training, and physical therapy quickly became incorporated in efforts to define new areas of investigation. In 1964, Dr. Bob Jackson, following his return from studying arthroscopy in Japan, introduced to North America the use of arthroscopy as a diagnostic tool for knee disorders. Commercial interests developed an appropriate sized camera, fiberoptic light source, and operative instruments which led to increased interest in and use of the procedure in the mid-1970s in the US. This advance in minimally invasive surgery progressed from diagnostic abilities to true surgical procedures with arthroscopic guidance. This endoscopic method not only revolutionized orthopaedic surgery but the entire field of surgery and its subspecialties. The American Academy of Orthopaedic Surgeons provided highly popular courses in arthroscopy and a generation of arthroscopists incorporated these procedures into their practices and education programs. I performed my first knee arthroscopic surgery in 1975. Internationally, similar efforts began with worldwide collaboration. Fellowships in orthopaedic sports medicine, often dominated by arthroscopic surgeries, were established. In the US, in 1991, there were 19 orthopaedic sports medicine fellowships based on an apprentice model. In 2000, there were 58 fellowships. This number almost doubled (93) by 2009 with 224 fellows that year. Forty-three percent of current US graduating orthopaedic residents take orthopaedic sports medicine fellowships. A Certificate of Added Qualification examination in orthopaedic sports medicine was initiated a decade ago. In addition to orthopaedic sports medicine fellowships, there are accredited sports medicine fellowships in Internal Medicine, Rehabilitation, Emergency Medicine, Pediatrics and, Family Medicine, the one with the largest percentage (80 %) of such fellowships. The field of pediatric and adolescent sports medicine was essentially ignored for some time due to the then held notions that "children do not get significant sports injuries" and, "children heal any injury without difficulty". It always seemed to this author that scholastic athletes accounted for the largest number of athletes in the country and athletes in this vast population do indeed get sports injuries, usually not serious, but enough did have injuries, especially about the knee, that had long-term negative outcomes. This view was not incorporated into the general orthopaedic sports medicine milieu at that time nor was treatment of these young athletes considered by pediatric orthopaedic surgeons to be true pediatric orthopaedics, e.g., treatment of club foot, scoliosis or Perthes' disease. In 1972, in the US there were 4 million senior school (grades 9–12) athletes. In 2010, there were an estimated 25 million athletes, the major increase reflecting the governmental Title IX program requiring equal opportunities for participation in sports by girls/women as for boys/men. Sports were readily embraced by girls and women. A wide variety of individual and team sports are now available for this group of athletes. Twenty million pediatric and adolescent athletes take part in community based programs, primarily in soccer, baseball, basketball, swimming, and softball. There has been a significant rise in individual youth "extreme" sports with skate boards, bicycles, snow boards, and skis. Sports related injuries in patients <18 years old as extrapolated from emergency room visits in the US were estimated to be ∼1.2 million injuries in 2008–2009.

In addition to the technological developments that led to improved arthroscopic systems, other aspects of medical technology began to play increasing roles in sports medicine. Imaging techniques using CT and MRI became revolutionary aids in diagnosis. Anesthetic methods in pain management led to a huge increase in out-patient/same day discharge surgeries. Rehabilitation protocols which emphasized accelerated recovery with resultant diminished return to play time were developed to stem the negative effects of misuse and disuse.

Establishment of a sports medicine clinic devoted to pediatric and adolescent athletes was a pioneering effort by my mentor, colleague, and friend, Dr. Lyle Micheli, who began such a venue in the mid-1970s at Boston's Childrens' Hospital. This clinic became a model for a multi-disciplinary approach to care, clinical and epidemiologic research, and injury prevention program development. Since that time, other clinics with such a focus have arisen throughout the country and the world. There are now multiple national and international courses and symposia as well as textbooks which address this subspecialty area. A core of young US orthopaedic surgeons who are fellowship educated in pediatric orthopaedics and orthopaedic sports medicine will provide the leadership for future endeavors.

The initial reported overuse sports injury was a pediatric one, "little league elbow", described by Adams in 1965 in young boy baseball pitchers in California. Numerous overuse injuries occur at various anatomic sites. These are associated with intrinsic factors—gender, laxity, flexibility, strength, anatomic alignment and, extrinsic factors—training methods/coaching/supervision, practice and competition times, equipment/venues. The overuse conditions are often manifestations of rapid growth at junctional tendon-bone interfaces, e.g., Osgood–Schlatter's Disorder, Sever's calcaneal apophysitis.

Major injuries occur with increasing frequency with age of the athletes given their increased size and speed. Senior schools athletes' injuries accounted for ~ 40 % of sports injuries with 15 % of those requiring surgical treatment. In the junior school group of athletes, which represented ~ 15 % of injuries, only 5 % necessitated surgical management.

Growth must be considered as the pediatric orthopaedic surgeons "fourth dimension" given its impact on normal development and response to injury. This is especially important about the knee, the most common significant injury site, where physeal and intra-articular injuries occur. Musculoskeletal growth is variable in its onset, magnitude, intensity, and duration. Attendant with growth are changes in the athlete's co-ordination, strength, flexibility, and endurance. In assessing immature athletes, one must consider the physiologic age of the patient and not their chronological age. Negligence of this leads to lack of distinction between a child who is 100 pounds of mustache and muscle versus another child who is 100 pounds of facial peach fuzz and baby fat. This is especially true in the "never–never land" of adolescence. It is important to assess the problems of the early maturing athlete versus the late maturer, each of whom will have issues regarding choice of sports. In the US there is a major emphasis on sports requiring throwing, catching, and hitting a ball. The young athlete who does not excel in these skills may consider themself an athletic failure. Directing such an athlete into sports such as soccer, track and field, swimming, wrestling, or crew will provide a venue for achievement.

Structured, organized team sports beginning at ages 6–7 have replaced unstructured free play for many children in the US. There are now earlier competitions with prolonged seasons, sports camps, elite travel teams, and focus on a single sport year around. In contrast to this team regimen, extreme sports appeal to individuals. In response to the intense, competitive atmosphere surrounding some youth sports programs, there is a move afoot in the US of non-competitive sports programs with no scores being kept and no one declared a winner or looser but all a "participant". Children readily see through this by ages 9–10 and very much know who won or lost.

Sports are big business with massive finances driven by media contracts at elite collegiate athletic programs and in the professional ranks. Media coverage has increased the awareness of injuries sustained by these celebrity athletes and their recovery from them or the lack of the athlete's return to prior superstardom. The public's expectations of treatment and outcomes following injury in the scholastic athlete are often based on these cases. Such high profile role models often drive parents and young athletes to feel almost assured that they (the athlete), too, can have such success leading to the development of "premature professionals" with exaggerated expectations. Such attitudes cause a loss of focus and purpose of youth sports. In the US, ~ 5 % of senior school athletes go on to participate in collegiate athletics and of those, only 2 % do so on an athletic scholarship. Of the collegiate athletes, between 1 % and 9 % become professional athletes. Despite such daunting data, many youth sport athletes insist that their future lies in professional athletics.

Involvement in athletics may have negative effects on some participants including psychological "burn-out", eating disorders, and use of performance enhancing medications. The overall effects of sports participation in the appropriate setting are, however, highly positive and include improved physical health with lower rates of obesity, diabetes, heart disease and osteoporosis, and enhanced psychosocial health as seen with lower rates of teen pregnancy, recreational drug use, and higher self-esteem.

Injury prevention is a necessary part of all orthopaedic sports medicine programs and includes assessment of intrinsic and extrinsic factors as etiologic agents of injury. The focus of youth sports programs needs to remain on learning skills, teamwork, fair play, and fitness while enjoying the sport. Despite a large number of youth who remain involved in organized sport, the significant drop out rate (~ 70 %) of youth sports participants in the US by ~ 13 years of age needs to be reversed by innovative programs. Adoption of the European model of the non-school-based community sports club which provides life-long opportunities for sport and fitness and an active life style would go a long way to provide athletic longevity and health in the US.

The above commentary represents reflections on over 60 years of involvement in pediatric and adolescent sports. This has been as a player (little league, senior school, college), a coach (senior school), a parent of 3 high level collegiate athletes, an official/referee, and a sports orthopaedic surgeon and team physician for little leaguers, scholastic, collegiate, and professional athletes. It also incorporates information gained during years of interactions with sports medicine practitioners in numerous fields during faculty participation in national and international meetings and courses. Major changes have occurred over these past 6 decades in diagnosis and management of sports related injuries as well as the establishment of sports medicine as a recognized field of study. The emergence of pediatric and adolescent sports medicine as an acknowledged sub-specialty is gratifying to see.

I thank my colleague, academic collaborator, and friend, Dr. Vincenzo Guzzanti, for the honor of presenting this information and these observations. I congratulate him for bringing his more than two decades of experience in pediatric and adolescent sports medicine to the development, along with other sports medicine experts, of this excellent textbook. This monograph will serve as a valuable reference and overview of the field as well as a stimulus to the readers for additional study in this field.

Carl L. Stanitski
Emeritus Professor of Orthopaedic Surgery
Medical University of South Carolina
Charleston, SC, USA

Preface

At the ending of a clinical and academic career, one reflects on what one has done and also asks if one left a mark in their field. This text was designed to give witness of my study and of research in sports injuries in young athletes. Some topics in the book reflect a personal experience. Other chapters are presented by colleagues selected for their recognized international standing in clinical and scientific expertise.

Over the past 20 years, an increased number of children and adolescents became involved in a wide spectrum of sports. For these athletes immersed in beginning or competitive levels of sport, there is a need for available information to reassure parents of the children's physical, mental, and social development and to provide sports medicine specialists with data for prevention, diagnosis, and management of athletic disorders to prevent delayed or unsuitable treatment. It is also important to not have sports associations lose the major focus of development of young athletes, that is, in addition to learning and enjoying the game(s), and to generate interest in long-term fitness and participation in sports. The various demands on the young, developing athlete must be understood on the basis of normal growth and development of the skeletally immature individual on the way to adulthood, especially in the physiologic "never-never land" of adolescence.

It is well known that very young children have muscle fiber numbers, types, and distribution ratios similar to adults. Since growth can be characterized by a protein anabolic state to support tissue synthesis, children's musculoskeletal systems are much more dynamic than in adults. Developing tissues—bone, articular cartilage and, especially, bone–tendon junctions—are more susceptible to such developmental dynamics. At particular risk is the immature physis. Physeal and epiphyseal damage may cause damage of greater consequences because of the potential negative impact of prolonged growth at the site of injury. More specific discussion of various injuries will be presented in subsequent chapters.

Controversy exists regarding management of capsular and ligamentous tears about the knee and ankle and the consequences of nonoperative or surgical treatment on later joint stability and development. Specific chapters are devoted to algorithms for diagnosis and treatment of ligamentous tears at these sites in children's and adolescents as well as discussion about patellar instability.

Overuse syndromes of the musculoskeletal system due to training and competition and specialized rehabilitation methods for young athletes are also presented. The text contains a specific chapter about orthopaedic disorders which must be considered in the differential diagnosis of sports related conditions to avoid delayed diagnosis and treatment.

Acknowledgments

I would like to thank Dr. Carl Stanitski for honoring me by writing a foreword to the text, the authors for their excellent chapters, and my colleagues in the Department of Orthopaedic and Trauma Surgery at Hospital Bambino Gesù IRCCS of Rome (in the photo), for their direct and indirect scientific contributions. My heartfelt thanks go to the editorial staff of Springer. Special thanks also to Alessandro Adducci of the Eventi Formativi ECM and to Gabriele Bacile of the Servizio Relazioni Esterne, Comunicazione e Marketing, Hospital Bambino Gesù IRCCS, Rome, for their superb photography.

I am very pleased to acknowledge the generous help and patience of my resident contributors to this work. Special acknowledgement goes to Laura Deriu, Rossella Lavanga and Giusy Caruso.

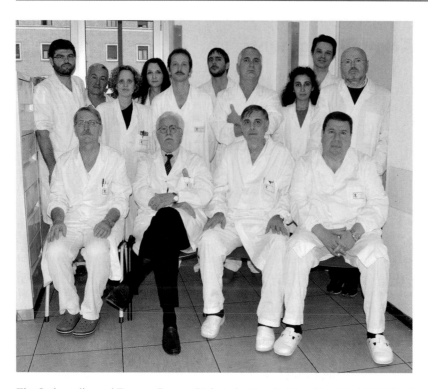

The Orthopedics and Trauma Surgery Unit at the Hospital Bambino Gesù IRCCS of Rome: standing in the back row, from the left, Dr. Angelo Gabriele Aulisa, Dr. Francesco Falciglia, Dr. Susanna Rivelli, Dr. Alessia Poggiaroni, Dr. Pietro Savignoni, Dr. Fabio Massimo Pezzoli, Dr. Rossella Lavanga, Dr. Giuseppe Mastantuoni, Dr. Fortunato Testa; sitting in the front row, from the left, Dr. Renato Maria Toniolo, Prof. Vincenzo Guzzanti (Head of the Unit), Dr. Antonio Di Lazzaro, and Dr. Antonio Lembo.

Contents

The Shoulder

The Elbow

Wrist and Hand

The Hip

The Knee

Ankle and Foot

Orthopedic Diseases

Imaging

Basic Science and Injury in Growing Athletes: Cartilage, Menisci, and Bone

Cosimo Tudisco, Flavia Botti, Salvatore Bisicchia
and Ernesto Ippolito

In the last few years, competitive sports participation among western children has increased [1–3], with a rise in related injuries [4] because top-ranking young competitors undergo rigorous training for many hours a day [5, 6].

1.1 Articular Cartilage

1.1.1 Basic Science

Articular cartilage covers the surfaces of synovial joints and plays an important role in load distribution, shock absorption, and reducing friction during motion. Articular cartilage is composed of hyaline cartilage and has no blood or lymphatic vessels and no innervations, so its healing potential after an injury is very limited [7]. Nourishment for the articular cartilage comes mainly from the synovial fluid. Maroudas has demonstrated that there is no permeability of the bone/cartilage interface to water and solutes in adults and no detectable material transfer occurs across this zone; in the child, on the other hand, the bone/cartilage interface is permeable

to water and solutes [8]. Although articular cartilages in the human body have the same structure and function, some properties, such as cartilage thickness, cellular density, composition of the extracellular matrix, and mechanical features, may vary between different joints and between different areas of the same joint. Articular cartilage consists of one cellular type, the chondrocytes, surrounded by the extracellular matrix [7].

The extracellular matrix is made up of a variety of structural macromolecules and fiber components that give the cartilage its biomechanical properties of rigidity, elasticity, and resiliency. The extracellular matrix is composed of 80 % water, which can move in and out of the tissue during compression and relaxation. Volume, concentration, and behavior of the water within the tissue depend mainly on interaction with the structural macromolecules (i.e., proteoglycans) that keep the fluid within the joint by regulating the concentration of electrolytes. The fluid of the extracellular matrix also contains gases, small proteins, metabolites, and a high concentration of cations to counterbalance the negatively charged proteoglycans. Structural macromolecules of the cartilage, namely collagen, proteoglycans, and non-collagenic proteins, are about 20 % of the dry weight of the tissue: collagen accounts for 55–60 %, proteoglycans for 25–35 %, and non-collagenic proteins for 15–20 %. Collagen is a glycoprotein representing the fibrous part of the extracellular matrix; its fibers are mainly Type II (90–95 %) with

C. Tudisco (✉) · F. Botti · S. Bisicchia · E. Ippolito
Orthopedic Surgery, Department of Clinical Science
and Translational Medicine, University of Rome
"Tor Vergata", Viale Oxford 81, 00133, Rome,
Italy
e-mail: cosimo.tudisco@uniroma2.it

V. Guzzanti (ed.), *Pediatric and Adolescent Sports Traumatology*,
DOI: 10.1007/978-88-470-5412-7_1, © Springer-Verlag Italia 2014

small amounts of Types VI, IX, X, and XI. Proteoglycans can be preset as small chains (i.e., decorin, biglycan, and fibromodulin) or large complexes (aggrecan); the most important non-collagenic proteins are fibronectin and tenascin.

Collagen fibers form a tridimensional scaffold of fibrils that give resistance and rigidity to cartilage. Proteoglycans are macromolecules with a protein core, and many lateral glycosaminoglycans (GAGs), which are long unbranched chains of amino sugars and acid monosugars, that have a negative charge. More than 100 proteoglycan molecules can be connected to a single chain of hyaluronic acid by small junction proteins, forming a big complex called aggrecan. Hyaluronic acid is a long chain of glucuronic acid and N-acetylglucosamine without any protein core, with a high hydration that helps in load distribution and protects chondrocytes from mechanical stress. Proteoglycans, hyaluronic acid, and aggrecan are highly hydrated and interwoven and entrapped into the scaffold of collagen fibers. As water volume in the extracellular matrix increases due to hydration of the macromolecules, the collagen fibers tighten, thereby avoiding swelling and softening of the cartilage and maintaining its biomechanical properties.

There are three different regions in the extracellular matrix of the cartilage [9, 10] (Fig. 1.1):

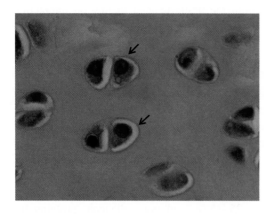

Fig. 1.1 Chondrocytes embedded in the cartilage matrix. The thin layer of pericellular matrix (*arrows*) is surrounded by the territorial and interterritorial matrix (Alcyan-PAS; x 100 objective)

- the pericellular matrix is a thin layer around the chondrocyte, rich in proteoglycans and non-collagenic proteins, but without collagen fibers;
- the territorial matrix is located around the pericellular matrix and is formed of thin collagen fibrils;
- the interterritorial matrix, which forms most of the extracellular matrix, has large collagen fibers and many proteoglycans.

In articular cartilage, there are four different highly organized regions, and each one has distinct composition, mechanical properties, cellular density, and morphology [11–15] (Fig. 1.2). The most superficial is the tangential superficial zone that, although very thin, is made up of two layers. The first one is lamina splendens that has thin fibrils, few polysaccharides and no chondrocytes. The second layer is also composed of thin fibrils but has few elliptically shaped chondrocytes, with the major axis parallel to the articular surface. The extracellular matrix is very rich in collagen fibrils parallel to the articular surface and poor in proteoglycans.

The subsequent region is the intermediate or transitional zone (superior and inferior) that has features of both the superficial zone (superior) and the underlying deep zone (inferior). It is thicker than the superficial zone and has many round-shaped chondrocytes that are very active metabolically, producing a considerable amount of extracellular matrix with large and irregularly arranged collagen fibers, a higher concentration of proteoglycans and a lower content of water than the superficial zone.

In the deep zone, known as radial zone, the chondrocytes are round-shaped, even more active metabolically and tend to form columns of 4–8 elements perpendicularly to the articular surface. The extracellular matrix is made up of very thick collagen, high content of proteoglycans, and very low content of water. The collagen fibers are arranged obliquely to the articular surface in the superior radial zone and perpendicularly in the inferior radial zone.

Collagen fibers cross the calcification area, called the tidemark, a basophilic line that separates the deep zone from the underlying calcified

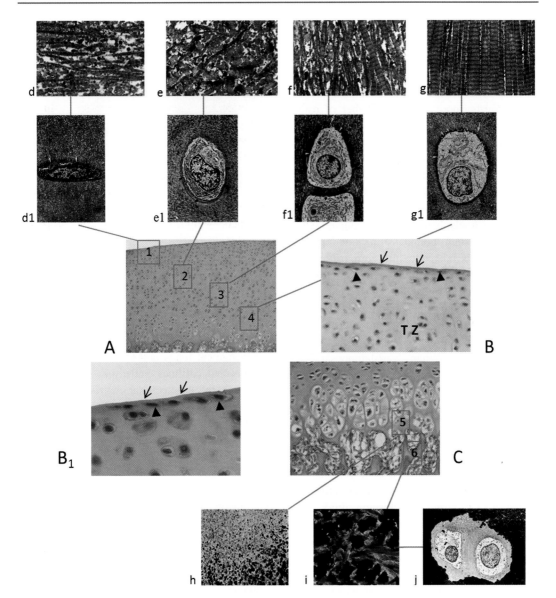

Fig. 1.2 A Microphotograph of normal articular cartilage obtained from a rabbit femoral head (H and E, x 2.5 objective). **B–B₁** High magnification of the most superficial tangential zone with its "lamina splendens" (*arrows*) and the underlying elliptically shaped chondrocytes (*arrowheads*); the area below is the intermediate or transitional zone with its round-shaped chondrocytes (TZ), (x 40; x 100 objective); **C** deep and calcified zone with the perpendicular columns of round-shaped chondrocytes and the underlying hypertrophic chondrocytes (x 40 objective). **d–j** Electron microphotographs from articular cartilage. **d–d1** tangential zone (zone 1 in **A**) with the longitudinally oriented collagen fibers (**d**) and the elliptic chondrocytes (**d1**); **e–e1** Transitional zone (zone 2 in **A**) with the oblique collagen fibers and the round-shaped chondrocytes; **f–f1** Superior radial zone (zone 3 in **A**) showing the slightly oblique collagen fibers and the chondrocytes in the radial columns; **g–g1** Inferior radial zone (zone 4 in **A**) with the collagen fibers vertically oriented and the hypertrophic chondrocytes; **h** matrix in the tidemark (zone 5 in **C**); **i–j** mineralized matrix and the mineralized chondrocytes (zone 6 in **C**)

cartilage, thereby joining two tissues with different rigidity. The calcified cartilage separates the articular cartilage from the underlying subchondral bone; it has fewer chondrocytes than the deep zone, but they are hypertrophic and less active. Furthermore, a small number of osteoblasts and osteoclasts, Type I and X collagen fibers and small blood vessels coming from the subchondral bone are present in this region (Fig. 1.2). The immature cartilage is characterized by the absence of calcified cartilage.

Articular cartilage is subject to various mechanical loads, both static and dynamic. The ability to sustain compression, traction, and shear forces is related to the composition and integrity of the extracellular matrix; in particular, rigidity and permeability are related to proteoglycans, collagen fibers and their interaction, while resistance to tension and elasticity are related to the tridimensional configuration of collagen fibers. When cartilaginous tissue undergoes compression, the fluid of the extracellular matrix tends to leave the reticulum of proteoglycans, reducing the hydration of the negative charges of these macromolecules that repel one another, thereby increasing the rigidity of the cartilaginous tissue and reducing its deformation. Water allows a homogeneous distribution of loads from the superficial to the deep layers; in fact, during compression, fluids cross the cartilage up to the articular surface. Although fluid movements across the cartilage are not easy, this tissue behaves as a sponge: the greater the speed of deformation, the greater the resistance of the tissue, because water cannot flow away very fast. This phenomenon has led to the concept that cartilage has two phases, the solid phase formed of proteoglycans, collagen fibers, and cells; and the fluid phase made up of water that can move across the extracellular matrix. The solid phase is elastic and uncompressible and absorbs just 5 % of the loads applied to the joint, while the fluid phase is compressible and non-viscous and absorbs the remaining 95 % (Fig. 1.3). After an impact, the whole cartilage behaves as a solid uncompressible phase, because fluid has no time to flow across the solid phase [16, 17].

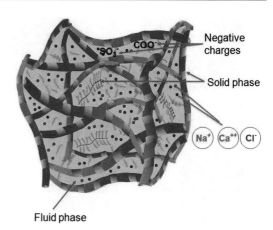

Fig. 1.3 Articular cartilage has two phases: the solid phase is uncompressible and is made up of proteoglycans, collagen fibers, and cells. The fluid phase is compressible and non-viscous and is formed of water and ions that can move across the extracellular matrix

Mechanical loads and the subsequent deformations that cartilage undergoes cause modifications in the extracellular matrix and cellular metabolism. Compression of 25–30 % can be a threshold after which chondrocytes may be permanently deformed, perhaps owing to breakage or reorganization of the cytoskeleton. Static compression forces are able to downregulate gene expression and production of Type II collagen, aggrecan, and non-collagenic proteins; on the other hand, cyclic loads upregulate protein production, in particular aggrecan. Finally, long-term immobilization or reduced loading leads to a decrease in proteoglycans synthesis and softening of the cartilage (chondromalacia) [18].

1.1.2 Injury

Injuries to the articular cartilage with or without involvement of the subchondral bone represent a serious problem, because cartilage has a low healing potential. The reparation process leads to fibrocartilage, rather than hyaline cartilage, which has different biomechanical properties that cannot deal with the stress applied to a joint [19]. It is well known that only small lesions can

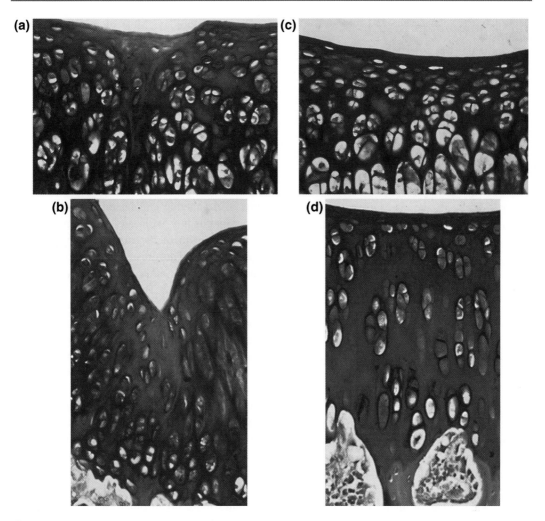

Fig. 1.4 Microphotographs of experimentally induced lesions in the articular cartilage of the femoral trochlea in skeletally immature Wistar rats taken 14 (**a**) and 50 (**b**) days after surgery. Microphotographs of the non-operated knee (control group) 14 (**c**) and 50 (**d**) days after surgery (Alcyan-PAS; x 40 objective)

heal; larger lesions and full-thickness lesions rarely heal spontaneously [20] (Fig. 1.4).

In the young population, two mechanisms of chondral lesions are possible: an acute lesion (chondral or osteochondral fracture) or a chronic overload or overuse (osteochondritis dissecansand microtrauma). Several classifications of articular cartilage lesions have been described in the literature, but the two most popular are the Outerbridge [21] and the International Cartilage Research Society (ICRS) classifications [22, 23]. The Outerbridge classification [21] was published in 1961 to describe chondral and osteochondral lesions of the patella. Nowadays, it is widely applied to all the compartments of the knee and also to other joints. Lesions are divided into 4 grades:

1. softening and swelling of the cartilage,
2. fragmentation and fissuring in an area half an inch or less in diameter,
3. the same as grade 2, but an area more than half an inch in diameter is involved,
4. erosion of cartilage down to bone.

The ICRS classification can be applied to osteochondritis dissecans [22] or to cartilage lesions [23]. It comprises four grades and several subgroups (Table 1.1).

Table 1.1 ICRS classification [22] for articular cartilage lesions

Grade 0	Normal
Grade 1	Nearly normal—superficial lesions
	a. Soft indentation
	b. Superficial fissures and cracks
Grade 2	Abnormal—lesions extending down to <50 % of cartilage depth
Grade 3	Severely abnormal
	a. Cartilage defects extending down >50 % of cartilage depth
	b. Down to calcified cartilage
	c. Down to but not through the subchondral bone
	d. Blisters
Grade 4	Severely abnormal—cartilage defects extending down to the subchondral bone

1.2   Menisci

Several menisci are present in the body: in the temporomandibular, acromioclavicular and sternoclavicular joints, and knees. In these joints, the menisci increase the contact surfaces between incongruent bones, improving load distribution and stability.

The knowledge of their gross and microscopic anatomy and biochemical composition is fundamental for understanding their function and their pathology. Most of the literature has been written on the menisci of the knee.

1.2.1   Basic Science

The characteristics and properties of the medial and lateral meniscus of the knee are acquired during prenatal development, and then, they change throughout growth. The ratio of areas of the medial and lateral tibial plateau and of the area of the medial and lateral meniscus do not vary significantly with age, implying relatively uniform growth of the menisci compared with tibial growth. The gross and histological morphology, on the other hand, change progressively with age. The meniscus is already identifiable between 7.5 and 8 weeks of gestation. In the embryonic and early fetal development of the human knee, the meniscus is composed of densely packed fibroblasts, with a large nucleus-to-cytoplasm ratio, without a definite arrangement of the meniscal cells. Vessels are extremely numerous, traversing the horizontal width of both menisci, and they look more prominent in the coronary and capsular ligaments that represent the principal site of meniscal blood supply (Fig. 1.5).

During fetal life, the collagen fiber bundle becomes more organized with time, with a circumferential orientation in the middle and an oblique orientation at the attachment sites,

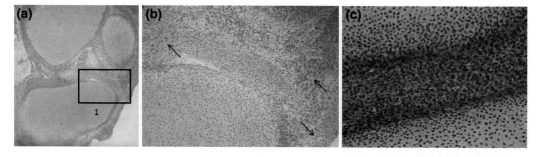

Fig. 1.5 Microphotographs of a developing knee obtained from a 17-week human fetus. **a** embryonic cartilage of the distal end of the femur, proximal end of the tibia, menisci, and joint cavity (H and E x 1.5 objective); **b** a higher magnification of area 1 shows the medial meniscus with blood vessels prominent along the peripheral margin of the meniscus (*arrows*), (x 20 objective); **c** a higher magnification of the medial meniscus shows the densely packed fibroblasts with a large nucleus-to-cytoplasm ratio (Masson trichrome; x 40 objective)

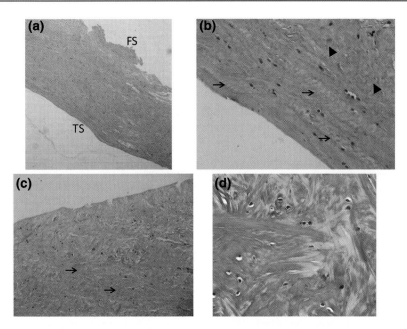

Fig. 1.6 Longitudinal section through a human meniscus of a 9-year-old child. **a** full-thickness section showing both the tibial side (*TS*) and the femoral side (*FS*) of the inner part of the meniscus (H and E x 4.5 objective); **b** tibial side with the radially oriented collagen fibers (*arrows*); the meniscal cells are uniformly distributed without a definite arrangement. The aforesaid collagen fibers change direction and run vertically (*arrowheads*) (x 40 objective). **c** peripheral part of the meniscus with the circumferentially distributed collagen fibers (*arrows*) (x 20 objective). **d** high magnification showing the area where the collagen fibers change their orientation (Masson trichrome; x 40 objective)

where fibrocartilage starts to be present. The intercellular matrix gradually becomes more collagenous and the nucleus-to-cytoplasm ratio decreases.

After birth, the menisci show a higher collagen content. The fibroblasts look more mature, with relatively smaller nuclei, and they are arranged in a more orderly fashion. The blood vessels are less represented in the menisci and appear to be predominantly located in the peripheral part.

In the toddler age, vascularity continues to progressively decrease, proceeding from the inner to the outer part of the meniscus, with a reduction in cellularity and an increase in collagen content. The fiber pattern progresses to the vertical direction of the radial fibers in relation to the weight-bearing stresses. From a biomechanical point of view, circumferentially arranged fibers withstand tension force, while the radially oriented fibers resist longitudinal splitting of the meniscus. Growth of each meniscus follows

enlargement of the distal femoral and proximal tibial epiphysis.

In the childhood and in the adolescence, the menisci are similar to those of adults, but with vessels still represented, exclusively in the outer one-third of the periphery, adjacent to the coronary ligaments, and with an abundant intercellular matrix (Fig. 1.6).

In adult life, the menisci are fibrocartilaginous semicircular-shaped structures made up of collagen (75 %) and non-collagenic proteins (8–13 %), namely glycoproteins and GAGs. Type I collagen is the most frequent (90 % of all collagen chains). Type II collagen is also present in the inner avascular portion of the meniscus. Type III, V, and VI collagen fibers have been described in small quantities. This last one seems to connect different proteins of collagen I fibers, thereby creating a net among collagen fibers.

Proteoglycans, a non-collagenic protein, are 1 % of the dry weight of the meniscus. They are made up of a polypeptide, hyaluronic acid,

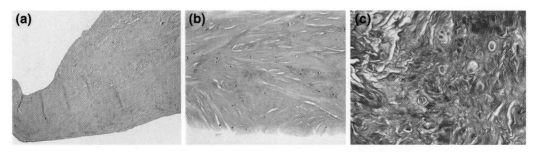

Fig. 1.7 Microphotographs of human menisci in the adult age. **a** meniscus of a 35-year-old man at low magnification (H and E; x 4 objective); **b** higher magnification (H and E; x 10 objective); **c** higher magnification (Masson trichrome; x 20 objective). All the samples have a similar appearance: the fibrocartilaginous cells are surrounded by an abundant extracellular matrix with different orientation of the collagen fibers. No blood vessels are present

linked by a covalent link with polysaccharides (GAGs), negatively charged amino sugars that attract water in the matrix. The most represented proteoglycan is aggrecan, but decorin (a smaller proteoglycan) has also been described. Fibromodulin and thrombospondin, on the other hand, are the glycoproteic component; they can be linked to the proteoglycan aggregates stabilizing the matrix organization.

At histological examination, fibroblasts and fibrocartilaginous cells are surrounded by an extremely abundant extracellular matrix of collagen fibers that have a circumferential direction, ideal for load distribution during compression. Radial fibers are also present to increase structural integrity and probably to prevent longitudinal tears [24]. Elastic fibers (0.6 % of the dry weight of the meniscus) seem to improve the return to the original shape after a deformation [25] (Fig. 1.7).

Every meniscus covers about two-thirds of the articular surface of the joint. In section, the meniscus is triangular-shaped; it is thicker on the peripheral part and adherent to the joint capsule, and thinner on the free edge. Blood vessels are present only in the one-third of the peripheral menisci, adjacent to the coronary ligaments.

The meniscus has important biomechanical functions. It is important in the transmission and absorbance of mechanical stresses. Moreover, because of its heterogenic composition, it has a fundamental role in sustaining compression (inner avascular part) and tension forces (outer vascularized zone).

1.2.2 Injury

Meniscal lesions are extremely frequent in sports players. Men are more affected than women (2.5–1); the medial meniscus (74 %) and the right knee (52 %) are more often involved. The meniscal lesion is usually the consequence of an incorrect movement of the menisci in the flexion–extension of the knee joint mainly due to lack of synchronism during the range of motion of the knee, knee traumas, or knee hyperflexion with a sudden extension. In these cases, the menisci are torn by vertical compression forces and/or horizontal rotational forces.

Different classifications are used for meniscal lesions. One is related to the presence of the lesion in one of the 3 different zones of vascularization of the meniscus: the red/red zone, the most peripheral one, with abundant vascular support; the red/white zone, the intermediate zone, with scanty vascularization; and the white/white zone, the central one, completely avascular. This classification has a prognostic value for the possible healing of the lesions in relation to the presence of vascular supply [26] Meniscal sutures should be systematically performed in children and adolescents with meniscal tears; meniscal resection, even if partial, should be avoided, to prevent the development of degenerative osteoarthritis [27] (Fig. 1.8a).

Another classification is based on the type of lesion [28]. Vertical lesions are the longitudinal and the radial lesions. A neglected radial tear,

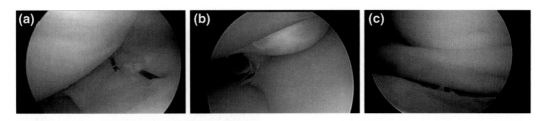

Fig. 1.8 **a** Arthroscopic suture of a longitudinal peripheral lesion of the medial meniscus. **b** Flap lesion of the medial meniscus. **c** «Bucket-handle» lesion of the medial meniscus

usually an oblique one, may try to heal itself and round off into a rounded beak like a parrot's beak (the parrot-beak or flap tear), and this can catch in the joint (Fig. 1.8b). "Bucket-handle tears" are particular longitudinal lesion running from the anterior to the posterior horns, causing the central portion of the meniscus (the bucket handle) to displace into the joint (Fig. 1.8c). Horizontal lesions, on the other hand, are those with a horizontal opening of the meniscus that can be complete or partial. There are also complex lesions that are a combination of the foregoing ones.

1.3   Bone

In the growing athlete, bone is composed of cartilaginous and bone tissues. Bone growth occurs by several mechanisms that differ from long bones to short and flat bones. Furthermore, particular mechanisms are involved in epiphyseal and apophyseal growth and development (Table 1.2). Genetic, hormonal, and environmental factors modulate bone growth during childhood and adolescence, and knowledge of the morphofunctional aspects of the epiphysiometaphyseal growing cartilage mechanisms and speed of bone growth is important for understanding the treatment and prognosis of many injuries in these patients.

1.3.1   Basic Science

1.3.1.1 Long Bones
Long bones are basically composed of two epiphyses separated by the diaphysis, which have different growth mechanisms. Diaphyseal growth

Table 1.2 Mechanisms of enchondral ossification

Type 1	Columns of proliferating and degenerating cartilaginous cells
	a. Growth plates of long bones
	b. Triradiate cartilage of the pelvis
Type 2	Clusters of proliferating and degenerating cartilaginous cells
	a. Epiphyseal aspect of the secondary ossification centers of long bones
	b. Growth cartilage of short bones
	c. Growth plates of vertebral bodies up to 4 years
Type 3	Clusters of proliferating and degenerating cartilaginous cells separated by septa with thick collagen fibers
	a. Growth cartilage of the iliac crest
	b. Growth plates of vertebral bodies after 4 years
Type 4	Direct ossification from cartilage
	a. Metaphyseal aspect of secondary ossification centers of long bones
	b. Apophyseal ossification nuclei (iliac crest, vertebral plates, tuberosity of the calcaneus, etc.)
Type 5	Ossification from fibrocartilage
	a. Insertions of ligaments and tendons

occurs both longitudinally (increased length) and radially (increased diameter). The growth in length of the long bones is the consequence of enchondral ossification of the epiphyseal-metaphyseal centers located at the extremities of the long bones, whereas radial growth is due to enchondral ossification of the periosteum.

Epiphyses have particular growth mechanisms. After birth, the epiphysis of long bones is made up of a cartilaginous scaffold that increases its diameters by interstitial growth. In a given age range (that is typical of each epiphysis), a secondary ossification center appears in the epiphyseal cartilage, and this nucleus grows by enchondral ossification of the surrounding cartilaginous layer. The epiphyseal cartilage is formed of two qualitatively different portions, one toward the joint and one toward the metaphysis (lamina or placca terminale).

The articular portion of the epiphyseal cartilage is made up of two different layers:

1. A peripheral one is the articular cartilage that will be present all through life
2. A deeper one is the epiphyseal cartilage that will grow by interstitial enchondral ossification until adolescence (the end of skeletal growth).

It is possible to differentiate these two parts only by particular immunohistochemical stainings. On the articular surface, chondrocytes are stretched and parallel to the surface. In the deeper layers, they are round shaped and distributed regularly. Near the secondary ossification center, there are clusters of chondrocytes that undergo the same processes of maturation, hypertrophy and degeneration as the chondrocytes of the growth plates. These clusters are separated by thick septa of mineralized matrix, forming a scaffold for osteoblasts to produce bone matrix. The new bone trabeculae have a direction that is parallel or oblique to the ossification center, whereas in the metaphyseal growth, plate trabeculae are perpendicular to the growth center (Fig. 1.9).

These histological differences can explain why the growth rate of the epiphysis is much slower than that of growth plates. The same enchondral ossification observed on the articular side of the epiphysis of long bones is present in short bones and vertebrae up to the age of 4 [29, 30].

The metaphyseal side of the cartilaginous layer around the secondary ossification center bone seems to ossify directly from cartilage. Chondrocytes do not undergo hypertrophy and degeneration, and the extracellular matrix is not degraded. Bone formation is anticipated by loss of its staining with Alcyan Blue , but it is

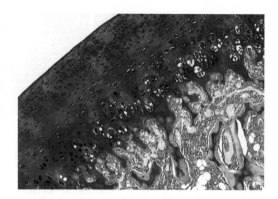

Fig. 1.9 Microphotograph of the articular portion of the epiphyseal cartilage obtained from a rabbit femoral head (Alcyan-PAS; x 20 objective). The chondrocytes differ in shape and distribution from the articular surface to the deep zone. The different histochemical affinities in this area can be observed. (Masson trichrome; x 40 objective)

strongly PAS positive. In this area, it is possible to observe cells that are located between bone and cartilaginous matrixes, with features in between osteocytes and chondrocytes. This enchondral ossification model, that is even slower, is also observed in the ossification center of the iliac crest, in the epiphyseal center of the vertebrae and in the accessory centers of the acetabulum [31, 32] (Fig. 1.10).

The metaphyseal growth cartilage (growth plate) is adjacent to the metaphyseal portion of the epiphyseal cartilage, toward the diaphyseal side. Different layers of cartilagineous cells can be observed in the growth plate:

• Germinal layer: it is close to the epiphysis, and chondroblasts are arranged in the extracellular matrix in a jumble. An injury to this layer results in a halt in growth.
• Proliferation and maturation layer : chondrocytes duplicate and are typically arranged in columns.
• Hypertrophic and degenerating layer : chondrocytes increase their volume and die.
• Ossification layer: this is the terminal part of the cartilage, where vessels arrive and provide oxygen and preosteoblasts at the level of longitudinal and transverse septa.

In this particular cartilage, chondrocytes are arranged in columns, each cell separated from the other by thin transversal septa, while the

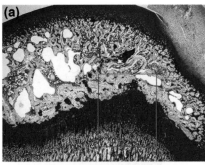 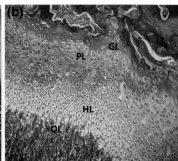

Fig. 1.10 **a** Microphotograph of a proximal femoral epiphysis of a skeletally immature rabbit (Alcyan-PAS; x 10 objective). **b** Higher magnification of area 1 showing the cartilagineous metaphyseal layer. Near the secondary ossification center the condrocytes do not change their aspect; the underlining growth plate shows 4 different layers: germinal layer (*GL*); proliferation layer (*PL*); hypertrophic layer (*HL*); ossification layer (*OL*) (Masson trichrome; x 40 objective)

columns of chondrocytes are separated by thick longitudinal septa. Histochemical staining and ultrastructural observations have shown a different structural organization of the longitudinal septa compared with the transversal ones [33]. They also perform different functions. The transversal septa are progressively reabsorbed at the level of the degenerating layer to allow blood vessel penetration. The longitudinal septa, on the other hand, are the cartilaginous model on which ossification by the osteoblasts, coming from the new vessels, starts to take place (Fig. 1.10).

In conclusion, during skeletal growth, in the epiphyseal cartilage, with the chondroblasts organized in clusters, and in the metaphyseal cartilage, with the chondroblasts organized in columns, we can observe the following processes with different morphological expressions:

1. Matrix degradation of the thin transversal septa
2. Mineralization of the matrix of the longitudinal septa and of the thick transversal septa
3. Blood vessel penetration into the space obtained by the matrix degradation of the thin transversal septa
4. Calcium deposit on the calcified septa by the osteoblasts coming from the blood vessels.

These phenomena are strictly related to one another, and the growth rate of the skeleton is regulated by their speed.

1.3.1.2 Perichondrial Groove

The perichondrial groove (groove of Ranvier) is located around the boundaries between the epiphysis and the metaphysis and is responsible for remodeling the epiphyso-metaphysis of long bones. It is composed of a group of cells and vessels proliferating and differentiating in several ways. Different types of cells are present in the perichondrial groove:

a. The "bone mark": this is a deep, thick layer of cells that will differentiate into osteoblasts that will make the cortical bone surrounding and sustaining the metaphysis. This shell surrounds the metaphyseal cartilage and takes part in bone remodeling of the metaphyseal region of the bone, due to an osteoclastic resorption of its inner part.
b. A superficial layer of cells that will differentiate into chondroblasts, which are responsible for the radial growth of the epiphyses.
c. A more superficial layer of cells that will differentiate into fibroblasts, which will make an external fibrous shell, continuous with the perichondrium and the periosteum [34] (Fig. 1.11). A trauma of the perichondrial groove during skeletal growth could be responsible for the final altered shape and volume of the metaepiphysis of that particular long bone.

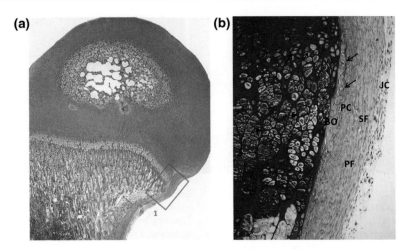

Fig. 1.11 **a** Microphotograph of a proximal femoral epiphysis of a skeletally immature rabbit (H and E; x 2.5 objective). **b** Perichondral groove (high magnification of area *1*): (Alcyan-Pas; 40 x objective). The growth plate is surrounded by the ring of Ranvier. Bone layer (*BO*); osteoblasts (*thin arrows*); prechondroblasts (*PC*); prefibroblasts (*PF*); superficial fibrous layer (*SF*); joint capsule (*JC*); Between the chondrocytes, in the growth plate, the transversal cartilaginous septa (*thick arrows*) and the longitudinal cartilaginous septa (*arrowheads*) can be observed

1.3.1.3 Vascularization

Metaepiphyses have 3 different types of vascularization.

1. Diaphyseal-endosteal vessels that supply blood to the ossification process of the metaphyseal cartilage.
2. Perichondrial vessels that supply blood to the perichondrium and also to the perichondrial groove.
3. Epiphyseal vessels that supply blood to the different ossification centers of the epiphysis: the superficial layers of the metaphyseal cartilage and the epiphyseal cartilage toward the metaphyseal side and toward the articular side.

The superficial cells of the articular cartilage get their nourishment by diffusion of the synovial fluid from the articular space. It has been confirmed, in experimental models, that an interruption of the blood supply of the epiphyseal vessels causes distress for the osteogenetic processes of the epiphyseal ossification center and of the metaphysis growth plate but not for the chondrogenetic process of the articular cartilage [35].

The epiphyseal vessels of growing long bones reach the nucleus of ossification first through the joint ligaments and capsula and then through the peripheral cartilaginous epiphysis, initially following an extra-articular pathway, without crossing the metaphyseal growth plate (type B vascularization). The epiphyseal vessels of the proximal femoral epiphysis and of the proximal radial epiphysis, on the other hand, are mainly intra-articular and reach the cartilaginous epiphyseal nucleus by crossing the metaphyseal growth plate (type A vascularization). These last epiphyses are more exposed to vascular lesions as a consequence of traumatic injury of the metaepiphyseal complex (Fig. 1.12).

1.3.1.4 Short and Pelvic Bones

The growth of short bones of the tarsus and carpus is regulated by the cartilaginous envelope around the ossification nucleus. Chondrocytes closer to the nucleus are arranged in clusters as occurs in the epiphyseal cartilage of long bones, but the organization of the cartilage is the same all around the nucleus because the metaphyseal cartilage is missing. The most external part of the cartilaginous envelope forms the articular cartilage.

In vertebrae, the growing cartilage has a structure similar to that of the other short bones up to the age of 4. The vertebral body grows with an enchondral mechanism around the

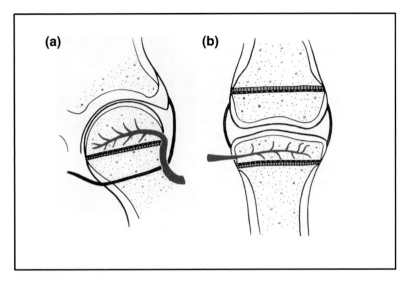

Fig. 1.12 Different types of vascularization of the epiphyseal vessels in growing long bones. **a** Type **a** vascularization: the epiphyseal vessels reach the nucleus of ossification by crossing the metaphyseal growth plate. **b** Type **b** vascularization: the epiphyseal vessels reach the nucleus of ossification without crossing the metaphyseal growth plate

ossification nucleus. At the age of 4, the growing cartilage disappears and the radial growth of the vertebral body occurs by intramembranous ossification from the periosteum.

In the superior and inferior parts of the vertebral body, a hyaline cartilage disk is present. This last one is made by two different structures: the vertebral plate, where the annulus fibrosus is inserted, and the vertebral growth plate. The first one is important to contrast the mechanical loads, whereas the second one, made by short columns of chondrocytes separated by thick extracellaluar matrix septae, is responsible for the longitudinal vertebral growth.

humeral contributing 80 % to upper extremity growth, the distal radial 75 % and the distal ulnar 80 % [36].

It is also important, as Green and Anderson [37] reported in their tables, that the amount of growth of the long bones is not constant but varies with age: it is quite rapid in the lower extremities, especially distally, during childhood and then slows down until the pubertal period, when the growth plates are under the stimulus of sex hormones . At the pubertal growth spurt, vertebral and pelvis plates are especially active, while the limb growth plates tend to reduce their contribution to growth.

1.3.1.5 Functional Aspects

The metaepiphyseal complexes of the long bones do not participate with the same percentage in the growing process. In the lower extremity, the knee metaphyses are more active regarding lower extremity growth than the hip and the ankle metaphysis, with the distal femoral metaphysis contributing 70 % and the proximal tibial metaphysis 55 %. In the upper extremity, on the other hand, the metaphyses away from the elbow are the more active ones, with the

1.3.2 Injury

The longitudinal growth of the bone can be temporarily or permanently damaged by traumatic, vascular, metabolic, infectious, thermal, or iatrogenic factors. Traumatic lesions of the epiphyso-metaphyseal area have an unpredictable prognosis. In fact, the traumatic lesion involves the metaepiphysis but sometimes the articular cartilage as well, with bone growth disorders and also degenerative changes of the joint. It is also impossible to determine qualitatively and quantitatively how much each of these anatomical components have been damaged by the trauma. A few long-term follow-up studies of traumatic lesions of growing cartilages have concluded that it is impossible to predict the outcome of these lesions.

An experimental histological study on induced metaepiphyseal lesions in rabbits showed that the fracture line reaches the articular cartilage, the epiphyseal growing center and then the metaphyseal cartilage, dividing, at this level, the cellular columns at the hypertrophic or degenerative layer, but there are reports of propagation of the fracture line into the germinal layer with devascularization of this layer [38]. A lesion of the vessels at the fracture line produces a hematoma with a consequent inflammatory reaction. Necrotic cartilage cells are present around this area.

In areas where the blood supply was interrupted or the physis was incorrectly aligned, trabecular bone will eventually replace the cartilage and form a bony bridge between metaphysis and epiphysis (Fig. 1.13).

Regardless of the type of fracture, if the epiphyseal blood supply is interrupted as a consequence of the fracture, the subsequent ischemia of the germinal cells of the affected physis can lead to serious growth disorders.

Experiments demonstrating damage to the physis after epiphyseal vessel occlusion were reported by Trueta and Amato [39] and more recently by Kim and Su [40]. In experimentally induced ischemia of the proximal femoral epiphysis in rabbits, Tudisco et al. [35] showed that an ischemic insult to the femoral capital epiphysis results in necrosis of the epiphyseal growth plate which is more severe if the ischemia is induced before the appearance of the secondary ossification center. Small ectopic centers of ossification in the epiphyseal cartilage, around the epiphyseal ossification nucleus, are the result of the revascularization process after the ischemic insult; their presence jeopardized the uniformity of the proximal femoral epiphysis causing the femoral head deformity (Fig. 1.14).

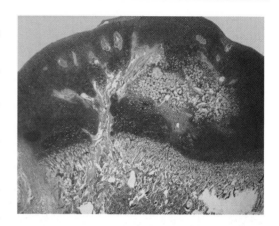

Fig. 1.13 Microphotograph of the proximal femoral epiphysis in a skeletally immature rabbit after interruption of vascular supply. In the ischemic and then revascularized areas, trabecular bone replaced the cartilage and formed a bony bridge between metaphysis and epiphysis

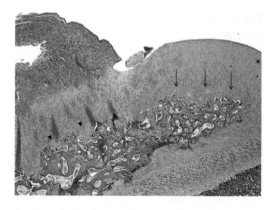

Fig. 1.14 Microphotograph of experimentally induced ischemia in the proximal femoral epiphysis in a skeletally immature rabbit. Small ectopic centers of ossification in the epiphyseal cartilage (*arrows*), around the epiphyseal ossification nucleus (*arrowheads*), are the result of the revascularization process after the ischemic insult

The incidence of physeal fractures in relation to the totality of fractures in children is around 15 %, but some authors think this number could be closer to 30 % [41–43]. Regarding the age at occurrence, it is a well-known fact that the incidence is higher in ages close to puberty, and therefore, chronologically slightly sooner in girls than in boys [41, 44], and these fractures are more frequent in boys than in girls. The two most

(a)   **(b)**   **(c)**

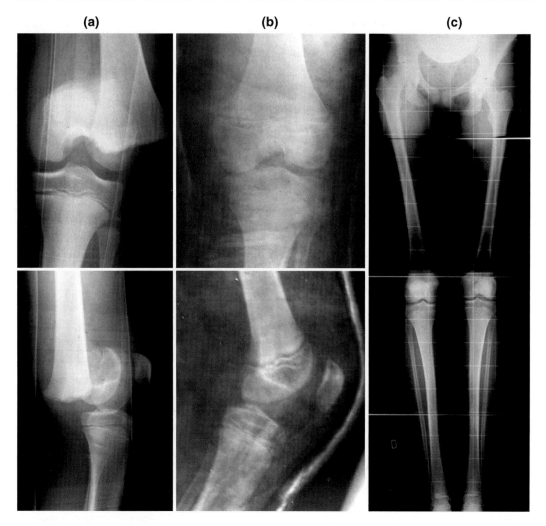

Fig. 1.15 a X-rays of a Salter–Harris type 2 left distal femoral physeal fracture in an 8-year-old girl. **b** The fracture was treated by a very good closed reduction and immobilization by a long-leg cast with flexed knee and without weight-bearing for 5 weeks, followed by a straight long-leg cast for additional 5 weeks. **c** The X-rays taken after 5 years showed a leg length discrepancy due to a left femur shortening of almost 4 cm

widely used classifications of fractures of the growth plate are from Salter and Harris [43] and Ogden et al. [45].

The prognosis for physeal fractures depends on a series of factors: the type of fracture, the amount of growth remaining, the displacement of the fragments, the anatomical reduction, and the severity of the injury. The most common sequelae of physeal fractures are partial or total cessation of bone growth, due to a premature physeal closure, or a delay in growth, with a consequent shortening and/or angular deformity of the bone segment involved (Figs. 1.15 and 1.16). In certain types of fractures, a stimulus of the growth plate closest to the fracture can occur.

Fig. 1.16 **a** X-rays of a Salter–Harris type 3 right distal tibial physeal fracture in a 9-year-old boy. The fracture was treated by closed reduction and immobilization with a short-leg cast for 5 weeks. **b** The X-rays taken after 12 years showed a very severe varus deformity of the ankle

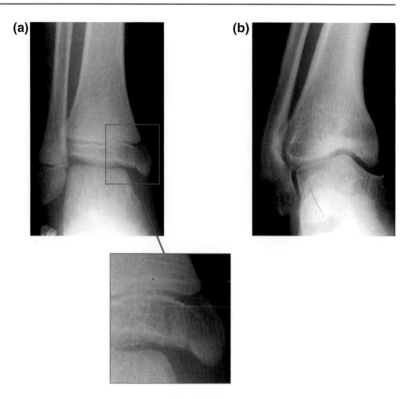

References

1. Hallal PC, Victora CG, Azevedo MR, Wells JC (2006) Adolescent physical activity and health: a systematic review. Sports Med 36:1019–1030
2. Strong WB, Malina RM, Blimkie CJ, Daniels SR, Dishman RK, Gutin B, Hergenroeder AC, Must A, Nixon PA, Pivarnik JM, Rowland T, Trost S, Trudeau F (2005) Evidence based physical activity for school-age youth. J Pediatr 146:732–737
3. Biddle SJ, Asare M (2011) Physical activity and mental health in children and adolescents: a review of reviews. Br J Sports Med 45:886–895
4. Luke A, Lazaro RM, Bergeron MF, Keyser L, Benjamin H, Brenner J, d'Hemecourt P, Grady M, Philpott J, Smith A (2011) Sports-related injuries in youth athletes: is overscheduling a risk factor? Clin J Sport Med 21:307–314
5. Bruns W, Maffulli N (2000) Lower limb injuries in children in sports. Clin Sports Med 19:637–662
6. Brenner JS, American Academy of Pediatrics Council on Sports Medicine and Fitness (2007) Overuse injuries, overtraining, and burnout in child and adolescent athletes. Pediatrics 119:1242–1245
7. Buckwalter JA, Mankin HJ (1998) Articular cartilage: tissue design and chondrocyte-matrix interactions. Instr Course Lect 47:477–486
8. Maroudas A, Bullough P, Swanson SA, Freeman MA (1968) The permeability of articular cartilage. J Bone Joint Surg Br 50(1):166–177
9. Guilak F, Alexopoulos LG, Upton ML, Youn I, Choi JB, Cao L, Setton LA, Haider MA (2006) The pericellular matrix as a transducer of biomechanical and biochemical signals in articular cartilage. Ann N Y Acad Sci 1068:498–512
10. Poole CA (1997) Articular cartilage chondrons: form, function and failure. J Anat 191:1–13
11. Hollander AP, Dickinson SC, Kafienah W (2010) Stem cells and cartilage development: complexities of a simple tissue. Stem Cells 28:1992–1996
12. Simon WH (1970) Scale effects in animal joints. I. Articular cartilage thickness and compressive stress. Arthritis Rheum 13:244–256
13. Modl JM, Sether LA, Haughton VM, Kneeland JB (1991) Articular cartilage: correlation of histologic zones with signal intensity at MR imaging. Radiology 181:853–855
14. Bullough P, Goodfellow J (1968) The significance of the fine structure of articular cartilage. J Bone Joint Surg Br 50:852–857
15. Waldschmidt JG, Rilling RJ, Kajdacsy-Balla AA, Boynton MD, Erickson SJ (1997) In vitro and in vivo MR imaging of hyaline cartilage: zonal anatomy, imaging pitfalls, and pathologic conditions. Radiographics 17:1387–1402
16. Becerra J, Andrades JA, Guerado E, Zamora-Navas P, López-Puertas JM, Reddi AH (2010) Articular

cartilage: structure and regeneration. Tissue Eng Part B Rev 16:617–627

17. Lu XL, Mow VC (2008) Biomechanics of articular cartilage and determination of material properties. Med Sci Sports Exerc 40:193–199

18. Buckwalter JA, Einhorn TA, Simon SR (2000) Orthopaedic basic science, 2nd edn. American Academy of Orthopaedic Surgeons, Rosemont

19. Browne JE, Branch TP (2000) Surgical alternatives for treatment of articular cartilage lesions. J Am Acad Orthop Surg 8:180–189

20. Hjelle K, Solheim E, Strand T, Muri R, Brittberg M (2002) Articular cartilage defects in 1,000 knee arthroscopies. Arthroscopy 18:730–734

21. Outerbridge RE (1961) The etiology of chondromalacia patellae. J Bone Joint Surg Br 43-B:752–757

22. International Cartilage Research Society 3rd Meeting (2000) Gotenborg, Sweden

23. Brittberg M, Winalski CS (2003) Evaluation of cartilage injuries and repair. J Bone Joint Surg Am 85-A(Suppl 2):58–69

24. Renström P, Johnson RJ (1990) Anatomy and biomechanics of the menisci. Clin Sports Med 9:523–538

25. Walker PS, Erkman MJ (1975) The role of the menisci in force transmission across the knee. Clin Orthop Relat Res 109:184–192

26. Arnoczky SP, Warren RF (1982) Microvasculature of the human meniscus. Am J Sports Med 10:90–95

27. Noyes FR, Chen RC, Barber-Westin SD, Potter HG (2011) Greater than 10-year results of red-white longitudinal meniscal repairs in patients 20 years of age or younger. Am J Sports Med 39:1008–1017

28. Easley ME, Cushner FD, Scott N (2001) Arthroscopic meniscal resection. In: Insall JN, Scott WN (eds) Surgery of the knee, 3rd edn. Churchill Livingstone, Philadelphia, pp 473–520

29. Cooper RR (1978) Clinical roentgenographic and laboratory studies of epiphyseal-metaphyseal dysplasias. Residents lecture. Department of Orthopaedic Surgery, University of Iowa, Iowa

30. Ippolito E, Postacchini F, Scola E (1983) Skeletal growth in normal and pathological conditions. Ital J Orthop Traumatol 9:115–127

31. Ponseti IV, Pedrini-Mille A, Pedrini V (1968) Histological and chemical analysis of human iliac crest cartilage. I. Observations on trunk growth. Calcif Tissue Res 2:197–213

32. Kalayjian DB, Cooper RR (1972) Osteogenesis of the epiphysis: a light and electron microscopic study. Clin Orthop Relat Res 85:242–256

33. Ippolito E (1981) Histochemical study of human epiphyseal cartilage. Ital J Orthop Traumatol 7:223–234

34. Shapiro F, Holtrop ME, Glimcher MJ (1977) Organization and cellular biology of the perichondrial ossification groove of Ranvier: a morphological study in rabbits. J Bone Joint Surg Am 59:703–723

35. Tudisco C, Savarese E, Botti F, Febo A, Ippolito E (2005) Histopathologic changes in the growth plate cartilage of proximal femoral epiphysis following interruption of blood supply. An experimental investigation in immature rabbits. Abstract from 24th European Pediatric Orthopaedic Society (EPOS) Congress. Palma de Mallorca., Spain

36. Serafini-Fracassini A, Smith JW (1974) The structure and biochemistry of cartilage. Churchill Livingstone, Edinburgh

37. Anderson M, Green WT, Messner MB (1963) Growth and predictions of growth in the lower extremities. J Bone Joint Surg Am 45:1–14

38. Ogden JA (1993) The pathology of growth plate injury. Mapfre Medicina 4(Suppl. 2):8–14

39. Trueta J, Amato VP (1960) The vascular contribution to osteogenesis. III. Changes in the growth cartilage caused by experimentally induced ischaemia. J Bone Joint Surg Br 42:571–587

40. Kim HK, Su PH (2002) Development of flattening and apparent fragmentation following ischemic necrosis of the capital femoral epiphysis in a piglet model. J Bone Joint Surg Am 84:1329–1334

41. Mizuta T, Benson WM, Foster BK, Paterson DC, Morris LL (1987) Statistical analysis of the incidence of physeal injuries. J Pediatr Orthop 7:518–523

42. Mann DC, Rajmaira S (1990) Distribution of physeal and nonphyseal fractures in 2,650 long-bone fractures in children aged 0–16 years. J Pediatr Orthop 10:713–716

43. Salter R, Harris W (1963) Injuries involving the epiphyseal plate. J Bone Joint Surg Am 45:587–622

44. Morscher E (1968) Strength and morphology of growth cartilage under hormonal influence of puberty. Animal experiments and clinical study on the etiology of local growth disorders during puberty. Reconstr Surg Traumatol 10:3–104

45. Ogden JA, Ganey T, Light TR, Southwick WO (1993) The pathology of acute chondro-osseous injury in the child. Yale J Biol Med 66:219–233

Basic Science and Injury in Growing Athletes: Muscle, Tendon, and Ligament

Antonio Gigante, Alberto Busilacchi, Francesco Greco and Luigi de Palma

Children and adolescents should not be considered "small adults": this concept is also valid for the soft tissues of the locomotor apparatus. Since the young athlete is growing, anatomical structures are more flexible and somewhat weaker than those of an adult, which entail different injury risk factors. Despite that, it is quite rare to observe complete soft tissue tears, especially from an indirect mechanism of injury. Concerning the basic science of the musculoskeletal soft tissue healing in the young, it is important to point out that today very little literature is available. Thus, perhaps incorrectly, we assume that the healing in growing people undergoes the same phase as that in adults: however, higher concentrations of growth factors (GFs) and cell responsivity and tissue conditioning to external stimuli let us hypothesize a faster recovery period. This hypothesis arises only from preclinical studies and lacks direct evidence in human tissues [1]. However, it is also known that age influences the quality of scar tissue, mostly in joint capsules, in ligament and tendons: in children and adolescents up to 20 years scar is lax and rich in elastic proteins, leading to a higher risk of relapse [2–8].

2.1 Epidemiology

Commonly, pediatric injuries are wrongly discussed as a single group: in fact, there is wide variability in injuries based on size, speed, and strength among pre-adolescents, adolescents, and young adults. Wessel et al. [9] reviewed the pattern of intra-articular knee lesions in different pediatric age groups by evaluating post-traumatic hemarthrosis in patients up to 16 years of age. Patients with knee trauma were divided into three age-related groups which showed that the incidence of hemarthrosis increased with increasing age. The most common diagnosis in all groups was sprains without disruption of ligaments, which was presumed to be due to a synovial tear. Damore et al. [10] reported the relative frequency of sports-related injuries to be 41 % of all musculoskeletal injuries among 1,421 children and adolescents. They further stated that the injuries involved more commonly males (62 %), and the most common injury sites included the ankle and foot (20 %), followed by the forearm-wrist (17 %) and hand (17 %). Sprains and contusions were the most common types of injuries followed by fractures. Taylor and Attia [11] described the demographics and types of sports-related injuries in patients between the ages of 5 and 18 years who presented to the emergency department. An average age of 13.0 years for males and 12.4 years

A. Gigante (✉) · A. Busilacchi · F. Greco · L. de Palma
Clinical Orthopedics, Department of Clinical and Molecular Sciences, School of Medicine, Marche Polytechnic University, Via Tronto 10, 60126, Ancona, Italy
e-mail: a.gigante@univpm.it

A. Busilacchi
e-mail: albertobusilacchi@yahoo.it

for females was found, with the majority of traumas involving males (71 %). Sprains, strains,
fractures, contusions, and lacerations accounted
for 90 % of injury types. Even insurance compa-
nies commissioned a study to assess injury risk
among children, adolescents, males, and females
[12]: the Authors reported an increasing injury
ratio with increasing age and pointed out a relative
higher risk of females.

2.2 Risk Factors for Soft Tissue Injury in Growing Athletes

2.2.1 Growth and Histological Features

Growth is a crucial factor in the occurrence of
injuries, mostly overuse ones, in children and
adolescent athletes. Growing hyaline cartilage in
immature skeleton is found not only at the
growth plate but also in epiphyseal region (the
so-called osteo-chondro-epiphysis) (Fig. 2.1)
and at apophyseal insertions. In adolescents,
tendon and ligament insertions to bone are
mediated by a thick layer of cartilaginous tissue
(Fig. 2.2). In younger subjects, tendons and ligaments are directly inserted into hyaline cartilage
(Fig. 2.3). Both biomechanical and clinical evidences lead this growth cartilage to be considered weaker to direct and indirect trauma (such
as avulsion injuries) [13] and repetitive micro-
traumas than the mature adult counterpart [14].

Growth itself is a risk factor for injuries in the
young athletes: in fact, soft tissues passively
elongate in response to the longitudinal growth
of the bones, thus becoming progressively tigh-
ter, especially during periods of "rapid growth."
This decreased flexibility exposes the young,
and mostly adolescents, to injure.

2.2.2 Gender

For a number of years, several anatomic/physi-
ologic differences have been thought to

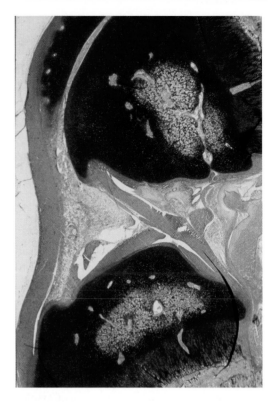

Fig. 2.1 Growing hyaline cartilage in immature skeleton is found not only at the growth plate but also in
epiphyseal region (the so-called osteo-chondro-epiphysis) and at apophyseal insertions

influence patterns of injury between males and
females, including degree of ligamentous laxity,
differences in muscle recruitment, pelvis structure, lower extremity alignment, mechanics of
jumping and landing, muscle strength and conditioning and hormonal regulation [15, 16].
Furthermore, changes in the number of females
participating in sports and the intensity of
training and competition have to be considered.
By comparing high school cross-country track
injuries between males and females, Rauh et al.
[17] found a higher risk of injury in girls. Girls
were twice as likely to get injured during a
competitive meet than boys.

2.2.3 Training Errors

Abrupt changes and unsound increases in
intensity of training clearly predispose a person

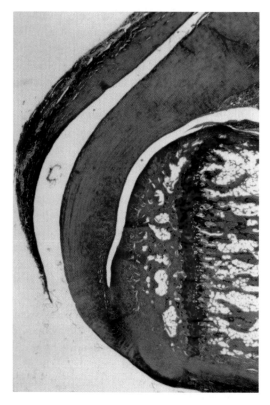

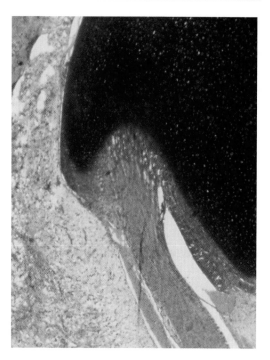

Fig. 2.3 In younger subjects, tendons and ligaments are directly inserted into hyaline cartilage

Fig. 2.2 In adolescents, tendon and ligament insertions to bone are mediated by a thick layer of cartilaginous tissue

to overuse injury [18]. Poorly trained coaches and overzealous parents must share the blame with the athletes in this regard. In general, increasing the duration or intensity of training by more than 10 % per week should be avoided because it increases fatigue significantly and is responsible for a higher risk of acute traumas and overuse injuries [19]. Furthermore, the wrong execution of technical gesture might determine injuries, in both upper and lower limbs. In fact, quick change of direction, uncontrolled kicks or throws are commonly associated with sprains or strains and insertional pain syndromes.

2.2.4 Muscle–Tendon Imbalance

Adolescent growth peak is normally accompanied by decreased flexibility [20] and an

increased risk of overuse injury. Traction apophysitis is another form of disease in which microtraumatic etiology unloads kinematic energy on apophyses rather than on the tendon.

Young throwing athletes seem prone to chronic anterior subluxation of the shoulder. This may reflect contracture of the posterior capsule as a result of chronic overhead use with secondary anterior laxity [14]. Similarly, today, lots of young athletes are showing more insertional overuse injuries and avulsion injuries because inappropriate training sessions are developing muscle mass when the tendons and mainly their bony insertions are still weak and unable to absorb the loads generated during movement [21, 22].

2.2.5 Anatomical Malalignment

Femoral anteversion, external tibial torsion, leg length discrepancies, patellofemoral incongruency, genu varum/valgum, and pes planus are all considered malalignment conditions. Excessive femoral anteversion is extremely common, mostly in females, as it may lead to patellofemoral joint problems whose symptoms at the beginning are referred to tendons or its bony insertions [23]. External tibial torsion may play a role as a predisposing mechanical factor in the onset of Osgood–Schlatter disease in male athletes [13]. However, since it may contribute to injury in young athletes, anatomical malalignment is generally well tolerated by the body, and thus, care must be taken not to overlook its role [18].

2.2.6 Footwear and Playing Surface

Proper shoes, specifically suitable for the young athlete's anatomy and activity, must provide support and impact absorption as well as protection from hyperpronation, chronic tendon, and muscle inflammation or ankle sprain. Too soft shoes and soles should be avoided because they modify the lower limb proprioception giving analog chronic inflammatory conditions in joint capsules, tendons, and ligaments. Relative hardness of the playing ground is also another factor that can lead to injury. In fact, a subtle change in hard surfaces has been reported to be significantly associated to overuse injury [24, 25] in children and mostly adolescents.

2.3 Muscle Injuries

Muscle damage is defined as the lesion of muscle fibers without involvement of the extracellular matrix, blood vascularization or innervation [26]. The severity of muscle injury is defined by the amount of muscle tissue involved and by the extent and location of the effusion. Numerous attempts to classify muscle injuries have been proposed for years [27–32]: various criteria should be taken into consideration which makes it difficult to set up a classification. Muscle injuries can be divided into subacute, acute, and chronic ones [31]. Subacute lesions are injuries that are mainly caused by an eccentric overload. Chronic lesions are the

development of acute and subacute lesions of considerable size, or the evolution of a pathological process of healing because of management errors. The first element to be considered in the classifications is the direct or indirect nature of the acute trauma [33]:

- *Muscle injury from direct trauma*, according to the classical interpretation, it implies the existence of a force acting from the outside. Frequently, these injuries are considered as minor pathological conditions, designed to heal quickly which have no consequences. Considering from an anatomic/pathologic viewpoint, the so-called "contusion" does not differ from a muscle injury due to other mechanisms. From a functional point of view, the state of muscle contraction, resulting from a trauma, causes a limitation in the articular range of movement due to a reduced extensibility of the muscle. Therefore, in agreement with Reid [34, 35], muscle injuries by direct trauma can be divided into three degrees, depending on the severity, indirectly indicated by practicable range of motion:

1. Mild muscle injury: it allows more than half of the range of motion;
2. Moderate degree muscle injury: it allows less than half but more than one-third of the range of motion;
3. Severe muscle injury: the range of motion allowed is less than one-third.

  - *Muscle injury from indirect trauma* requires more complex mechanisms of action, which involves the intrinsic detrimental forces that develop within the muscle itself or the musculoskeletal system. In indirect trauma, it is possible to assume a neuro-muscular dysfunction, such as a sudden passive stretch of the muscle due to a tensile force applied during the contraction phase, or a very rapid contraction of the muscle from a state of complete relaxation. This type of injury is very often localized in proximity to the muscle–tendon junction, although it can also be localized in the middle of the muscle. Some variants of indirect trauma are usually described as:

1. *Twitching:* It presents with muscle pain that occurs almost always a certain period of time after doing a sport, with a variable latency (few hours/days). It is poorly localized due to widespread alteration of the muscle tone which, in the absence of anatomical lesions detectable macroscopically or with an optical microscope, is attributable to a state of muscle fatigue.

2. *Strain:* It is always the consequence of an acute painful episode that occurs during sports, which is very often well localized. The patient is forced to stop activities, while not necessarily leading to immediate functional impotence. There are no pathologic macroscopic lacerations of the muscle fibers: the disorder may be attributed to alteration of the myofibrils function, a neuro-muscular alteration in conduction or submicroscopic lesions at the level of the sarcomere.

3. *Tear:* It is characterized by violent acute pain due to a lesion of a variable number of muscle fibers. The muscle tear is always accompanied by a hemorrhage, depending on the amount and location of the lesion. The classification in degrees is related to the quantity of muscle tissue going from grade I (laceration of the few myofibrils within a muscle bundle, but not the whole bundle) to grade III, or rather to complete muscle rupture.

Although muscle trauma has several etiologies and mechanisms to occur, the healing phases are the same in all types of injury. However, the time occurring for complete recovery may vary. It has been shown that the pathophysiological processes in muscle injury (necrosis/degeneration, inflammation, repair, and formation of fibrous scar tissue) are interrelated and time-dependent [36].

The healing process of muscle lesion has well-defined phases [33]. The initial degeneration/necrosis phase is characterized by the formation of hematoma. The subsequent inflammation phase and the phase of repair fibrosis are correlated and time-dependent, followed by scar tissue remodeling. Because of mechanical trauma, the muscle fibers are damaged in the integrity of the plasmatic membrane and basal lamina, allowing extracellular calcium to enter the cell. These fibers undergo necrosis and apoptosis mediated by intrinsic proteins. Small newly and locally formed vessels bring neutrophils, monocytes, and macrophages, which invade the lesion. Then, T cells come to the injured tissue, which by their chemotactic powers, activate and attract GFs. Then, the secretion of adhesion molecules (P-selectin, L-selectin, and E-selectin), cytokines (IL-8, IL-6, and IL-1) and of TNF-α and TNF-β influence the local blood supply and vessel permeability [37].

Several GFs, including fibroblast growth factor (bFGF), insulin-like growth factor I (IGF-1), vascular endothelial growth factor (VEGF), and platelet-derived growth factor (PDGF), have been tested to potentiate tissue healing. Specific GFs also have a fundamental role in accelerating the repair processes and in facilitating a quicker and more complete muscle repair. However, the mechanism of action has been only partially clarified [38]. The role played by macrophages in the early hours after muscle injury (promote inflammation through their chemotactic power, but also promote muscle regeneration by the release of GFs) is also clear, while the action of neutrophils is still not clear.

Despite literature that shows that neutrophils might cause damage to muscle tissue due to the relaxation of free radicals and other oxidants, which significantly slow muscle regeneration, it has been confirmed that the deprivation of these cells in the first phase of inflammation causes an increase in fibrosis within the regenerated muscle [39].

Insulin-like growth factor (IGF), *hepatocyte growth factor* (HGF), *epidermal growth factor* (EGF), and *platelet-derived growth factor* (PDGF-AA and PDGF-BB) are all able to regulate the proliferation and differentiation of cells called "myoblasts" to regenerate and repair muscle fiber: these cells are responsible for the proliferative phase of the healing. TGF-β is active during inflammation and influences the regulation of cell migration and proliferation, while VEGF is produced at the highest levels only after the inflammatory phase, since it is a potent stimulator of angiogenesis in all the soft tissues.

The HGF and *leukemia inhibitory factor* (LIF) are two known examples of stimulators of satellite cells: HGF activates satellite cells quiescent in skeletal muscle. However, the injection of HGF directly into a damaged muscle does not promote its repair. Preliminary data indicate that LIF can improve muscle healing, but there is need for further experimental research to study this effect [40]. Myosatellite cells have the potential to heal muscle lesions, providing additional myonuclei to their parent muscle fiber; otherwise, they return to a quiescent state [41]. More specifically, upon activation, satellite cells can re-enter the cell cycle to proliferate and to differentiate into myoblasts [42]. The release and activation of satellite cells is due to rupture of the plasma membrane and basal lamina. Afterward, under the influence of GFs, these cells proliferate and differentiate into multinucleated myotubes and eventually mature muscle [33, 37]. These satellite cells probably come from somatic lineage and are normally in a dormant state. They are located between the basal lamina and the plasma membrane of each myofiber [37]. The regenerated cells have a central nucleus and are easily identified histologically. In most cases, this process leads to the formation of a new muscle with a fibrous scar tissue variable in size, depending on the degree of primary lesion [43, 44]. Frequently, an incomplete recovery of functional capacity of damaged muscle is observed, which is directly proportional to the area involved by the trauma. Other GFs, like bFGF and PDGF, improve the proliferation of satellite cells, but IGF-1 appears to be crucial in mediating the growth of skeletal muscle. The systemic regulation of IGF-1 results in an increased protein content of the muscle and in a decreased degradation of the tissue. On the other hand, IGF-1 is a potent mitogen for fibroblasts: thus, it also increases the production of matrix components (e.g., collagen), decreasing the expression of enzymes like collagenase or metalloproteinases with consequent development of muscle fibrosis. However, age-related changes in muscle cannot be overlooked: age determines changes in the muscle tissue, within which the motor units undergo a rearrangement consisting in the re-innervation of muscle fibers in which the aging process has determined the denervation. The survivor motor units, therefore, constitute a greater number of muscle fibers, so with more difficulty in graduate the intensity of the force [45]. Both collagen synthesis and cross-linking, such as elastic fibers, change in muscle structure over time, giving a more elastic/lax scar in young experimental animals than adult ones [4, 46].

2.4 Tendon

Mature tendon is constituted of rare elongated flattened fibroblasts (Fig. 2.4), while immature growing tendon is constituted of numerous rounded (chondral-like) cells arranged in long columns (Fig. 2.5). In children and adolescent athletes, complete tendon tears are quite rare. On the other hand, increasing functional demand and technical difficulty in sports gestures lead more frequently to chronic impairment, or rather to overuse injuries and tendon degeneration [47–49]. Effective repair of short and intra-capsular tendons (e.g., rotator cuff tendons) often relies on tendon-to-bone integration [50], whereas the repair of long and sheathed tendons often depends on the prevention of repair site gapping and maintenance of tendon gliding, recurring to its early mobilization [51, 52]. Albeit, any

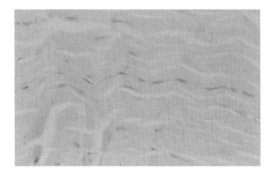

Fig. 2.4 Mature tendon is constituted of rare elongated flattened fibroblasts

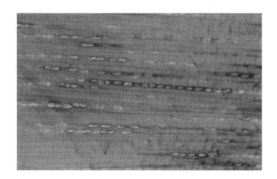

Fig. 2.5 Immature growing tendon is constituted of numerous *rounded* (chondral-like) cells arranged in long columns

specific or faster tendon-healing process has been never demonstrated in children and adolescents, and commonly, it is presumed it followed the adult healing phases: an initial inflammatory phase (first week/s), followed by a proliferative phase (order of weeks) and followed by a remodeling phase (of months/about a year). The inflammatory phase is characterized by increased vascular permeability and a diapedesis of inflammatory cells, or rather, granulocytes, monocytes, and also platelets. These latter release cytokines and GFs acting as recruiters for fibroblasts and tenocytes. Subsequently, during the proliferative phase, fibroblasts at the lesion site multiply and begin producing extra cellular matrix, and in particular, collagen I and elastic proteins [53]. During the remodeling phase, cellularity decreases while collagen is cross-linked assume the orientation along the force vectors. Cells might populate the repairing site from the surrounding environment: fibroblasts from the endotendon and epitendon, inflammatory cells from the vasculature, and synoviocytes from the sinovial sheaths. Osteoclasts are also attracted to the repair site, and resorption of bone at the repair site can impair recovery [54].

Anitua et al. [55, 56] have demonstrated in vitro that the levels of VEGF and HGF increase significantly upon contact with the pool of GFs physiologically released, suggesting that accelerate the proliferation of tendon cells as stimulate the synthesis of type I collagen. PDGF

is produced as a result of damage to the tendon: it helps to stimulate the production of other GFs and plays a role in tissue remodeling by promoting replication of mesenchymal stem cells, production of osteoid, replication of endothelial cells and the synthesis of new collagen. It is likely that it may be the first growth factor localized in wound, acting as a "primer" in connective tissue healing. Furthermore, in vitro and in vivo studies have shown that bFGF is a potent stimulator of angiogenesis and a regulator of cell migration and proliferation. It was found to be highly expressed during the initial inflammatory phase in a series of experimental animals, probably assisting fibroblast proliferation and migration, and increasing the production of new collagen [57, 58].

2.5 Ligament Injuries

From a biomechanical point of view, ligaments are considered as static joint stabilizers and can be exposed to injury, as a consequence of both indirect and direct trauma. It is also known that in young subjects a hyperlax pattern might be associated with a higher risk of injury, like in the knees or elbows [59, 60]. It is also true that partial tears or insertional bony (tibial) avulsion occur more frequently in children than in young adolescents, being one of the most common ligament injuries [61–63] at that age. Concerning the complete midsubstance ACL disruption in the skeletally immature patient, it has been the focus of several clinical studies [64–68].

Nowadays, the literature shows a high agreement in surgical indications for young athletes reporting ligament lesions. For instance, the goals of treatment for the ACL-deficient knee include prevention of functional instability, acute or chronic meniscal derangement, chondral pathology, and joint deterioration. Flynn et al. [68] designed a study to objectively measure knee laxity in children. Physical examination and the KT1000 arthrometer were used to test knee laxity in 150 healthy, uninjured children between 6 and 18 years of age. Data were analyzed to determine the change in laxity with age, laxity differences between boys and girls, and the correlation between KT1000 measurements and subjective tests for laxity. There was no statistical difference in knee laxity between boys and girls of similar ages. Knee laxity, determined by using the arthrometer, was significantly greater in younger children. Furthermore, the same author stated a familiar predisposition in ligament tearing [69].

When a tear occurs immediately after a trauma, healing process starts. Hemathrosis (in intra-articular ligaments) or hematoma (in extra-articular ligaments) and post-traumatic inflammation are responsible for the necrosis of cells and degradation of the damaged tissue. Then, similar to tendon healing, midsubstance torn ligament undergoes a subsequent proliferation and then remodeling phases. Actually, no proper study has been performed on the biology of ligament healing in pediatric age. In fact, only the clinical and biomechanical outcomes after conservative treatment in skeletally immature patients have been investigated [70]. The Authors observed poor and unacceptable results with joint instability and "giving way" sensation and gathered that the healing process cannot provide is the so-called "restitutio ad integrum" in such cases.

Thus, surgical indication in the presence of ligament tear (e.g., ACL) is recommended, but with extreme care, avoiding any damage to the open physes [70]. In this case, the healing is properly called "ligamentization".

Ligamentization is a process that involves the grafted tendon in the role of neo-ligament, which consists of three stages: sinovialization or peri-legamentous phase, intra-legamentous phase with cell proliferation, and the phase of the reconstruction of the architecture of the ACL with the rearrangement of the collagen fibers along the vectors of the forces, which include not just one direction but several others including torsional movements.

The process starts immediately after surgery with hemarthrosis. In hemarthrosis, GFs, released from platelet α-granules and cytokines, give initial stimulation to tissue repair. Increasing knowledge about GFs, above all those regarding the origin of platelets, is opening up new therapeutic approaches to accelerate both *graft* sinovialization and osteo-integration [71]. Furthermore, starting from hemarthrosis, the so-called mesenchymal stromal cells, responsible for osteo-integration process since its earliest stages, are released through bone tunnels [72]. Making distinctions, Morito et al. introduced the expression "*sinovial fluid mesenchymal stem cells*" (SF-MSC) to define the cells of the sinovial fluid that tend to settle the site of injury and set up the healing process [73].

According to Janssen [74], who made a comparison between arthroscopic and histological findings, complete tendon ligamentization takes place in two years. In the intra-articular environment, the *graft* is "sinovialized" by the adhesion of the sinoviocytes and the sinovial mesenchymal cells floating in the articular fluid that proliferate on the top layer covering the entire graft. In the early phases of integration, *graft* viability depends on the diffusion of sinovial fluid nutrient as well as on sinoviocytes, which metabolically interact with the *graft*.

At the same time, the inner part of the *graft* undergoes a weakening because of the atrophy of tissues and the necrosis of the tenocytes. The inner part of the *graft* is gradually repopulated by cells from fibroblastic line about 4–6 months later: this second phase, called the intra-legamentous phase, lasts for at least 6 months. After that, the last phase takes place, which is the remodeling of the collagen structure, for which a time limit is not yet unanimously accepted. As nutrient substances do not initially reach the inner part of the graft, the central role of the sinovialization phase for the success of the process of ligamentization is clear.

The importance of peri-legamentous connective tissue was explained by an experimental study on rats: removing this tissue coating from the *graft*, revitalization had a later start compared to the group with preserved peritenon, in which it was already observed on the second day. After 15 weeks, the neo-ligament completely depends on the vessels, which envelop the *graft* as a result of a neo-angiogenic process [75].

Through histological samples, Yamakado et al. [76] asserted that ligamentization is not a uniform phenomenon, since the central region of the *graft*, in the longitudinal direction of the structure, seems to be constantly late compared to the ends that are in contact with bone tunnels. Analyzing human and sheep samples of neo-ACL, Scranton et al. demonstrated that the ossification of the *graft* ends is carried out through a cartilagineous callus at the tunnels; that Sharpey fibers of osteo-tendineous and osteo-ligamentous junctions appear in both sample series as early as six weeks after surgery. During the phase of ligamentization in the *graft*, there are both myoblasts and smooth muscle cells that are not found in the native ACL which tend to disappear during the process of maturation of the neo-ligament (4).

Falconiero et al. [77] analyzed 48 biopsies from patellar tendon *graft* and *hamstring*, from 3 to 120 months after surgery. After analyzing the results, they established that remodeling could be considered as concluded only after 12 months. In fact, after this end-point, there were no significant changes in vascularization, spatial orientation, and concentration of collagen fibers. These results are used by the same Authors to justify an early rehabilitation protocol aimed at accelerating the return to full physical activities.

In 2005, Marumo et al. [78] set up a study to investigate the differences of cross-linking between the native ACL, the reconstructed one with *bone–tendon–bone* (BTB) and *hamstring*, which demonstrated that the cross-links (dihydroxy-lisino-leucine/hydroxy-lisino-leucine/ratio) increased statistically significantly in the treated specimen, confirming that the neo-ligament is normally stronger than the native ACL. Differently and earlier compared with others [79], by the exceedance of the normal cross-link ratio with both autografts, they defined the process of ligamentization as "complete" within one year.

By using Transmission Electron Microscopy (TEM) analysis, Zaffagnini et al. demonstrated that the maturity of the remodeled *graft* is achieved within two years after surgery [80].

The only animal study concerning the role played by the ACL reconstruction on growth plates is the one by Guzzanti et al. [81]. Limited metaphyseal damage and possible valgus axial deviations but not a complete epiphysiodesis after drilling to place the graft was demonstrated. This reduced, at least from a biological point of view, the big concerns about the potential damage of ACL surgery in skeletally immature patients.

2.6   Conclusion

This chapter described what today is known about soft tissue healing. No proper studies have till date investigated in children and adolescents from the initial phase up to complete recovery in terms of basic science. However, a lot of indirect data regarding the quality of healing have been taken from clinical and radiological results. A recurrent finding is that in muscle, tendon, and ligament, the healing process leaves a lax and ineffective repairing scar some months after injury, when treated conservatively. Age-related changes in connective architecture show an increase in rates of collagens, as cross-linking rate, giving a progressively harder scar depending on age. Furthermore, soft tissue trauma influences cartilage surface integrity, limb axis but not physis premature closure.

Thus, in children and adolescent athletes, who are subjected to higher risk of injury during physical activities, soft tissue traumas should be promptly treated in order to avoid laxity, muscle imbalance, joint instability, and relapse of injury.

References

1. Gigante A, Del Torto M, Manzotti S et al (2012) Platelet rich fibrin matrix effects on skeletal muscle lesions: an experimental study. J Biol Regul Homeost Agents 26:475–484
2. Fujii K, Tanzer ML (1974) Age-related changes in the reducible crosslinks of human tendon collagen. FEBS Lett 43:300–302

3. Amiel D, Kuiper SD, Wallace CD et al (1991) Age-related properties of medial collateral ligament and anterior cruciate ligament: a morphologic and collagen maturation study in the rabbit. J Gerontol 46:B159–165

4. Kovanen V, Suominen H (1989) Age- and training-related changes in the collagen metabolism of rat skeletal muscle. Eur J Appl Physiol Occup Physiol 58:765–771

5. Mays PK, Bishop JE, Laurent GJ (1988) Age-related changes in the proportion of types I and III collagen. Mech Ageing Dev 45:203–212

6. Mohan S, Radha E (1980) Age-related changes in rat muscle collagen. Gerontology 26:61–67

7. Bailey AJ (1975) Age-related changes during the biosynthesis and maturation of collagen fibres. Biochem Soc Trans 3:46–48

8. Listrat A, Lethias C, Hocquette JF et al (2000) Age-related changes and location of types I, III, XII and XIV collagen during development of skeletal muscles from genetically different animals. Histochem J 32:349–356

9. Wessel LM, Scholz S, Rusch M (2001) Characteristic pattern and management of intra-articular knee lesions in different pediatric age groups. J Pediatr Orthop 21:14–19

10. Damore DT, Metzl JD, Ramundo M et al (2003) Patterns in childhood sports injury. Pediatr Emerg Care 19:65–67

11. Taylor BL, Attia MW (2000) Sports-related injuries in children. Acad Emerg Med: Official J Soc Acad Emerg Med 7:1376–1382

12. Shea KG, Pfeiffer R, Wang JH et al (2004) Anterior cruciate ligament injury in pediatric and adolescent soccer players: an analysis of insurance data. J Pediatr Orthop 24:623–628

13. Gigante A, Bevilacqua C, Bonetti MG, Greco F (2003) Increased external tibial torsion in osgood-schlatter disease. Acta Orthop Scand 74(4):431–436

14. O'Neill DB, Micheli LJ (1988) Overuse injuries in the young athlete. Clin Sports Med 7:591–610

15. Rauh MJ, Macera CA, Ji M, Wiksten DL (2007) Subsequent injury patterns in girls' high school sports. J Athletic Training 42:486–494

16. Rauh MJ, Nichols JF, Barrack MT (2010) Relationships among injury and disordered eating, menstrual dysfunction, and low bone mineral density in high school athletes: a prospective study. J Athletic Training 45:243–252

17. Rauh MJ, Margherita AJ, Rice SG et al (2000) High school cross country running injuries: a longitudinal study. Clin J Sport Med: Official J Can Acad Sport Med 10:110–116

18. Micheli LJ, Klein JD (1991) Sports injuries in children and adolescents. Br J Sports Med 25:6–9

19. Micheli LJ (1995) Sports injuries in children and adolescents. Questions and controversies. Clin Sports Med 14:727–745

20. Falciglia F, Guzzanti V, Di Ciommo V, Poggiaroni A (2009) Physiological knee laxity during pubertal growth. Bull NYU Hosp Jt Dis 67(4):9–325

21. Venturelli M, Schena F, Zanolla L, Bishop D (2011) Injury risk factors in young soccer players detected by a multivariate survival model. J Sci Med Sport/ Sports Med Aust 14:293–298

22. Vandervliet EJ, Vanhoenacker FM, Snoeckx A, Gielen JL, Van Dyck P, Parizel PM (2007) Sports-related acute and chronic avulsion injuries in children and adolescents with special emphasis on tennis. Br J Sports Med 41(11):827–831

23. Micheli LJ, Slater JA, Woods E, Gerbino PG (1986) Patella alta and the adolescent growth spurt. Clin Orthop Relat Res:159–162

24. Menant JC, Steele JR, Menz HB et al (2009) Rapid gait termination: effects of age, walking surfaces and footwear characteristics. Gait Posture 30:65–70

25. Menant JC, Steele JR, Menz HB et al (2009) Effects of walking surfaces and footwear on temporo-spatial gait parameters in young and older people. Gait Posture 29:392–397

26. Benazzo F, Al E (1989) Attuali orientamenti nella patogenesi, evoluzione e trattamento degli ematomi muscolari negli atleti. IJ Sports Traumatol 4:273

27. Chan O, Del Buono A, Best TM, Maffulli N (2012) Acute muscle strain injuries: a proposed new classification system. Knee Surg Sports Traumatol Arthrosc: Official J ESSKA 20:2356–2362

28. Kullmer K, Sievers KW, Rompe JD et al (1997) Sonography and MRI of experimental muscle injuries. Arch Orthop Trauma Surg 116:357–361

29. du Plessis MP (1979) [Muscle injuries] South African Med J Suid-Afrikaanse tydskrif vir geneeskunde 55:633–634

30. Kvist M, Jarvinen M (1982) Clinical, histochemical and biomechanical features in repair of muscle and tendon injuries. Int J Sports Med 3(1):12–14

31. Huard J, Li Y, Fu FH (2002) Muscle injuries and repair: current trends in research. J Bone Joint Surg Am 84-A:822–832

32. Korenyi-Both AL, Korenyi-Both I (1986) Physical injuries, contractures and rigidity of skeletal muscle. J Med 17:109–120

33. Crisco JJ, Jokl P, Heinen GT et al (1994) A muscle contusion injury model. Biomechanics, physiology, and histology. Am J Sports Med 22:702–710

34. Reid MB, Haack KE, Franchek KM et al (1992) Reactive oxygen in skeletal muscle. I. Intracellular oxidant kinetics and fatigue in vitro. J Appl Physiol 73:1797–1804

35. Reid MB, Shoji T, Moody MR, Entman ML (1992) Reactive oxygen in skeletal muscle. II. Extracellular release of free radicals. J Appl Physiol 73:1805–1809

36. Jarvinen TA, Jarvinen TL, Kaariainen M et al (2005) Muscle injuries: biology and treatment. Am J Sports Med 33:745–764

37. Hurme T, Kalimo H, Lehto M, Jarvinen M (1991) Healing of skeletal muscle injury: an ultrastructural

and immunohistochemical study. Med Sci Sports Exerc 23:801–810

38. Menetrey J, Kasemkijwattana C, Day CS et al (2000) Growth factors improve muscle healing in vivo. J Bone Joint Surg Br 82:131–137

39. Tidball JG (2005) Inflammatory processes in muscle injury and repair. Am J Physiol Regul Integrative Comparative Physiol 288:R345–353

40. Molloy T, Wang Y, Murrell G (2003) The roles of growth factors in tendon and ligament healing. Sports Med 33:381–394

41. Kadi F, Charifi N, Denis C et al (2005) The behaviour of satellite cells in response to exercise: what have we learned from human studies? Pflugers Arch: Eur J Physiol 451:319–327

42. Siegel AL, Kuhlmann PK, Cornelison DD (2011) Muscle satellite cell proliferation and association: new insights from myofiber time-lapse imaging. Skeletal Muscle 1:7

43. Li Y, Pan H, Huard J (2010) Isolating stem cells from soft musculoskeletal tissues. J Visualized Experiments: JoVE 41

44. Huard J (2008) Regenerative medicine based on muscle stem cells. J Musculoskelet Neuronal Interact 8:337

45. Khattak MJ, Ahmad T, Rehman R et al (2010) Muscle healing and nerve regeneration in a muscle contusion model in the rat. J Bone Joint Surg Br 92:894–899

46. Best TM, Hunter KD (2000) Muscle injury and repair. Phys Med Rehabil Clin North Am 11:251–266

47. Belechri M, Petridou E, Kedikoglou S, Trichopoulos D (2001) Sports injuries among children in six European union countries. Eur J Epidemiol 17:1005–1012

48. Maffulli N, Longo UG, Spiezia F, Denaro V (2011) Aetiology and prevention of injuries in elite young athletes. Med Sport Sci 56:187–200

49. Kriz P (2011) Overuse injuries in the young athlete. Med Health, R I 94:203, 206–208

50. Weiss JM, Arkader A, Wells LM, Ganley TJ (2012) Rotator cuff injuries in adolescent athletes. J Pediat Orthop Part B

51. Al-Qattan MM (2010) Zone I flexor profundus tendon repair in children 5–10 years of age using 3 "figure of eight" sutures followed by immediate active mobilization. Ann Plastic Surg 68:29–32

52. Al-Qattan MM (2011) A six-strand technique for zone II flexor-tendon repair in children younger than 2 years of age. Injury 42:1262–1265

53. Gigante A, Specchia N, Rapali S et al (1996) Fibrillogenesis in tendon healing: an experimental study. Boll Soc Ital Biol Sper 72:203–210

54. Cadet ER, Vorys GC, Rahman R et al (2010) Improving bone density at the rotator cuff footprint increases supraspinatus tendon failure stress in a rat model. J Orthop Res: Official Publ Orthop Res Soc 28:308–314

55. Anitua E, Sanchez M, Nurden AT et al (2007) Reciprocal actions of platelet-secreted TGF-beta1 on the production of VEGF and HGF by human tendon cells. Plast Reconstr Surg 119:950–959

56. Anitua E, Andia I, Sanchez M et al (2005) Autologous preparations rich in growth factors promote proliferation and induce VEGF and HGF production by human tendon cells in culture. J Orthop Res: Official Publ Orthop Res Soc 23:281–286

57. Thomopoulos S, Das R, Sakiyama-Elbert S et al (2010) bFGF and PDGF-BB for tendon repair: controlled release and biologic activity by tendon fibroblasts in vitro. Ann Biomed Eng 38:225–234

58. Thomopoulos S, Zaegel M, Das R et al (2007) PDGF-BB released in tendon repair using a novel delivery system promotes cell proliferation and collagen remodeling. J Orthop Res: Official Publ Orthop Res Soc 25:1358–1368

59. Larson RV, Ulmer T (2003) Ligament injuries in children. Instr Course Lect 52:677–681

60. Sanders WE, Wilkins KE, Neidre A (1980) Acute insufficiency of the posterior cruciate ligament in children. Two case reports. J Bone Joint Surg Am 62:129–131

61. Chen WT, Shih TT, Tu HY et al (2002) Partial and complete tear of the anterior cruciate ligament. Acta radiol 43:511–516

62. Song EK, Seon JK, Park SJ, Yoon TR (2009) Clinical outcome of avulsion fracture of the anterior cruciate ligament between children and adults. J Pediatr Orthop Part B 18:335–338

63. Lo PA, Drake JM, Hedden D et al (2002) Avulsion transverse ligament injuries in children: successful treatment with nonoperative management. Report of three cases. J Neurosurg 96:338–342

64. Hawkins CA, Rosen JE (2000) ACL injuries in the skeletally immature patient. Bulletin 59:227–231

65. Finlayson CJ, Nasreddine A, Kocher MS (2010) Current concepts of diagnosis and management of ACL injuries in skeletally immature athletes. Physician Sports Med 38:90–101

66. Arbes S, Resinger C, Vecsei V, Nau T (2007) The functional outcome of total tears of the anterior cruciate ligament (ACL) in the skeletally immature patient. Int Orthop 31:471–475

67. Schachter AK, Rokito AS (2007) ACL injuries in the skeletally immature patient. Orthopedics 30:365–370; quiz 371–362

68. Steadman JR, Cameron-Donaldson ML, Briggs KK, Rodkey WG (2006) A minimally invasive technique ("healing response") to treat proximal ACL injuries in skeletally immature athletes. J knee Surg 19:8–13

69. Flynn RK, Pedersen CL, Birmingham TB et al (2005) The familial predisposition toward tearing the anterior cruciate ligament: a case control study. Am J Sports Med 33:23–28

70. Mizuta H, Kubota K, Shiraishi M et al (1995) The conservative treatment of complete tears of the

anterior cruciate ligament in skeletally immature patients. J Bone Joint Surg Br 77:890–894

71. Fleming BC, Spindler KP, Palmer MP et al (2009) Collagen-platelet composites improve the biomechanical properties of healing anterior cruciate ligament grafts in a porcine model. Am J Sports Med 37:1554–1563

72. Ju YJ, Muneta T, Yoshimura H et al (2008) Synovial mesenchymal stem cells accelerate early remodeling of tendon-bone healing. Cell Tissue Res 332: 469–478

73. Morito T, Muneta T, Hara K et al (2008) Synovial fluid-derived mesenchymal stem cells increase after intra-articular ligament injury in humans. Rheumatology (Oxford) 47:1137–1143

74. Janssen RP, van der Wijk J, Fiedler A et al (2011) Remodelling of human hamstring autografts after anterior cruciate ligament reconstruction. Knee Surg Sports Traumatol Arthrosc 19:1299–1306

75. Sckell A, Leunig M, Fraitzl CR et al (1999) The connective-tissue envelope in revascularisation of patellar tendon grafts. J Bone Joint Surg Br 81:915–920

76. Yamakado K, Kitaoka K, Nakamura T et al (2001) Histologic analysis of the tibial bone tunnel after anterior cruciate ligament reconstruction using solvent-dried and gamma-irradiated fascia lata allograft. Arthroscopy 17:32

77. Falconiero RP, DiStefano VJ, Cook TM (1998) Revascularization and ligamentization of autogenous anterior cruciate ligament grafts in humans. Arthroscopy 14:197–205

78. Marumo K, Saito M, Yamagishi T, Fujii K (2005) The "ligamentization" process in human anterior cruciate ligament reconstruction with autogenous patellar and hamstring tendons: a biochemical study. Am J Sports Med 33:1166–1173

79. Scheffler SU, Unterhauser FN, Weiler A (2008) Graft remodeling and ligamentization after cruciate ligament reconstruction. Knee Surg Sports Traumatol Arthrosc 16:834–842

80. Zaffagnini S, De Pasquale V, Marchesini Reggiani L et al (2010) Electron microscopy of the remodelling process in hamstring tendon used as ACL graft. Knee Surg Sports Traumatol Arthrosc 18:1052–1058

81. Guzzanti V, Falciglia F, Gigante A, Fabbriciani C (1994) The effect of intra-articular ACL reconstruction on the growth plates of rabbits. J Bone Joint Surg Br 76:960–963

82. Flynn JM, Mackenzie W, Kolstad K et al (2000) Objective evaluation of knee laxity in children. J Pediatr Orthoped 20:259–263

83. Kocher MS, Garg S, Micheli LJ (2005) Physeal sparing reconstruction of the anterior cruciate ligament in skeletally immature prepubescent children and adolescents. J Bone Joint Surg Am 87:2371–2379

The Preparticipation Examination: Evaluation of the Pediatric and Adolescent Athlete

3

Paolo Zeppilli and Massimiliano Bianco

Health care of healthy pediatric–adolescent population is an item of great concern, due to social, economic, and emotional burden of adverse, sometime dramatic events in young subjects. For these reasons, several national organizations, in the last decades, have developed preventive care guidelines and measures focused specifically on adolescents [1–10]. Despite that, adherence to these preventive care guidelines remains generally low.

The only systematic medical screening of apparently healthy young population appears to be nowadays the pre-participation physical examination (PPE). The number of school-age children and adolescents practicing sports activity increases, in fact, every year and by now, in most of the countries, these young athletes are required to receive a medical examination. In some cases, this medical examination is the only health examination that some children ever receive.

3.1 Purpose of Pre-Participation Sports Examination

The purpose of the PPE has undergone significant transition in the last decades. A general consensus exists that, in general terms, the first goal of the examination is to ensure the health and safety of athletes by detecting conditions that may predispose to injury, disability, or death and to meet legal and insurance requirements. Secondary, PPE could be intended as a comprehensive medical examination to evaluate the general health and physical maturation of school-age individuals, to counsel them on health-related issues and indicate which sports are safer for each individual. Usually, however, there is no time for this kind of evaluation [11]. Finally, PPE could be focalized in obtaining performance measurements to optimize the training regimen or determining child's predisposition for different sports and roles.

3.2 Content, Frequency, and Set-up of Pre-Participation Sports Examination

The importance of PPE is widely recognized, despite there is an ongoing debate regarding the optimal approach to screen young competitive athletes. A great heterogeneity exists, in fact, regarding content, frequency, and organizational set-up of the PPE [12] with only a few countries

P. Zeppilli (✉) · M. Bianco
Sports Medicine Unit, Università Cattolica del
Sacro Cuore, Largo Agostino Gemelli 8, 00168,
Rome, Italy
e-mail: p.zeppilli@rm.unicatt.it

M. Bianco
e-mail: massimiliano.bianco@fastwebnet.it

V. Guzzanti (ed.), *Pediatric and Adolescent Sports Traumatology*,
DOI: 10.1007/978-88-470-5412-7_3, © Springer-Verlag Italia 2014

(like Italy) requiring pre-participation medical clearance before participation in official competitive events [13]. Surely, it is known for a long time that the main causes of adverse events in young competitive (or not competitive) athletes are cardiovascular diseases [14–16]. Since 1996, in USA, the Sudden Death and Congenital Defects Committee of the American Heart Association (AHA), following the recommendations of the 36th Bethesda Conference, recommend a personal/family history and a physical examination focused on the detection of cardiovascular abnormalities [17]. AHA guidelines do not include a 12-lead ECG or other testing, which are requested largely at discretion of the examining physician. This guideline, moreover, suggests that a complete physical examination has to be performed to the athlete upon entering high school or college, and then every 2 years.

The European Society of Cardiology (ESC), instead, underlines the role of an annual examination which includes (in addition to history taking and physical examination) a systematic 12-lead ECG at rest [4]. The European model is based on the believing that the addition of 12-lead ECG enhances the sensitivity of the screening process for detection of cardiovascular diseases with risk of sudden death, first of all hypertrophic cardiomyopathy [18], as suggested by the long-lasting Italian experience [16, 19].

Regarding the personnel allowed to perform the PPE, the AHA and ESC guidelines underline that athletic screening should be performed by physicians who are knowledgeable about cardiovascular diseases, with medical skills and background to reliably obtain a detailed cardiovascular examination.

More differences exist on the organizational set-up, with three types of PPE [11]:
1. *Office-based examination*: the doctor visits the athlete in his/her office. The pros are that physician is familiar with the patient and may have more time and privacy for counseling about sensitive issues. The cons include a lack of continuity from year to year if the athlete changes physicians, longer times,

higher costs and, eventually, difficulties in reaching the office.
2. *Assembly line examination*: a large number of athletes are examined by a single physician in sequence, usually nearby the athletic field, requiring less time, lower costs, and fewer logistical problems. Disadvantages include possible communication problems, lack of individual attention, a lower level of privacy, and possible poor history taking.
3. *Station examination*: multiple examiners perform discrete examinations in a sequence of stations. This is a cost-effective and efficient method and specialized expertise of single doctors is met. On the other hand, noise and confusion are frequent with possible compromised care, lack of privacy, short time for each investigation and possible communication problems when some health issue rises.

However, whichever type is chosen, the PPE should be performed in an appropriate medical office, with all the necessary medical instruments, in a clean and quite environment, with a comfortable temperature and lighting. The athletes should be advised to dress sports shoes and gym clothes to ease the examination, particularly when other diagnostic tests can possibly be performed.

3.3   Medical History

An accurate medical history is fundamental in every medical field and represents the first important step to discover unknown illness or achieve the correct medical diagnosis.

In PPE, exists the particular problem of the accuracy and truthfulness of the information given by athletes. The physician has to remember that athletes may omit to refer symptoms, past illnesses, or injuries they fear might exclude them from sport. A past history of denied or restricted sports participation by another medical doctor is often omitted by the athletes. For all these reasons, it is better to ask the athletes or, when underage, his/her parent to subscribe the anamnesis itself. Moreover, athletes may not deem significant something that may in fact be essential and/or they may not know important information about their own or their family medical history. It has been observed that only 19–39 % of athlete's responses match info from their parents [20], so that the presence of parents is recommended during PPE and should be obligatory for minors.

Many authors have formulated medical history form including the items they feel important. This questionnaire should be easily understood, even by children, including, if necessary, examples. If possible, one may ask the athlete to complete the medical history form in advance, even if with illiteracy quite high in some areas, and the increasing number of foreign athletes, this can be a significant problem. In each case, however, the physician should reevaluate the different items during the examination, to be sure the athletes, or their parents, have correctly understood and answered to the different questions of the form.

Although medical history form may vary in the different healthcare organizations, there are several areas widely considered important in its structure. First of all, the medical questionnaire should investigate the *family history*. The majority of conditions at risk of sudden death during sports, especially in the young, are genetically determined diseases with an autosomal dominant pattern of inheritance, hence, the importance of family history in identifying affected athletes. The family history is considered positive when close relative(s) had experienced a premature heart attack or sudden death (<55 years of age in males and <65 years in females), or in the presence of a family history of cardiomyopathy, Marfan syndrome, long or short QT syndrome, Brugada syndrome, severe arrhythmias, coronary artery disease, or other disabling cardiovascular diseases [21]. Family history is also important to screening individuals, even children, at risk of diabetes, hypertension, lipid abnormalities, bleeding disorders [9, 22–25].

A good medical history has then to inquire about all of the different systems of the body. *Cardiovascular diseases* are the main killer in apparently health young athletes, then specific questions have to be strictly done about the presence and the characteristics of cardiovascular symptoms such as chest pain/discomfort, syncope (or near syncope), irregular heartbeat/palpitations, dyspnea or fatigue out of proportion with exercise. Moreover, the past detection of a heart murmurs or high blood pressure should be investigated, as the previous request of second-(ultrasound, ECG stress test, Holter monitoring, etc.) or third (MRI, electrophysiological study, angiography, etc.)-level cardiologic examinations or previous medical ban from sports practice. Particular attention has to be taken also concerning virus and/or bacterial infections that could involve cardiac structures (recent history of mononucleosis, pneumonia, toxoplasmosis, Epstein Barr, adenovirus, streptococcus, etc.). Moreover, particularly for athletes coming from or with recent trips to foreign countries (Africa, Asia, Central/South America, etc.), the examining doctor should take in the due count possible contacts with specific local infective diseases (malaria, dengue, leishmaniasis, etc.).

The *musculoskeletal history* is also critical in athletes, so that the physician should investigate eventual past recurrent injuries (sprain, strains, dislocations, ligament injuries, stress fractures). Musculoskeletal injury patterns of concern vary by sport: fractures and ligament injuries are more common in high-contact or collision sports. Low-contact or endurance athletes are more likely to have a history of overuse injury, tendonitis, or stress fractures.

Neurologic history of headaches, head injuries with loss of consciousness, previous diagnoses of concussions or seizure disorders are also of utmost importance and have to be investigated, especially in contact sports. If any of these neurological symptoms are present, a neurologic clearance should be required before starting the sport activity or return to play decision. In these cases, a computerized neuropsychological evaluation may be helpful. Moreover, in case of a recent concussion, the young athlete should avoid sport practice (both competitions and training sessions) until clinical and instrumental clearance, to prevent the risk of dramatic "second-impact syndrome," reported to be more frequent in the young [26].

Any other ongoing medical condition or chronic medical problems requiring constant monitoring should be investigated. Eventually, previous hospitalizations or surgical procedures should be recorded; if any are recent, a proper release should be obtained from the consultant doctor or surgeon who treated the athlete, to be included in the athlete's record.

History of asthma or cough with exercise has to be investigated. Asthma is one of the most common chronic illnesses of the young, afflicting an estimated 7 million (9.4 %) children in the United States [27]. In more than 85 % of cases, it is associated with exercise-induced bronchospasm. The prevalence of exercise-induced bronchospasm is believed to be from 10 to 35 % of athletes and it should be suspected in any athlete with history of wheezing during sports [28, 29].

History of *allergies or anaphylactic* reactions to medications, insects, foods, and exercise also [30], have to be investigated, especially in open space sports activities.

History of only a single normally paired organ (single kidney or monocular subjects), history of bleeding disorder, or other hematological diseases are also of great concern. Collision sports, actually, should be discouraged in subjects with single normally paired organ, due to the unbearable risk to lose the only functioning organ. In case of bleeding and hematological diseases, a consultant release should be obtained and included in the athlete's record. However, contact sports should be avoided in the presence of bleeding disorders.

The athlete should be current on immunizations against tetanus, measles, hepatitis B, and varicella. Immunization against human papilloma virus should be recommended in both sexes (possibly at the age of 11–12 years).

A *physiological anamnesis* should investigate eating habits, use/abuse of coffee, tea, or other stimulants (coke), abuse of candies or licorice (with possible water and salt metabolism changes and hypertensive effect), kind of sleep, diuresis, and defecation. After gaining the confidence of the young athlete, *forbidden habits* , such as chemical or substance abuse (alcohol, illicit drugs, tobacco, steroid, or other hormones), or dangerous sexual practices, have to be investigated, possibly asking the parents to leave the medical room for a few minutes. If tobacco is admitted, numbers of cigarettes per day and years of smoking has to be inquired. Use of *drugs/supplements* is also critical.

The medical history should also include questions about the *menstrual function* in female athletes, which is strictly linked with bone mineral density and important for the prevention of osteoporosis. Primary amenorrhea (absence of menstrual bleeding and secondary sexual characteristics in a girl by age of 14 years or the absence of menses with normal development of secondary sexual characteristics in a girl by age of 16 years) or secondary amenorrhea (absence of periods for more than three cycles) are quite common among high-level female athletes and could suggests the feared female athlete triad (eating disorders, amenorrhea, and osteopenia). The potential presence of *eating disorders*, possibly part of the triad, has also to be investigated. Problems with body perception are most prevalent in sports that have weight classes or emphasize appearance or leanness for improved performance. Some studies have shown that as many as 25–31 % of female athletes have an eating disorder [31, 32]. On the other side, obesity is nowadays a social problem in many civilized areas and is often linked with psychological discomfort as depression and bulimia.

Finally, *sports anamnesis* is critical concerning the number of training sessions the athlete is involved in a week, how many hours a single workout lasts, and in what kind of exercise it consists. The competitive level and the best results in the athletic career should also be recorded.

3.4   Physical Examination

Physical examination, general and apparatus specific, is the fundamental second step of the PPE. The examining physician should start from general data and continue analyzing all the body systems in a systematic way, noting his/her findings in the athlete's record.

3.4.1 General Data

The main anthropometric parameters as height and weight have to be always carefully measured. From these parameters, body mass index (BMI = weight in kilograms/height in meters square) could be derived and plotted on appropriate local BMI centile charts.

In case of extreme thinness, information about eventual recent loss of weight and eating habits must be taken. If the suspicious of growth deficit and/or eating disorders exists, further diagnostic examinations must be requested with the support of consultant pediatric endocrinologists. If recent loss of weight is associated to increased thirsty, type 1 diabetes mellitus must be ruled out (urinalysis and serum glucose may solve the doubt). In case of obesity, advice on a correct diet and lifestyle must be given and the presence of stigmata of syndromes associated with obesity must be searched (developmental delay, dysmorphism, hypogonadism in males, manifestations of hyperandrogenism in females, purple abdominal striae, and acanthosis nigricans).

If possible, body fat determination (by means of plicometer or bio-electrical impedance analysis) and waist circumference are of great importance especially in sports with weight categories and in case of overweight or underweight athletes. The waist measurement has to be taken at the end of the normal expiration at the narrowest part of the torso at the level of the natural waist between the last touchable rib and the iliac crest, with the tape parallel to the ground; the child should stand erect with the abdomen relaxed, arms at the sides, and the feet together.

3.4.2 Skin

Skin examination should be carried out with great accuracy, during PPE screening as well as before the game in the competition place. The presence of suspect moles requiring further dermatologic evaluation is mandatory as melanoma is a very aggressive malignancy, not rare in the young.

The skin evaluation, moreover, should be carried out looking for rashes, infections, and infestations. In case of active skin lesions (impetigo, molluscum contagiosum, herpes simplex, tinea corporis, scabies), direct skin contact or mat activities like wrestling (herpes gladiatorum), gymnastics, and martial arts should be avoided or allowed only with protective clothing/covering.

3.4.3 Head, Eyes, Ears, Nose, Oral Cavity, or Throat

The athlete should have adequate vision and visual acuity measurement (using standard Snell's vision chart) must be at least 20/40 in each eye. Athletes who are functionally one-eyed (defined as having less than 20/40 corrected vision in one eye), or athletes who had undergone major eye-surgical procedures or severe ocular injuries, should dress proper eye protection in case of sports at high risk of eye injuries (basketball, baseball, racquetball and all the other sports using a ball, puck, bat, or racquet); very high-risk sports with full contact (boxing, wrestling, contact martial arts) where protections are not allowed should be strongly discouraged. However, due to the high defensive potential of eye-protectors, these devices should always be dressed when available.

Evaluation of the equality of pupils is also important, since a small or even important difference in pupils diameter may be present even in normal eyes. This characteristic (anisocoria) must be known, since in case of head injuries the new onset of anisocoria can be a sign of cerebral damage.

The physical examination should carry on with a general examination of the ears, nose, oral cavity, and neck. Oral ulcer, poor gum, or dentition may indicate an eating disorder, such as bulimia; oral lesions like leucoplachia, rise the suspicion of heavy tobacco smoking; a high, arched palate can be a sign of Marfan syndrome; a bifid uvula or history of a cleft palate can rise the suspicion of Loeys-Dietz syndrome (characterized by aortic root aneurisms and bicuspid aortic valve); metal braces require an oral protection during contact sports activity, to prevent wounds in case of traumatic events. Auditory canal or tympanic membrane scars due to past infections, surgical procedures or traumatic events, should be investigated and may require proper protection in case of aquatic sports; if needed, a consultant certification may be requested, particularly for sports like diving, martial arts with full contact among competitors, and gun shooting disciplines.

Nasal benign tumor or septal deviations should be recognized and, if the case, corrected. Nasal ulcers rise the suspicion of cocaine use. Submandibular, occipital, or laterocervical adenopathies must be searched, since the risk of infective diseases or neoplastic processes.

3.4.4 Cardiovascular System

Physical examination should emphasize the assessment of cardiovascular system, since structural cardiac or cardiovascular problems are the first cause of sudden death in athletes. In the cardiovascular examination, 3 steps are recommended:
1. brachial artery blood pressure measurement (sitting), preferably in both arms,
2. femoral pulses assessment and
3. heart murmur auscultation.

Brachial blood pressure and pulse measurement are the first to be detected. Blood pressure must be measured in a relaxed environment, with a cuff of appropriate size for the anthropometric characteristics of the child (it should encircle at least two-thirds of the arm). The most common cause of an abnormal value in children, actually, is improper cuff size. Stressing factors must be avoided, as a recent heavy meal, physical activity, coke or tobacco use, full urinary bladder. If the initial value is elevated, two or three subsequent readings should be obtained

and, if the case, after 10–15 min of rest. Hypertension in the adolescent can be a marker of hormonal, renal, cardiovascular or central nervous system abnormalities or substance abuse. Extensive data on blood pressure for children are poor, but standards have been developed by National High Blood Pressure Education Program Working Group on High Blood Pressure in Children and Adolescents in 2004 when charts were published based on child's age and sex [33].

When examining pulses, a rapid or irregular radial pulse should be correlated with the cardiac and general examination to determine its clinical significance. A feeble, absent, or tardus femoral artery pulse should be correlated with aortic coarctation and, in this case, the examining doctor must search for the presence of an interscapular murmur.

Heart auscultation is critical to rise the suspicion of primitive or secondary heart valve problems (the most common being mitral valve prolapse and bicuspid aortic valve) or cardiac defects (i.e., shunts, patent ductus arteriosus, patent foramen ovalis, interatrial or interventricular septum defects). Attention must be paid to the presence of any murmur and its characteristics, such as intensity (loudness), frequency (pitch), quality, duration, configuration, primary location (point of maximum intensity), and site(s) of radiation.

Heart auscultation should be always done with the athlete supine and standing, since murmurs consistent with dynamic left ventricular outflow obstruction (in hypertrophic cardiomyopathy) increases upon standing.

Usually, innocent murmurs, not rarely detachable in children, have a low intensity (less than grade 3/6), are early- or mid-systolic and vibratory (Still's murmur). Normal variants in an "athlete's heart" include an S3, from increased ventricular filling due to the exercise-induced bradycardia and mild cardiomegaly, or a systolic murmur due to increased stroke volume. Heart murmurs requiring referral before cardiac clearance are generally of grade 3/6 or more, holosystolic or late systolic, diastolic, systo-diastolic, ejective clicks, or every murmur whose intensity increases with Valsalva maneuver.

A variety of physiologic maneuvers that alter cardiovascular hemodynamics can be used to aid in characterizing and differentiating cardiac murmurs, as the sudden transit from a lying to standing position or, even more, from a squatting to a standing position, deep breathing, passive leg raising, the Valsalva maneuver or an isometric handgrip exercise. Squatting increases the venous return to the heart, and consequently the left ventricular volume, stroke volume, and the systemic vascular resistance. The transition from squatting to standing reverses these changes. Valsalva maneuver and isometric exercise have opposite effects, since they decrease the venous return to the heart.

Usually, innocent murmurs' intensity increases when squatting and decreases with Valsalva maneuver or isometric handgrip, similarly to what happens in aortic stenosis. However, it is quite easy to suspect an aortic stenosis, due to systolic murmur's characteristics (typically harsh or rough), louder intensity (usually grade 2, 3, or 4/6), with crescendo-decrescendo configuration and a low to medium pitch, distinctive localization (aortic areas), and irradiation (toward carotid arteries). To further differentiate innocent from pathologic murmurs:

- in case of hypertrophic cardiomyopathy, the doctor can hear an apical systolic murmur that increases in standing position, becomes softer if the athlete performs a sustained handgrip or a squatting position (due to the reduction of left ventricular outflow obstruction and, so, of the murmur intensity), while becomes louder if the athlete performs a Valsalva maneuver (due to the increase of left ventricular outflow obstruction);
- in case of mitral valve prolapse, the physician can hear a mid-systolic apical click with late systolic murmur that increases while standing and if the athlete performs a sustained handgrip.

Physical examination in young athletes must include a look for the stigmata of Marfan syndrome as disproportionately tall stature (mainly depending on the upper body segment), arm span greater than height, thoracic and spine deformities (pectus excavatum, kypho-scoliosis), joint contracture or laxity, flat feet, myopia. In the suspicion, particularly when familiar history is positive for Marfan syndrome, due to high risk of sudden death to aortic aneurism dissection, the boy/girl must be screened with echocardiogram (to rule out ascending aorta enlargement and mitral valve prolapse), slip-lamp examination (searching for lens' subluxation/ectopia) and, eventually, spine MRI (to exclude dural ectasia). A diagnosis can be made following the revised Ghent criteria [34], even if in people below the age of 18 the syndrome is often expressed incompletely [35].

Finally, ankle swelling and/or pulmonary crackles must be ruled out as they may be a sign of a cardiovascular disease.

3.4.5 Chest and Lungs

The patient should be in the proper position, i.e., sitting up on the examining table or bed, ensuring that his/her chest is not leaning against anything. Skin, nails, and lips should be inspected, noting whether cyanosis or pallor is present, as they may be signs of respiratory (or heart) disorders. The doctor should then note shape and symmetry of the chest, looking at one side as a comparison for the other, observing how the chest expands during breathing (palpation may be useful at this purpose). The antero-posterior diameter is usually less than the lateral. The so-called barrel chest results from compromised respiration as occurs in chronic asthma, emphysema, or cystic fibrosis. In this case, the ribs are more horizontal and the spine is usually kyphotic.

Other changes in chest wall shape and symmetry may be the result of structural problems in the spine (kyphosis, scoliosis), rib cage, or sternum. Two common structural problems are pigeon chest (pectus carinatum), with a prominent sternal protrusion, and funnel chest (pectus excavatum), with an indentation of the lower sternum.

The second step in chest examination is palpation, mainly oriented to note the quality of the tactile fremitus. The doctor should ask the patient to say a few words ("99" or, in children, "Mickey Mouse") while systematically palpating the chest with the palmar surfaces of the fingers or with the ulnar aspects of the hand, comparing both sides simultaneously and symmetrically. Decreased or absent fremitus may indicate excess air in the lungs (it happens in bronchial obstruction, emphysema, or pneumothorax). Increased fremitus occurs in the presence of fluids or a solid mass within the lungs (it happens in lung consolidation, heavy but non-obstructive bronchial secretions, compressed lung, or tumors). More gentle, tremulous fremitus occurs with some inflammatory and infectious processes.

Percussion is another important phase of chest physical examination. All the examined areas have to be compared symmetrically, using one side as a control for the other. Resonance, the expected sound, can usually be heard over all areas of the lungs. Increased resonance is associated with hyperinflation and may be a sign of asthma, emphysema, or pneumothorax. On the contrary, reduced resonance (dullness or flatness) suggests pneumonia, atelectasis, or pleural effusion.

The final step is auscultation. The doctor should listen systematically at each position throughout inspiration and expiration, comparing symmetrically both sides. Broncho-vesicular (usually heard over major bronchi) and bronchial (usually heard over the trachea) breathing sounds have not to be heard over the peripheral lung tissue where vesicular sound is expected, or it can be sign of lung consolidation. In these cases, actually, breath sounds are easier to be heard as the sound transmission is easier. If fluid has accumulated in the pleural space, a foreign body (or secretions) obstructs the bronchi or the lungs are hyperinflated, breathing sounds are relatively more difficult to hear.

The following sounds should be considered abnormal:

- Crackles or crepitations (named rales in the past): usually heard during inspiration, are caused by the "popping open" of small airways and alveoli collapsed by fluid, exudate, or lack of aeration during expiration. Fine crackles usually indicates an interstitial process (pulmonary fibrosis or congestive heart failure), while coarse crackles indicate an airway disease, as bronchiectasis.
- Rhonchi: heard as deep, gurgling noises, usually prolonged and continuous during expiration, they are caused by the passage of air through an airway obstructed by thick secretions, muscular spasm (asthma), tumors, or external pressure (lymph nodes or other masses). Contrary to crackles, in general, rhonchi tend to disappear after coughing.
- Wheezes (or sibilant rhonchi): heard as continuous, coarse, whistling sounds, they are caused when some part of the respiratory tree is narrowed or obstructed, the most frequent cause in the young being asthma attacks and, in the baby, bronchiolitis. A special type of wheeze is stridor. When heard solely in the expiratory phase, it usually indicates a lower respiratory tract obstruction, as with aspiration of a foreign body. Stridor in the inspiratory phase is usually heard with obstruction in the upper airways (trachea, epiglottis, or larynx) and is a medical emergency.
- Friction rubs: these sounds originate outside the lungs and can be heard in both inspiration and expiration. They may be a sign of pleurisy or, when heard in the heart area and without disappearing holding the breath, of pericarditis.

3.4.6 Abdomen

Abdominal examination should be led with the athlete in supine position, free of clothes, looking for surgical scars or other skin abnormalities, abdominal masses, abnormal abdominal pulsations, hernias, soreness, rigidity, or enlargement of liver or spleen; all these conditions require further diagnostic examinations. If splenomegaly is suspected, ultrasound should be used to evaluate the size of the spleen and a recent history of infectious mononucleosis should be investigated, since the risk of splenic rupture. In this case, any contact or strenuous sports participation is contraindicated for a minimum of 3 weeks after the onset of systemic illness. Hepatomegaly also requires the same diagnostic work-up, since active hepatitis is a contraindication to contact and strenuous sports due to increased risk of liver injury and contagion. Sometimes, the abdominal examination allows to discover an inguinal or umbilical hernia, which should be repaired if large or if patients are symptomatic, in order to minimize the risk of incarceration. This assessment, finally, checks for pregnancy in female athletes.

3.4.7 Genitourinary System

In young males, the genitourinary system examination should mainly assess the presence of undescended or abnormal testicles and inguinal hernia; in case of testicular active problems, the athlete must be referred to a consultant and exercise (especially contact sports) should be avoided.

Testicle cancer is the main cause of death for malignant disease among young males (aged 18–35 years), and the PPE gives the possibility to explain to the young athlete the value of testicle self-evaluation.

In female, the PPE screening usually does not include a genitourinary system examination. However, it must be recommended and postponed to appropriate place and time if the clinical history or the physical examination raises a suspicion of any problem.

In both sexes, history of urinary recurrent infections should be the sign of ureter reflux due to an anomalous ureter/bladder junction. If the case, ultrasound examination of urinary tract and consultant referral can be requested.

3.4.8 Musculoskeletal System

The nature and duration of the musculoskeletal system examination during PPE is a subject of debate, and there are no absolute guidelines on this focus. The examiner must choose the best method based on athlete's traumatic history, eventual presence of musculoskeletal symptoms or signs, type of sports, available tools and time, personal experience, and skills. It has been observed that musculoskeletal examination is of poor value in asymptomatic athletes with no traumatic injuries history, while history alone is much more sensitive in detecting significant musculoskeletal lesions. Accordingly, a reasonable approach could be to use a simplified general examination in asymptomatic athletes with no history of previous traumatic events. On the other hand, if the clinical history or the general examination detects the presence of sport specific complaints, constant joint or muscle pain, previous, recurrent or recent musculoskeletal injuries, joint instability or locks, muscular weakness or atrophy, etc., a thorough, specific to the problem, musculoskeletal examination becomes necessary. Constant pain in one joint/area for more than 3 weeks is generally considered an indication for further work-up, either by imaging or specialist consultation.

A general musculoskeletal examination should look at quickly identifying joint stability and range of motion, muscle strength, eventual presence of asymmetries, or clinically relevant lesions.

During a general musculoskeletal examination, the following maneuvers should be performed [11]:

1. inspection, with the athlete standing in face of the examiner, to evaluate pose and trunk/arms symmetry;
2. observation of neck range of motion through the extension and forward/lateral flexion;
3. resisted shoulder shrug (to evaluate trapezius strength);
4. internal and external rotation of the shoulders (glenohumeral joint range of motion; it should be 90 degrees in external rotation);
5. resisted shoulder abduction (to evaluate deltoid strength);
6. elbows' extension and flexion (elbow range of motion; it should be 150 degrees);

7. elbows' pronation and supination, with arms in 90 degree flexion (elbow and wrist range of motion);
8. fist clench and finger spread (to evaluate hand/finger range of motion and deformities);
9. inspection of the back (to evaluate shoulder, chest and upper limbs symmetry, scoliosis);
10. back extension with straight knee (spondylolysis e spondylolisthesis);
11. back flexion with straight knee (to evaluate thoracic and lumbar spine range of motion, scoliosis, hip motion, hamstring tightness, thigh flexor muscles flexibility);
12. inspection of the lower extensors, asking the athlete to tighten and relax the quadriceps (to evaluate legs' symmetry and lengths, ankle or knee effusions);
13. toe and heel walking (to evaluate calf symmetry, leg strength, balance);
14. duck walking (to evaluate hip, knee and ankle motion and suspect meniscal lesions).

The physician should consider, however, that this examination does not allow to determine an exact diagnosis or the precise severity of a musculoskeletal, tendon or joint lesion. If appropriate, the examiner must complete the examination with further specific joint or muscle tests, request instrumental examinations (ultrasound, Rx, MRI), and/or refer the athlete to an orthopedic consultant.

3.4.9 Neurological System

In most cases, a normal musculoskeletal examination implies normal neurologic functions. During PPE, therefore, a neurologic examination should be performed if something abnormal has been noted in the musculoskeletal system or if the patient has positive familiar history of hereditary neurologic disorders, an history of concussion, or seizures.

Any athlete with history of an isolated or recurrent concussive event needs an accurate investigation of his/her motor, cognitive, and behavioral functions, as well as coordination.

This is of great importance, since the risk of a potentially fatal condition known as second-impact syndrome, a rapid cerebral swelling which can result if the athlete has a second concussion before recovering from the first one [26]. Concussion [also called mild traumatic brain injury (MTBI)] is a complex pathophysiological process affecting the brain induced by traumatic biomechanical forces [36]. As concussion is often underreported or unreported among athletes and coaching staff [37], the PPE is a unique moment for the doctor to educate the athletes on the health consequences linked with MTBI and to make them reflect whether any concussion has occurred (and when) in their athletic career. It should be important to ask the athletes, especially if engaged in contact sports, if they ever suffered from headache, dizziness, nausea, "foggy" or "slow" feeling, visual or balance disturbances, amnesia, irritability, loss of consciousness, or convulsions. These concussion symptoms typically spontaneously improve within minutes from the impact and resolve by about five to seven days, although, in some cases, they may persist from weeks to months (post-concussive syndrome).

If the athlete has never suffered a concussion, it could be very useful to evaluate his/her cognitive functions during PPE by means of a computerized neuropsychological test or other tests investigating different cognitive domains (balance, visual attention, etc.). This will be his/her baseline record, which will be helpful in case of any future concussion to evaluate his/her recovery.

In case of a previous concussion, especially if the doctor is asked to take the return to play decision, a valuable tool is the Sport Concussion Assessment Tool (SCAT2) [36]. The SCAT2 provides a standardized scoring system that takes into account symptoms, physical examination findings, cognitive function, balance and coordination, as well as Glasgow Coma Scale scores. The return to play decision, however, is symptoms driven and should take place in a stepwise fashion, to safeguard at most athletes' health [36, 38, 39].

Another point of concern in the PPE is history of seizure disorder. This is not an absolute contraindication to sports if well-controlled. Regular participation in physical activity can improve physical and psychosocial outcomes in these patients, and they may be allowed to participate in team sports or even contact or collision activities wearing the appropriate protective gear. The International League Against Epilepsy suggests restriction only from sports that involve extreme risk if a seizure should occur, such as hang-gliding, scuba-diving, downhill skiing, free climbing, and car/motorbike racing [40]. In water sports, however, careful supervision should be requested.

Despite several theoretical risks of a lower seizure threshold when engaged in sport activities (i.e., stress, hyperventilation), there seems to be no increased risk of injury or seizure activity as the result of such participation. However, any recent epileptic fit should require a neurological check, especially when the athlete is engaged in water sports, archery, shooting, etc.

References

1. Goodwin MA, Flocke SA, Borawski EA et al (1999) Direct observation of health habit counseling of adolescents. Arch Pediatr Adolesc Med 153:367–373
2. American Academy of Pediatric Committee on Practice and Ambulatory Medicine (2000) Recommendations for pediatric preventive healthcare. Pediatrics 105:645–646
3. Bethell C, Klein J, Peck C (2001) Assessing health system provision of adolescent preventive services: the young adult healthcare survey. Med Care 39:478–490
4. Corrado D, Pelliccia A, Bjørnstad HH, Vanhees L, Biffi A, Borjesson M, Panhuyzen-Goedkoop N, Deligiannis A, Solberg E, Dugmore D, Mellwig KP, Assanelli D, Delise P, van Buuren F, Anastasakis A, Heidbuchel H, Hoffmann E, Fagard R, Priori SG, Basso C, Arbustini E, Blomstrom-Lundqvist C, McKenna WJ, Thiene G (2005) Study group of sport cardiology of the working group of cardiac rehabilitation and exercise physiology and the working group of myocardial and pericardial diseases of the European society of cardiology. Cardiovascular pre-participation screening of young competitive athletes for prevention of sudden death: proposal for a common European protocol. Consensus statement of the study group of sport cardiology of the working group of cardiac rehabilitation and exercise physiology and the working group of myocardial and pericardial diseases of the European society of cardiology. Eur Heart J 26(5):516–524
5. Haney EM, Huffman LH, Bougatsos C, Freeman M, Steiner RD, Nelson HD (2007) Screening and treatment for lipid disorders in children and adolescents: systematic evidence review for the US preventive services task force. Pediatrics 120(1):e189–e214
6. Nemet D, Eliakim A (2009) Pediatric sports nutrition: an update. Curr Opin Cli Nutr Metab Care 12(3):304–309
7. Baker JL, Farpour-Lambert NJ, Nowicka P, Pietrobelli A, Weiss R (2010) Childhood obesity task force of the European association for the study of obesity. Evaluation of the overweight/obese child–practical tips for the primary health care provider: recommendations from the childhood obesity task force of the European association for the study of obesity. Obes Facts 3(2):131–137
8. Expert Panel on Integrated Guidelines for Cardiovascular Health and Risk Reduction in Children and Adolescents; National Heart, Lung, and Blood Institute (2011) Expert panel on integrated guidelines for cardiovascular health and risk reduction in children and adolescents: summary report. Pediatrics 128(5):S213–256
9. Daniels SR (2011) Screening and treatment of dyslipidemias in children and adolescents. Horm Res Paediatr 76(1):47–51
10. Schneider LM, Schermbeck RM, Chriqui JF, Chaloupka FJ (2012) The extent to which school district competitive food and beverage policies align with the 2010 dietary guidelines for Americans: implications for federal regulations. J Acad Nutr Diet 112(6):892–896
11. Mick TM, Dimeff RJ (2004) What kind of physical examination does a young athlete need before participating in sports? Clevel Clin J Med 71(7):587–597
12. Glover DW, Maron BJ, Matheson GO (1999) The preparticipation physical examination. Steps toward consensus and uniformity. Phys Sportsmed 27(8):29–34
13. Decree of the Italian Ministry of Health February 18 (1982) Norme per la tutela sanitaria dell'attività sportiva agonistica (rules concerning the medical protection of athletic activity). Gazzetta Ufficiale March 5, 1982, p 63
14. Maron BJ, Roberts WC, McAllister MH, Rosing DR, Epstein SE (1980) Sudden death in young athletes. Circulation 62:218–229
15. Thiene G, Nava A, Corrado D, Rossi L, Pennelli N (1988) Right ventricular cardiomyopathy and sudden death in young people. N Engl J Med 318:129–133
16. Corrado D, Basso C, Rizzoli G, Schiavon M, Thiene G (2003) Does sports activity enhance the risk of sudden death in adolescents and young adults? J Am Coll Cardiol 42:1959–1963

17. Maron BJ, Thompson PD, Puffer JC et al (1996) Cardiovascular preparticipation screening of competitive athletes: a statement for health professionals from the Sudden Death Committee and Congenital Cardiac Defects Committee, American Heart Association. Circulation 1996, vol 94, pp 850–856 (addendum published in Circulation 1998, vol 97, p 2294)

18. Corrado D, Basso C, Schiavon M, Thiene G (1998) Screening for hypertrophic cardiomyopathy in young athletes. New Engl J Med 339:364–369

19. Corrado D, Basso C, Pavei A, Michieli P, Schiavon M, Thiene G (2006) Trends in sudden cardiovascular death in young competitive athletes after implementation of a preparticipation screening program. JAMA 296(13):1593–1601

20. Stanley K (1994) Preparticipation evaluation in the young athlete. In: Stanitski CL, DeLee JC, Drez D (eds) Pediatric and adolescent sports medicine. WB Saunders Co, Philadelphia

21. Bar-Cohen Y, Silka MJ (2008) Sudden cardiac death in paediatrics. Curr Opin Pediatr 20:517–521

22. Valdez R, Greenlund KJ, Khoury MJ, Yoon PW (2007) Is family history a useful tool for detecting children at risk for diabetes and cardiovascular diseases? A public health perspective. Pediatrics 120:S78

23. Luma GB, Spiotta RT (2006) Hypertension in children and adolescents. Am Fam Physician 73:1558–1568

24. McNiece KL, Poffenbarger TS, Turner JL, Franco KD, Sorof JM, Portman RJ (2007) Prevalence of hypertension and pre-hypertension among adolescents. J Pediatr 150(6):640–644

25. Sorof JM, Lai D, Turner J, Poffenbarger T, Portman RJ (2004) Overweight, ethnicity, and the prevalence of hypertension in school-aged children. Pediatrics 113:475–482

26. Thomas M, Haas TS, Doerer JJ, Hodges JS, Aicher BO, Garberich RF, Mueller FO, Cantu RC, Maron BJ (2011) Epidemiology of sudden death in young, competitive athletes due to blunt trauma. Pediatrics 128(1):e1–e8

27. http://www.cdc.gov/nchs/fastats/asthma.htm. Accessed Oct 2012

28. Wilber RL, Rundell KW, Szmedra L, Jenkinson DM, Im J, Drake SD (2000) Incidence of exercise-induced bronchospasm in Olympic winter sport athletes. Med Sci Sports Exerc 32(4):732–737

29. Haahtela T, Malmberg P, Moreira A (2008) Mechanisms of asthma in Olympic athletes-practical implications. Allergy 63(6):685–694

30. Byrne S, McLean N (2001) Eating disorders in athletes: a review of the literature. J Sci Med Sport 4:145–159

31. Romano A, Di Fonso M, Giuffreda F, Papa G, Artesani MC, Viola M, Venuti A, Palmieri V, Zeppilli P (2001) Food-dependent exercise-induced anaphylaxis: clinical and laboratory findings in 54 subjects. Int Arch Allergy Immunol 125(3):264–272

32. Sundgot-Borgen J, Torstveit MK (2004) Prevalence of eating disorders in elite athletes is higher than in the general population. Clin J Sport Med 14:25–32

33. National High Blood Pressure Education Program Working Group on High Blood Pressure in Children and Adolescents (2004) The fourth report on the diagnosis, evaluation, and treatment of high blood pressure in children and adolescents. Pediatrics 114(2)4th Report:555–576

34. De Paepe A, Devereux RB, Dietz HC, Hennekam RC, Pyeritz RE (1996) Revised diagnostic criteria for the Marfan syndrome. Am J Med Genet 62(4):417–426

35. Dean JC (2007) Marfan syndrome: clinical diagnosis and management. Eur J Hum Genet 15:724–733

36. McCrory P, Meeuwisse W, Johnston K et al (2009) Consensus statement on concussion in sport, 3rd international conference on concussion in sport held in Zurich, November 2008. Clin J Sport Med 19(3):185–200

37. Delaney JS, Lacroix VJ, Leclerc S, Johnston KM (2002) Concussions among university football and soccer players. Clin J Sport Med 12(6):331–338

38. Pellman EJ, Viano DC, Casson IR, Arfken C, Feuer H (2005) Concussion in professional football: players returning to the same game—part 7. Neurosurgery 56(1):79–92

39. McCrea M, Guskiewicz KM, Marshall SW et al (2003) Acute effects and recovery time following concussion in collegiate football players: the NCAA Concussion Study. JAMA 290(19):2556–2563

40. http://www.ilae.org/Visitors/Documents/epilepsyand-sports.doc. Accessed 30 Oct 2012

Overuse Injuries

4

Lyle J. Micheli and Albert M. Pendleton

Pediatric sports participation has increased worldwide over the last several decades. In addition, the amount of time spent training for one sport is becoming more common; consequently, overuse injuries, the result of repetitive training, are becoming more prevalent in the pediatric population. Most overuse injuries are the result of repetitive stress to the bones, tendons, or tendinous attachments to the bone. The repetitive stress can often be attributed to poor biomechanics from muscle imbalance of the adolescent, which may be due to their specific anatomy or constitutionally excessive ligamentous laxity or tightness. The repetitive motions of many sports often lead to the muscle imbalance that drives the process. Many children focus on one sport year-round rather than having a seasonal sport. For example, ballet dancers will frequently have a very strong vastus lateralis, a tight iliotibial band (IT band), and a weak vastus medialis obliquus (VMO) due to the fact that most ballet motions take the leg into the abducted and externally rotated position. This can contribute to patellofemoral maltracking problems and as well as Iliopsoas tendinitis. Also, many overuse syndromes manifest themselves as a traction apophysitis due to overuse in the growing child with unfused growth plates such as Osgood-Schlatter disease, Sever's disease, medial epicondylitis, or Sinding-Larsen-Johansson syndrome.

The general treatment for many of the overuse syndromes is often very similar. However, sport-specific treatment directed at their specific muscle imbalance and anatomic variation is vital to getting them back to sport and continuing pain free. Treatment involves rest from the offending activity and correcting the muscle imbalance that may contribute to pain. Also, correcting errors in biomechanics of the specific athletic motions is important to keep the patient pain free in the future in order to continue participation. Bracing is often useful to provide support to allow the tissues to heal, with a concomitant strengthening program to prevent atrophy while the healing occurs. Stretching to correct muscle contractures is often required and anti-inflammatory medication may be necessary in the acute phase to allow therapy to be successful.

In this chapter, we will review the etiology, diagnosis, and treatment of several common overuse injuries. Note that certain conditions such as spondylolysis and osteochondritis dissecans that are associated with repetitive trauma will be covered in depth in other chapters in this book.

L. J. Micheli (✉)
Department of Sports Medicine, Boston Children's Hospital, 19 Longwood Avenue (2nd floor), Boston, MA 02115, USA
e-mail: l.micheli62@gmail.commarkdjenkins@comcast.net

A. M. Pendleton
Department of Sports Medicine, Boston Children's Hospital, 319 Longwood Avenue, Boston, MA 02115, USA
e-mail: albert.pendleton@me.com

V. Guzzanti (ed.), *Pediatric and Adolescent Sports Traumatology*,
DOI: 10.1007/978-88-470-5412-7_4, © Springer-Verlag Italia 2014

4.1   Patellofemoral Syndrome

Patellofemoral syndrome is the most common cause of knee pain evaluated by primary care physicians, sports medicine physicians, and orthopedic surgeons in this age group [1]. One study reported a patellofemoral pain syndrome incidence of 20 % in adolescents [2]. The etiology of patellofemoral syndrome is likely due to maltracking of the patella in the trochlear groove due to a number of causes [3]. The primary causes include abnormal alignment, muscle imbalance, or overuse. Malalignment that leads to patellofemoral pain syndrome includes genu varum or valgum, abnormal rotation including femoral anteversion, tibial torsion, or miserable malalignment. Muscle imbalance that leads to patellofemoral pain syndrome includes VMO weakness combined with IT band, quadriceps, and hamstrings contractures [4]. Muscle imbalance is often due to sport-specific training that emphasizes strengthening of only specific muscle groups. Witvrouw et al. found that a shortened quadriceps muscle, an altered VMO reflex response time, a decreased explosive strength, and a hypermobile patella were all correlated with the incidence of patellofemoral pain in a study of 282 male and female students [5].

The typical patient is between 8 and 16 years of age who has recently increased his or her activities. Their pain is often bilateral, but can be unilateral. The location is often described as vague discomfort but can usually be localized to the medial side of the patella or beneath the patella. Specific questioning usually reveals patients have more pain going up stairs than down stairs, as well as pain after sitting for long periods. The diagnosis is made by excluding other causes of knee pain that are in the differential such as OCD of the medial or lateral femoral condyle or the patella, medial patellar plica syndrome, anterior meniscus tear, patellar tendon tendinitis, Osgood-Schlatters, Sinding-Larsen-Johansson syndrome, discoid meniscus, or tumor. In addition, these patients will usually have a precipitating [22] cause for patellofemoral

maltracking such as a recent growth spurt, malalignment, or muscle imbalance.

Physical examination should start with assessment of alignment and rotational abnormalities looking for causes of patella maltracking. A gait assessment is very useful to note the effect of their alignment on the patella. Muscle imbalance and flexibility are important to note as well, including a weak VMO, tight quadriceps (Ely test), tight hamstrings (popliteal angles), and tight IT bands (Ober test). Assessment of foot deformity (i.e., pes planus) is also important in treatment considerations. Swelling of the knee may indicate an internal derangement or arthritis and requires additional evaluation. Dynamic examination of patellar tracking is necessary to identify those patients who are tracking laterally. An assessment of joint line tenderness is also important to eliminate meniscal pathology as the source of pain.

Radiographs are not always necessary though any clinical symptoms not consistent with patellofemoral syndrome should warrant them such as swelling, night pain, pain going down stairs, mechanical symptoms, unilaterality, or sensations of instability. In addition, patients who are not improving with a trial of dedicated physical therapy should also warrant radiographic evaluation. Anterior-posterior, lateral, notch, and sunrise views will rule out tumor or OCD and may also yield helpful information regarding trochlear anatomy and patellar tracking. MRI may be helpful in cases where the history is inconsistent with the diagnosis in order to rule out chondral or meniscal pathology.

Treatment of patellar femoral syndrome includes relative rest from the offending activity and correcting the causes of patella maltracking. VMO strengthening is at the core of physical therapy as strengthening will usually improve patella tracking, protecting those patients with malalignment. Both open kinetic-chain exercises (straight leg raising and terminal short arc extension) and closed kinetic-chain exercises (mini-squats and stepping up and down) have been shown to be effective in the treatment of patellofemoral pain syndrome [6, 7]. Patients with a tight lateral retinaculum will benefit from lateral retinacular stretching. Therapy should also focus on a regaining flexibility of the hamstrings, quadriceps, IT band, and Achilles [3]. Modalities and anti-inflammatories can be helpful in the early stages to calm down inflammation to allow therapeutic exercise. An off-the-shelf foot orthotic may be helpful as well for patients with pes planus or pes cavus to improve lower extremity alignment during sports activities. Finally, many patients report feeling symptomatic improvement when wearing a patella stabilizing brace though CT and MRI studies have shown no change in patellar tilt or subluxation and no improvement in dynamic tracking when the patient uses a brace or patellar taping [8, 9].

Most sports medicine physicians who treat children and adolescents with patellofemoral pain report that 95 % of symptoms resolve with time, rest, a prescribed therapy program, bracing, and anti-inflammatories [3]. However, one of the largest studies focusing only on adolescents, a 14–20-year follow-up study of girls with anterior knee pain found that only 22 % of patients were completely asymptomatic, but 90 % still participated in sports on a regular basis, but approximately 25 % of patients still reported significant symptoms [10].

tendinitis, or internal impingement. The etiology of almost all maladies of the throwing shoulder is similar including poor throwing biomechanics, scapular dyskinesis, muscle imbalance, glenohumeral internal rotation deficit (GIRD), and excessive throwing.

Little League shoulder was first described in 1966 as shoulder pain in skeletally immature patients with radiographic changes of osteochondrosis of the proximal humeral physis [12]. The injury is due to repetitive microtrauma to the physis from the rotational forces of the throwing motion. Radiographic changes usually include physeal widening (Figs. 4.1 and 4.2) or fragmentation, but can early growth plate closure can be seen. Premature closure can lead to angular deformity or limb length discrepancy as well.

Diagnosis of the cause of shoulder pain in the adolescent throwing athlete should begin with a throwing history of pitches per week and type of pitches thrown as well as documenting the number of months a year the patient participates in throwing sports. Physical examination should be comprehensive paying attention to the location of the pain and any areas of tenderness. Range of motion should be documented and compared to the contralateral side to assess for deficits, paying particular attention to internal

4.2 Overuse Throwing Injuries

Shoulder and elbow injuries in the adolescent throwing athlete are extremely common and the incidence is increasing [11]. Children are often participating in multiple leagues and playing for multiple teams year-round without any dedicated rest. In addition, parents or coaches who do not have training in proper pitching mechanics coach most children and adolescents.

4.2.1 Shoulder Pain

Shoulder pain in the throwing athlete can be due to a variety of causes including "little league shoulder," glenohumeral instability, rotator cuff

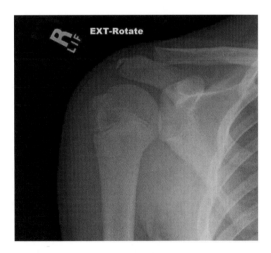

Fig. 4.1 Little league shoulder. Bilateral AP radiographs in external rotation. Note the physeal widening on the *right shoulder* compared to the *left shoulder*

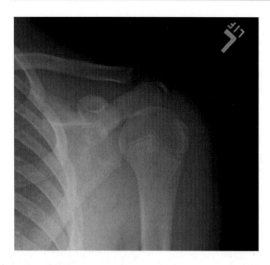

Fig. 4.2 Little league shoulder. Bilateral AP radiographs in external rotation. Note the physeal widening on the *right shoulder* compared to the *left shoulder*

rotation in abduction. Muscle atrophy should be noted as well, so as not to miss nerve impingement lesions. Provocative impingement maneuvers are important to assess for subacromial bursitis and impingement as well as assessing rotator cuff strength. Glenohumeral stability should be assessed along with generalized ligamentous laxity by the load and shift, sulcus sign, and modified Marshall test. A dynamic examination of scapular motion should be assessed with wall push-ups to evaluate for scapular dyskinesis or winging of the scapula.

Radiographs should be considered for patients with a history and physical examination consistent with little league shoulder. Radiographs should be taken AP in external rotation. Comparison to the contralateral side may be helpful in cases where physeal derangement is unclear.

Treatment for patients with a diagnosis of little league shoulder includes rest and activity modification for 2–3 months. Patients should refrain from pitching or playing catcher during this time. Patients then progress to a light tossing schedule and gradually progress with increasing distance and velocity. This protocol has shown excellent results with up to 91 % of patients remaining asymptomatic [13]. In addition, correcting errors in biomechanics is of vital

importance to prevent recurrence. Parents, coaches, and athletes should be aware of established guidelines for pitch counts and number of days per week allowed pitching for adolescent pitchers. Education of the athlete and parent is paramount to long-term success.

4.2.2 Prevention

Adolescent patients with shoulder pain and no radiographic changes require diagnosis-specific treatment. However, all throwing patients require an assessment of pitching mechanics. A stretching program is important to decrease pain and adaptive changes in throwing [14]. Posteroinferior capsular stretching has been shown to decrease GIRD and 90 % of patients with symptomatic GIRD (>25 degrees) respond to a dedicated posterior capsule stretching program [15]. Adolescent throwers with pain have been demonstrated to have greater relative strength of the dominant arm internal rotators and weaker relative strength of the supraspinatus and middle trapezius than athletes who do not have pain [16]. Consequently, a strengthening program focusing on strengthening the posterior musculature and rotator cuff is also important to help stabilize the shoulder and prevent injury.

4.2.3 Elbow Pain

Elbow pain in the adolescent throwing athlete is usually due to three main sources: medial-side tension, lateral-side compression, or posterior compartment shear [14]. Pain on the medial side of the elbow is often due to medial epicondyle apophyseal stress injury or avulsion "little league elbow" or tearing of the medial collateral ligament. Lateral compression injuries include capitellar OCD from repetitive microtrauma. Posterior compartment injuries include posteromedial impingement and olecranon stress fractures. Little league elbow results from repetitive stress and valgus overload of the medial structures. Repetitive contraction of the flexor pronator muscles stresses the chondro-osseous origin, leading to inflammation and apophysitis. Poor throwing mechanics increases the stress on the elbow driving the process. In addition, continuing to throw despite pain is counterproductive as decreases in velocity encourage overthrowing, which further stresses the elbow.

Patients are typically less than age 14 and report a triad of medial elbow pain, decreased throwing effectiveness and decreased throwing distance [13]. Physical examination should note the location of the pain, which is usually directly over the medial epicondyle. Swelling may be present and some patients may have a flexion contracture. Radiographic evaluation may be normal, though some patients will show irregular ossification, apophyseal enlargement, separation, and eventual fragmentation.

Treatment consists of rest followed by an assessment of throwing mechanics, strength, and flexibility. Correction of errors in throwing mechanics, strengthening of the rotator cuff and periscapular muscles, and eliminating contractures is of paramount importance to prevent recurrence of injury. Some recommend an initial period of rest of 2–4 weeks followed by a gradual return to throwing at 6 weeks if the athlete is symptoms free [17]. In those patients with medial epicondylar fragmentation documented on X-ray, recent evidence suggests improved return to throwing with a period of rest until elbow pain and tenderness of the medial epicondyle disappear [18]. Patients are then gradually permitted to perform limited throwing (30 % maximum strength) and then increase the distance and strength of throwing gradually.

4.3 Traction Apophysitis

4.3.1 Etiology

The etiology of all traction apophysitis is similar. The etiology is repetitive microtrauma to the physis from repeated contraction of the attached muscles. Apophysitis occurs when the body's capacity to heal is slower than the amount of rest

the athlete gives the body. In addition, growth spurts compound the problem by increasing the tension on the apophysis from muscle tightness and contractures.

4.4 Pelvic Apophysitis

Pelvic apophysitis can occur at any of the apophyseal insertions sites around the pelvis or hip including anterior superior iliac spine, anterior inferior iliac spine, greater trochanter, ischial tuberosity, or iliac crest. Pelvic apophysitis is common among distance runners and dancers as well as hockey, lacrosse, and football [19].

Patients complain of dull pain about the hip that is worse with activity and gets better with rest. Often, there is a history of a recent growth spurt as well as a recent increase in activity. Careful examination reveals local tenderness over the apophysis. Patients will often have tight and contracted IT bands, hamstrings, quadriceps, and abductors. Radiographs may show physeal widening or irregular ossification but are often normal. However, radiographs are necessary to rule out avulsion fracture.

Treatment involves rest from the offending activity for 3–4 weeks followed by an individual and sport-specific therapy program focused on modalities to decreased pain and inflammation as well as stretching to eliminate contractures in the early phases. Once the patient is pain free, a gradual strengthening of the muscles around the hip is begun including back and abdominal muscles.

4.5 Sinding-Larsen-Johansson Syndrome

Sinding-Larsen-Johansson syndrome is due to a traction apophysitis at the inferior pole of the patella. However, some reports attribute it to a traction tendinitis with de novo calcification in the proximal attachment of the patellar tendon, which has been avulsed [20]. It affects children aged 10–12 years, and the symptoms are aggravated by running, jumping, stair-climbing, and kneeling.

Patients present with point tenderness over the inferior pole of the patella. Contraction of the quadriceps mechanism reproduces the pain, as well as stretch of the quadriceps. Radiographs may be normal but often show irregular calcification at the inferior pole of the patella.

Treatment consists of rest from activity and modalities directed at the source of pain. Stretching should focus on the quadriceps, hamstrings, and IT band. In severe cases, a splint or cast can be used to calm down inflammation followed by physical therapy. Symptoms are usually self-limited. Rarely, a separate ossicle may persist and become symptomatic, requiring surgical removal.

4.6 Osgood-Schlatter Disease

Osgood-Schlatter disease is a traction apophysitis of the tibial tubercle. The etiology is repetitive microtrauma to the tibial tubercle apophysis from repeated contraction of the quadriceps complex. The combination of rapid growth with repeated tensile forces on the apophysis leads to this very common disease.

The pain usually occurs in adolescent athletes who participate in activities requiring repetitive extension and contraction of the knee. It is particularly common in gymnasts. Boys are affected more often than girls with the peak age being 13 for boys and 12 for girls. Patients report pain and swelling over the tibial tubercle. Physical examination reveals the triad of tenderness to palpation over the tubercle, pain over the tubercle on short arc extension and pain over the tubercle with Ely testing (prone stretching of the quadriceps by bringing the foot to the buttock). Radiographic evaluation is necessary to rule out tumor or other serious causes of knee pain. Radiographs are often normal but may reveal elevation of the apophysis or ossicle formation. A 15-degree internal rotation view will show the apophysis much more clearly (Fig. 4.3).

Treatment consists of rest, activity modification, and modalities to eliminate the acute-phase pain and swelling. A physical therapy regimen focused on quadriceps, hamstrings, and IT band

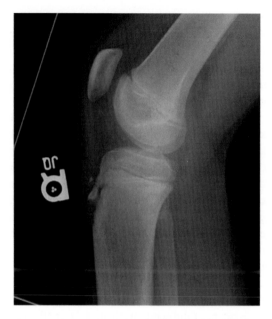

Fig. 4.3 Osgood-Schlatter Disease. Lateral radiograph of a child with Osgood-Schlatter disease, note the elevation of the tibial tubercle apophysis

stretching is then begun to decrease the forces applied on the tubercle. "Cho-pat" type braces can be used to help relieve the pain. Rarely, immobilization in a cast or removable brace is required, but may be helpful in recalcitrant cases. Symptoms are usually self-limited, though pain may persist until the apophysis closes. As many as 10 % of patients may experience pain after apophyseal closure due to formation of a separate ossicle, if non-surgical treatment fails, operative removal usually resolves the pain [21].

4.7 Sever's Disease

Sever's disease is a traction apophysitis of the calcaneus at the Achilles tendon insertion. It most commonly occurs in boys around age 12 and girls around age 11. The etiology is due to repetitive contraction of the plantar flexor muscles coupled with recent growth, tight plantar fascia, and a tight gastroc-soleus complex.

Pain is localized to the heel and exacerbated by running and standing for long periods. Compression of the calcaneus from the medial and lateral sides elicits pain. Foot position and heel cord tightness should be assessed during the examination. Radiographs are often not helpful but can help rule out calcaneal stress fracture and should be attained in cases of unilateral disease. MRI is seldom necessary unless the clinician is dealing with a prolonged course of pain not responsive to conservative measures or to rule out calcaneal stress fracture.

Treatment includes activity modification, ice, and anti-inflammatories to decrease pain in the acute period. Treatment then transitions to an Achilles and plantar fascia stretching program. Heel cups can be helpful to decrease the strain on the Achilles by elevating the heel, but can add to gastrocnemius tightness if the patient does not adhere to a stretching program [22]. An off-the-shelf foot orthotic can be helpful as well to keep the foot in more normal position for daily activities.

4.8 Iselin's Disease

Iselin's disease is a traction apophysitis of the base of the fifth metatarsal at the insertion of the peroneus brevis. Pain is exacerbated by running, jumping, and cutting sports.

Physical examination reveals pain at the base of the fifth metatarsal as well as pain with resisted eversion and extreme plantar flexion. Radiographs may show an enlarged apophysis but are necessary to rule out stress fracture.

Treatment involves activity modification or immobilization if symptoms are severe [21]. Patients should also work on peroneal and Achilles stretching, while strengthening the dorsiflexors and invertors.

4.9 Anterior Leg Pain

"Shin splints" or anterior leg pain is very common, especially in the running athlete. Shin splints include multiple diagnoses most commonly including medial tibial stress syndrome (MTTS), chronic exertional compartment syndrome (CECS), and tibial stress fracture [23].

The history usually reveals a recent increase in training in an unconditioned athlete. Patients usually complain of a gradual onset of pain that continues to worsen as training progresses eventually leading to an inability to compete. However, each syndrome may present in a different manner. It is imperative the clinician sort out the cause of the pain in order to implement the correct treatment plan and to rule out more serious diagnoses, such as tumor or infection.

4.9.1 Evaluation

Each patient should get a detailed history and nature of the symptoms. Does the pain start immediately with exercise or does it take several minutes? Does the pain worsen to the point where the activity has to be discontinued? Does the pain continue after exercise? Is there pain at night? In addition, the training history is important to document recent increases in training intensity or duration or changes in surface or footwear. Numbness or radiating pain suggests a neurologic origin where as night pain suggests an etiology within the bone.

Radiographs are necessary on all patients unless symptoms are minimal allowing the patient to play through the pain and the duration is less than 2 weeks. However, any red flag symptoms such as night pain, severe pain, point tenderness, or worsening symptoms warrant radiographic evaluation.

Physical examination should localize the site of maximal tenderness if it exists or document that the pain is diffuse. Percussion of the entire tibia can be helpful to identify a spot of maximal tenderness or if tenderness is diffuse. If tenderness is over the soft tissue, note if a mass is present. In addition, strength testing and sensory examination should be done to rule out nerve impingement lesions.

4.10 Medial Tibial Stress Syndrome

Medial tibial stress syndrome is thought to be a periostitis from excessive stress on the medial border of the tibia. The excessive stress can be from multiple factors including biomechanical factors such as tibia vara, sudden changes in training intensity, duration, footwear, and training surface, as well as soft tissue injuries such as muscle tightness and insertional tendinitis. Histologic specimens reveal an inflammatory process with vasculitis that is consistent with a periostitis [23]. MTSS is mostly attributed to the attachment of the soleus but the flexor digitorum longus and deep crural fascia also contribute to it [24]. Patients with excessive pronation of the hindfoot can lead to increased strain on the medial soleus as it eccentrically contracts during midstance to resist pronation. Bennett showed that there was positive correlation between patients with excessive pronation who had a higher incidence of MTSS [25]. However, other studies have not shown a correlation between MTSS and excessive pronation [26, 27].

Medial tibial stress syndrome usually presents as diffuse leg pain. Classically, the pain is located on the posteromedial aspect of the distal two-thirds of the tibia [28]. The pain is relieved by rest and exacerbated by activity. The pain usually progressively worsens to the point where the patient is unable to continue the activity. MTSS often occurs in patients who have a sudden increase in the frequency and intensity of athletic training. Physical examination often reveals hindfoot valgus and a pes planus deformity. Patients are generally tender to palpation along the posteromedial border of the distal third of the tibia. The area is often more diffuse than with tibial stress fracture, which should always be in the differential diagnosis. The tibial shaft is often not tender to percussion unless percussed posteromedially. Resisted plantar flexion may be painful as well, otherwise foot range of motion is usually non-tender. Imaging includes plain radiographs, which are usually normal, but some patients may show periosteal new bone formation with scalloping along the posteromedial border of the tibia [29]. MRI is often not helpful as a study of 19 patients with MTSS, only 5 showed periosteal edema on MRI [30]; however, it is helpful to rule out other diagnoses. Three-phase bone scan can be helpful to rule out stress fracture. In addition, 10 patients with shin splints underwent bone scan and the delayed images showed longitudinally oriented lesions along the posterior cortex of the tibia [31].

Management is non-surgical consisting of relative rest for up to 4 months with ice and modalities as an adjunct. Patients can participate in a cross-training program that does not involve stress on the tibia, swimming and cycling are good options. Once symptoms have abated treatment should focus on preventing recurrence. A dedicated triceps surae stretching program is an important part of treatment. Orthotics are also helpful to place the foot in a more suitable position for impact and may offload the soleus. Once the patient is ready to return to running, a program that allows a gradual increase in intensity and duration is important to prevent recurrence. Initially running on softer surfaces is also helpful as well. Surgery is generally not recommended though some authors have had good results with superficial posterior compartment fasciotomy [32].

4.11 Chronic Exertional Compartment Syndrome

Chronic exertional compartment syndrome is thought to be due to muscle ischemia during activity. The compartment is unable to expand to keep the pressure stabilized and consequently the compartment pressure increases. As the pressure increases, the muscles get decreased blood flow leading to ischemia.

Patients generally complain of pain during the first 30 min of exercise and the pain usually does not abate until several hours after exercise and may persist into the next day. Pain is often localized to the anterior and lateral compartments of the leg. Physical examination usually does not reveal any areas of palpable tenderness. Patients may also complain of parasthesias on the dorsum of the foot if CECS involves the lateral compartment or on the plantar surface if it involves the deep posterior compartment. The diagnosis of CECS is confirmed by measuring intra-compartmental pressure (ICP) pre- and post-exercise. Pedowitz et al. established guidelines for the diagnosis of CECS based on the ICP. The guidelines are as follows: pre-exercise compartment pressure greater than 15 mm Hg, 1 min post-exercise pressure greater than 30 mm Hg, and 5 min post-exercise pressure greater than 20 mm Hg [33]. Active research continues to search for a non-invasive reliable method to diagnose CECS such as MRI and near infrared spectroscopy (NIRS). A recent study reports an in-scanner exercise-based MRI examination to be 96 % sensitive and 87 % specific in the diagnosis of CECS confirmed by ICP measurement and clinical examination [34]. NIRS is a non-invasive method that measure tissue oxygenation at the site the probe is placed. Van den Brand et al. found that healthy volunteers had a significantly higher tissue oxygen saturation StO [2] than patients with CECS (56 versus 27, $P < 0.05$) during peak exercise. In addition, patients with CECS had a higher absolute and percentage change in their StO [2] between baseline and peak exercise (absolute 60 versus 35, $P < 0.05$; percentage 67 versus 38, $P < 0.05$). Finally, St0 [2] values in legs with confirmed CECS returned to normal after fasciotomy [35].

The treatment of CECS is surgical. Micheli et al. assessed multiple non-operative methods including ice, rest, electrostimulation, and stretching. Only prolonged rest with activity avoidance was effective [36]. Success of fasciotomy in the literature has ranged from 60 to 100 % [37]. The surgeon should address all compartments affected and ensure a complete fasciotomy is done at the time of surgery. Recurrence can occur after surgical treatment with reported rates as high as 17 % [37].

4.12 Tibial Stress Fracture

Tibial stress fractures are due to repetitive stresses on the tibia from repetitive loading. Intense exercise can lead to an imbalance in the body's ability to heal microscopic bone injuries. Bone healing lags behind bone injury leading to stress fracture [38, 39]. A recent increase in training is often the culprit, though other factors are important as well. If athletes increase their training too rapidly, then muscle fatigue sets in and leads to increased stresses as the muscles fail to absorb the shock. Consequently, increased force is transmitted to the bone. Anatomic variations in the tibia can contribute, including tibia vara and procurvatum of the tibia. In addition, poor nutrition, metabolic disorders, and hormonal imbalance can also lead to osteopenia or osteoporosis which can lead to stress fractures.

Patients usually present with activity-related pain that improves with rest. Patients can usually localize the pain to a specific spot on the tibia and pain usually persists after activity. Attaining the patients training history is important to determine whether the program has changed. Changes in terrain, footwear, duration, and intensity can all be causative factors. In addition, the athletes' general health, nutrition, eating habits, regular medications, and menstrual history (if female) are also important. Any suspicion of the female athletic triad (oligomenorrhea/amenorrhea, disordered eating, osteoporosis/osteopenia) should be evaluated with a metabolic bone work-up and referral to a specialist in this area. Treatment of the female athletic triad usually requires a multidisciplinary approach including sports medicine doctors, endocrinologists, psychiatrists, and nutritionists. Physical examination reveals swelling and focal tenderness to palpation. If this is not present, a bending or twisting force may elicit focal pain. The physician should also look for any possible causes of the stress fracture including malalignment (tibia vara, procurvatum, genu varum), rotational abnormalities, foot alignment, muscle tone, and leg length discrepancy.

Imaging should include plain radiographs to look for stress fracture and rule out tumor, though radiographs may be normal. Stress fractures can occur at any site along the tibia but the most frequent site is the posteromedial tibia (compression side). The fracture is usually transverse in orientation. However, patients can develop a stress fracture on the anterior cortex (tension side) in the middle one-third, which is

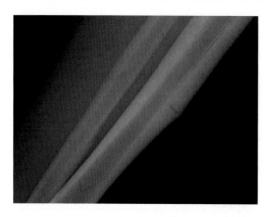

Fig. 4.4 Anterior tibial stress fracture: lateral radiograph of a gymnast with an anterior tension-sided tibial stress fracture

much more recalcitrant to treatment, and is often referred to as the "the dreaded black line" (Fig. 4.4). This type of fracture more often occurs in jumping and leaping activities like gymnastics, dance, or basketball. However, stress fractures are often diagnosed on subsequent imaging identified by periosteal thickening or sclerosis, cortical changes with initial decreased density and later callus formation or endosteal thickening and sclerosis [40]. Radiographs may also show alignment abnormalities such as tibia vara or procurvatum. The sensitivity of radiographs is 15–35 % initially and it may be several weeks before radiographic changes are evident [41]. Bone scan is excellent at picking up stress fractures with a high sensitivity (74–100 %) [42, 43], but will also be positive in cases of tumor or infection. MRI has replaced scintigraphy as the confirmatory test in most studies as its sensitivity is equal or better to scintigraphy but with a higher specificity [43, 44]. MRI can also detect reactive bone remodeling and early stress injury before fracture occurs [44]. Finally, MRI involves no radiation, which is advantageous especially in the adolescent population.

Treatment involves rest from the offending activity followed by gradual resumption of activity once the tibia is pain free. Typically, this process takes 3–4 months. Patients whose symptoms return after attempting to go back to activity must go back to a period of rest. Patients should be given a "return to running" program, emphasizing a slow return with leeway in the program that allows rest if pain returns. Changing to a softer running surface and a custom foot orthotic may be helpful as well. In addition, an evaluation of running mechanics can be helpful to correct running errors that cause increased impact. In addition, supplementation with calcium and vitamin D is also indicated. Current recommendations vary, though recent trends are toward superphysiolgic doses of calcium and vitamin D, 1,200–1,500 mg/d of calcium and 800–3,000 IU/d of vitamin D [45]. Anterior cortex stress fractures can be more challenging to heal due to decreased vascularity and due to the fact they are on the tension side of the bone. Casting for a period of 6–8 weeks is often appropriate followed by functional bracing. These patients often require a period of rest of a minimum of 4–6 months [46]. Mean time to return to sport is between 9 and 12 months [47]. Patients with a history of multiple stress fractures should get a work-up for metabolic bone disease from an endocrinologist. In addition, patients at risk for the female athletic triad (amenorrhea/oligomenorrhea, osteopenia/osteoporosis, and disordered eating) and a diagnosis of a stress fracture should also be referred to specialist in this area. Operative treatment is controversial in tibial stress fracture though some authors recommend intramedullary nailing for anterior cortex fractures with chronic changes and a wide fissure [48]. Borens et al. reported on anterior compression plating in high-performance female athletes with full return to sports at 10 weeks [49]. The role of pulsed ultrasound in the treatment of stress fractures has not been clearly defined though there is some evidence in the literature that they may hasten healing [50].

4.13 High-Risk Stress Fractures

4.13.1 Femoral Neck Stress Fracture

Femoral neck stress fractures can develop as the hip musculature becomes fatigued. Prolonged activity leads to a loss of the shock-absorbing effects of the muscles and increased stresses on the femoral neck. Coxa vara, osteopenia, and the female athletic triad are risk factors for femoral neck stress fracture. Patients usually present with groin pain. The pain is worse with weight bearing and straight leg raise is often painful.

Femoral neck stress fractures may be evident on plain radiographs as a lucent line, sclerosis, or callus formation (Fig. 4.5). However, X-ray may be negative. MRI is highly sensitive in identifying and delineating stress fractures in the

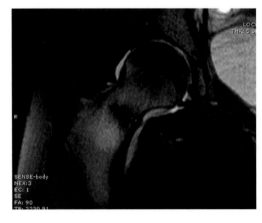

Fig. 4.6 Femoral neck stress fracture. MRI showing same fracture diagnosed on MRI 6 weeks earlier, radiographs were normal

femoral neck (Fig. 4.6). Femoral neck stress fracture can either be on the tension or the compression side of the bone. The compression type is the more common type and begins at the interior medial cortex of the femoral neck. These patients can usually be managed non-operatively. Tension-sided stress fractures start on the superior cortex and propagate inferiorly and medially across the femoral neck. These fractures have an increased chance of displacement compared to compression sided fractures with continued activity. Consequently, some authors recommend acute percutaneous fixation to avoid the potential risk of displaced fracture, while others report successful non-operative treatment [46]. Any patient with displacement requires urgent open reduction and internal fixation.

4.13.2 Navicular Stress Fractures

The tarsal navicular is susceptible to stress fracture as the central one-third has been identified as an area of maximum shear stress. In addition, the central zone of the navicular is devoid of a direct blood supply leading to delayed healing [51].

Patients often complain of vague foot pain though physical examination may reveal pain over the dorsal aspect of the navicular.

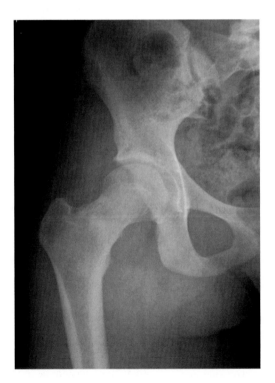

Fig. 4.5 Femoral neck stress fracture: AP hip radiograph showing callus formation at the and sclerosis of the femoral neck (*compression side*). This radiograph was taken 6 weeks after diagnosis, initial radiographs were normal

Diagnosis is made on plain X-rays or MRI evaluation revealing fracture in the central-third.

Aggressive management is important. Torg et al. performed a systematic review of surgical and non-surgical management and concluded that optimal initial treatment involved strict non-weight bearing for a minimum of 6 weeks [52]. Patients who did not undergo a minimum non-weight-bearing period of 6 weeks had a poor chance of returning to full activities. Average return to activities was between 4 and 6 months [53].

References

1. Thomeé R, Augustsson J, Karlsson J (1999) Patellofemoral pain syndrome: a review of current issues. Sports Med 28:245–262
2. Luhmann SJ, Schoenecker PL, Dobbs MB et al (2008) Adolescent patellofemoral pain: implicating the medial patellofemoral ligament as the main pain generator. J Child Orthop 2:269–277
3. Smith AD (2005) The skeletally immature knee: what's new in overuse injuries. In: Ireland ML (ed) Instructional course lectures sports medicine. American academy of orthopaedic surgeons, Rosemont, pp 371–378
4. Waryasz GR, McDermott AY (2008) Patellofemoral pain syndrome (PFPS): a systematic review of anatomy and potential risk factors. Dyn Med 7:9
5. Witvrouw E, Lysens R, Bellemans J et al (2000) Intrinsic risk factors for the development of anterior knee pain in an athletic population. A two-year prospective study. Am J Sports Med 28:480–489
6. O'neill DB, Micheli LJ, Warner JP (1992) Patellofemoral stress: a prospective analysis of exercise treatment in adolescents and adults. Am J Sports Med 20:151–156
7. Witvrouw W, Lysens R, Bellemans J et al (2000) Open versus closed kinetic chain exercises for patellofemoral pain: a prospective randomized sudy. Am J Sports Med 28:687–694
8. Gigante A, Pasquinelli FM, Paladini P et al (2001) The effects of patellar taping on patellofemoral incongruence: a computed tomograpy study. Am J Sports Med 29:88–92
9. Powers CM, Shellock FG, Beering TV et al (1999) Effect of bracing on patellar kinematics in patients with patellofemoral joint pain. Med Sci Sports Exerc 31:1714–1720
10. Nimon G, Murray D, Sandow M et al (1998) Natural history of anterior knee pain: a 14–20 year follow up of nonoperative management. J Pediatr Orthop 18:118–122
11. Adirim TA, Cheng TI (2003) Overview of injuries in the young athlete. Sports Med 33:75–81
12. Adams JE (1966) Little league shoulder: osteochondrosis of the proximal humeral epiphysis in boy baseball pitchers. Calif Med 105:22–25
13. Kocher MS, Waters PM, Micheli LJ (2000) Upper extremity injuries in the pediatric athlete. Sports Med 30:117–135
14. Vadasdi KB, Perez V, Ahmad CS (2010) Throwing injuries in adolescents. In: Ahmad CS (ed) Pediatric and adolescent sports injuries. AAOS, Rosemont, pp 71–85
15. Burkhart SS, Morgan CD, Kibler WB (2003) The disabled throwing shoulder: spectrum of pathology Part I. Pathoanatomy and biomechanics. Arthroscopy 19:404–420
16. Trakis JE, McHugh MP, Caracciolo PA et al (2008) Muscle strength and range of motion in adolescent pitchers with throwing-related pain: implications for injury prevention. Am J Sports Med 36:2173–2178
17. Chen FS, Diaz VA, Loebenberg M et al (2005) Shoulder and Elbow injuries in the skeletally immature athlete. J Am Acad Orthop Surg 13:172–185
18. Harada M, Takahara M, Hirayama T et al (2012) Outcome of nonoperative treatment of humeral medial epicondylar fragmentation before epiphyseal closure in young baseball players. Am J Sports Med 40(7):1583–1590
19. Frank JB, Jarit GJ, Bravman JT et al (2007) Lower extremity injuries in the skeletally immature athlete. J Am Acad Orthop Surg 15(6):357–366
20. Medlar RC, Lyne ED (1978) Sinding-Larsen-Johansson disease. Its etiology and natural history. J Bone Joint Surg Am 60(8):1113–1116
21. Outerbridge AR, Micheli LJ (1995) Overuse injuries in the young athlete. Clin Sports Med 14:503–516
22. Micheli LJ, Ireland ML (1987) Prevention and management of calcaneal apophysitis in children: an overuse syndrome. J Pediatr Orthop 7:34–38
23. Pell RF, Khanuja HS, Cooley GR (2004) Leg pain in the running athlete. J Am Acad Orthop Surg 12:396–404
24. Beck BR, Osternig LR (1994) Medial tibial stress syndrome: the location of muscles in the leg in relation to symptoms. J Bone Joint Surg Am 76:1057–1061
25. Bennett JE, Reinking MF, Pluemer B (2001) Factors contributing to the development of me- dial tibial stress syndrome in high school runners. J Orthop Sports Phys Ther 31:504–510
26. Hubbard TJ, Carpenter EM, Cordova ML (2009) Contributing factors to medial tibial stress syndrome: a prospective investigation. Med Sci Sports Exerc 41(3):490–496
27. Plisky MS, Rauh MJ, Heiderscheit B et al (2007) Medial tibial stress syndrome in high school cross-country runners: incident and risk factors. J Orthop Sports Phys Ther 37(2):40–47

28. Mubarak SJ, Gould RN, Lee YF et al (1982) The medial tibial stress syndrome. A cause of shin splints. Am J Sports Med 10:201–205

29. Michael RH, Holder LE (1985) The soleus syndrome: a cause of medial tibial stress (shin splints). Am J Sports Med 13:87–94

30. Anderson MW, Ugalde V, Batt M (1997) Shin splints: MR appearance in a preliminary study. Radiology 204:177–180

31. Holder LE, Michael RH (1984) The specific scintigraphic pattern of "shin splints in the lower leg": concise communication. J Nucl Med 25:865–869

32. Holen KJ, Engebretsen L, Grøntvedt T et al (1995) Surgical treatment of medial tibial stress syndrome (shin splint) by fasciotomy of the superficial posterior compartment of the leg. Scand J Med Sci Sports 5:40–43

33. Pedowitz RA, Hargens AR, Mubarak SJ et al (1990) Modified criteria for the objective diagnosis of chronic compartment syndrome of the leg. Am J Sports Med 18:35–40

34. Van den Brand JG, Verleisdonk EJ, van der Werken C (2004) Near infrared spectroscopy in the diagnosis of chronic exertional compartment syndrome. Am J Sports Med 32(2):452–456

35. Ringler MD, Litwiller DV, Felmlee JP et al (2012) MRI accurately detects chronic exertional compartment syndrome: a validation study. Skeletal Radiol Jul 13 (epub ahead of print)

36. Micheli LJ, Solomon R, Solomon J et al (1999) Surgical treatment for chronic lower-leg compartment syndrome in young female athletes. Am J Sports Med 27:197–201

37. Wittstein J, Moorman CT III, Levin LS (2010) Endoscopic compartment release for chronic exertional compartment syndrome: surgical technique and results. Am J Sports Med 38:1661–1666

38. Maitra RS, Johnson DL (1997) Stress fractures: clinical history and physical examination. Clin Sports Med 16:259–274

39. Boden BP, Osbahr DC, Jimenez C (2001) Low—risk stress fractures. Am J Sports Med 29:100–111

40. Ohta-Fukushima M, Mutoh Y, Takasugi S et al (2002) Characteristics of stress fractures in young athletes under 20 years. J Sports Med Phys Fitness 42(2):198–206

41. Lassus J, Tulikoura I, Konttinen YT et al (2002) Bone stress injuries of the lower extremity: a review. Acta Orthop Scand 73:359–368

42. Gaeta M, Minutoli F, Scribano E et al (2005) CT and MR imaging findings in athletes with early tibial stress injuries: comparison with bone scintigraphy findings and emphasis on cortical abnormalities. Radiology 235(2):553–561

43. Fredericson M, Bergman AG, Hoffman KL et al (1995) Tibial stress reaction in runners. Correlation of clinical symptoms and scintigraphy with a new magnetic resonance imaging grading system. Am J Sports Med 23(4):472–481

44. Ishibashi Y, Okamura Y, Otsuka H et al (2002) Comparison of scintigraphy and magnetic resonance imaging for stress injuries of bone. Clin J Sport Med 12(2):79–84

45. Shindel MK, Endo Y, Warren RF et al (2012) Stress fractures about the tibia, foot, and ankle. J Am Acad Orthop Surg 20:167–176

46. Boden BP, Osbahr DC (2000) High-risk stress fractures: evaluation and treatment. J Am Acad Orthop Surg 8:344–353

47. Rettig AC, Shelbourne KD, McCarroll JR et al (1988) The natural history and treatment of delayed union stress fractures of the anterior cortex of the tibia. Am J Sports Med 16(3):250–255

48. Chang PS, Harris RM (1996) Intramedullary nailing for chronic tibial stress fractures: a review of five cases. Am J Sports Med 24:688–692

49. Borens O, Sen MK, Huang RC et al (2006) Anterior tension band plating for anterior tibial stress fractures in high performance female athletes: a report of 4 cases. J Orthop Trauma 20(6):425–430

50. Brand JC, Brindle T, Nyland J et al (1999) Does pulsed low intensity ultrasound allow early return to normal activities when treating stress fractures? A review of one tarsal navicular and eight tibial stress fractures. Iowa Orthop J 19:26–30

51. Mann JA, Pedowitz DI (2009) Evaluation and treatment of navicular stress fractures, including nonunions, revision surgery, and persistent pain after treatment. Foot Ankle Clin 14(2):187–204

52. Torg JS, Moyer J, Gaughan JP et al (2010) Management of tarsal navicular stress fractures: conservative versus surgical treatment. A meta-analysis. Am J Sports Med 38(5):1048–1053

53. Shindel MK, Endo Y, Warren RF et al (2012) Stress fractures about the tibia, foot, and ankle. J Am Acad Orthop Surg 20:167–176

Physeal and Epiphyseal Cartilage Injuries

5

Onofrio Donzelli, Leonardo Marchesini Reggiani, Manuele Lampasi and Stefano Stilli

The growth plate is responsible for the longitudinal growth of the long bones [1, 2]. The growth plate is divided into two parts: an epiphyseal part with proliferative potential and a metaphyseal part without proliferative potential. The microstructural organization shows that the epiphyseal portion has more extracellular matrix than the cellular components. In the metaphyseal portion, the matrix reduces its volume and the cellular component increases. The cartilage cells also increase in volume and become ossified and mineralized.

The most metaphyseal layer is the critically injured point because the decrease in the extracellular matrix reduces its resistance to shear and bending forces. In the fractures involving the metaphyseal layers, the proliferative parts of the growth cartilage remain intact and adhere to the epiphysis and possibly no growth disturbance seems to occur.

In the trauma of the epiphysis, the proliferative layers are certainly involved and growth disturbance can occur.

As to the number of different layers of the growth cartilage, there are many theories [3]. Usually, four layers can be well identified (Fig. 5.1).

1. Undifferentiated or resting cartilage cells layer which lies immediately adjacent to the

O. Donzelli (✉) · L. M. Reggiani · M. Lampasi · S. Stilli
Pediatric Orthopedics and Traumatology, Istituto Ortopedico Rizzoli, Via Pupilli 1/10, 40136, Bologna, Italy
e-mail: Onofrio.donzelli@ior.it

L. M. Reggiani
e-mail: Leonardo.marchesinireggiani@ior.it

M. Lampasi
e-mail: Manuele.lampasi@ior.it

S. Stilli
e-mail: stefano.stilli@ior.it

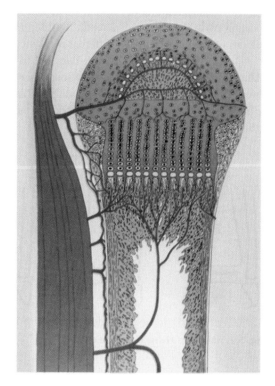

Fig. 5.1 Anatomy of the physeal cartilage

V. Guzzanti (ed.), *Pediatric and Adolescent Sports Traumatology*,
DOI: 10.1007/978-88-470-5412-7_5, © Springer-Verlag Italia 2014

epiphysis and shows irregularly scattered cartilage cells in a relatively quiescent state. This is the germinal layer that supplies the developing cartilage cells.

2. Zone of proliferating cartilage in which bone length is produced by the active growth of cartilage cells; chondrocytes assume a flattened appearance, begin to divide, and become organized into columns.

3. Hypertrophic cell zone (maturation zone) in which the chondrocytes begin to terminally differentiate; chondrocytes become enlarged, swollen, and vacuolated in the process of maturation leading to cell death; this is weakest portion of the epiphyseal plate.

4. Zone of provisional calcification in which chondrocytes prepare the matrix for calcification, which then serves as a template for osteoblastic bone formation. In this area, the extracellular chondroid matrix becomes impregnated with calcium salt.

The growth plate is supplied with three independent vascular systems: metaphyseal vessels, perichondral vessels, and epiphyseal vessels.

Growth plate maturation starts in an eccentric location of the physis, and potentially different regions of the plate can have different resistance to injuries. In adolescence period, two and triplane fractures (the so-called transitional fractures) can occur, especially in the distal tibia region due to the incomplete closure of the growth plate.

5.1 Classification

Salter and Harris physeal injury classification is used worldwide [4, 5]. Different classifications have been proposed, but this is very simple and repeatable. It is a descriptive classification but has also implication for the choice of treatment and for prognosis [6] (Fig. 5.2).

5.2 Salter and Harris I

The fracture is through the physis without involvement of the bone in the metaphysis or of the epiphysis. It is common in early childhood. It affects the proximal radius or the proximal humerus in upper extremity trauma and both proximal and distal femur or distal tibia in lower extremity trauma. The trauma produces shear or fracture lines that follow the growth plate, separating epiphysis from metaphysis. It usually happens in the metaphyseal side of the physis (large hypertrophying chondrocytes). It can show a minimum displacement. The articular surface and the germinative layer of the physis are not involved.

5.3 Salter and Harris II

The fracture involves both part of the physis and metaphysis. It usually occurs after age 10. The

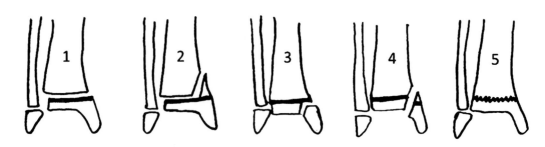

Fig. 5.2 Salter and Harris classification

bones most frequent involved are the humerus (especially the distal), the distal radius, the distal femur, and distal tibia. The mechanism is a shear trauma with angular force. It can be observed a failure of the physis in the tension side and a failure of the metaphysis on the compression side. As in Salter and Harris I, the germinative and proliferative layers of the physis are not injured.

5.4   Salter and Harris III

The fracture involves both parts of the physis and epiphysis. It usually occurs after age 10. This type of fracture generally occurs when the physis is partially ossified. This type of fracture passes through the germinative layer and the articular surface, inevitably damaging the reproductive layer of the physis.

5.5   Salter and Harris IV

The fracture involves epiphysis, physis, and metaphysis. The most frequent sites are the lateral condyle of the distal humerus under age 10 and the distal tibia over age 10. A fracture line divides into two portions the epiphysis–physis–metaphysis unit. The injury crosses all the growth cartilage layers and extends to the articular surface.

5.6   Salter and Harris V

The fracture involves only the physis with a compression mechanism and deforms the growth plate. It can be present in association with all of the other Salter–Harris fractures. It can be suspected in hard trauma with axial load injury. This fracture is difficult to diagnose and in most cases is a retrospective diagnosis where angulation or growth arrest development without radiological evidence of a growth plate injury [7].

5.7   Salter and Harris Types VI–IX (Rare)

Type VI: injury to the perichondral structures [8].

Type VII: isolated injury to the epiphyseal plate.

Type VIII: isolated injury to the metaphysis with a potential injury related to endochondral ossification.

Type IX: injury to the periosteum that may interfere with membranous growth.

5.8   Imaging

Usually, through a standard radiography, it is possible to diagnose Salter and Harris I to IV [9]. Opposite site X-rays can be useful for Salter and Harris I with little displacement. After a plain radiography, it can sometimes be recommended to perform an additional study: A CT scan with multiplanar reconstruction better clarifies the fracture and can help make a management decision. It is typically used for planning surgery in the Salter and Harris III and Salter and Harris IV fracture or to follow a conservative management. For Salter and Harris V, MR imaging can identify hemorrhage and hematoma within the growth plate immediately after injury but cannot be routinely used [10]. Some authors proposed bone scintigraphy to monitor the Salter and Harris V trauma. Technetium bone scan results are positive, showing different uptake in damaged physis, 6 months after trauma, and can used to evaluate growing potential (prognostic data) [11].

5.9   Transitional Fractures (Two-Plane and Tri-Plane Fractures)

The ossification of the growth plate of the distal tibia starts eccentrically from the anterolateral region of the medial malleolus [12–15]. Then, the mineralization process proceeds

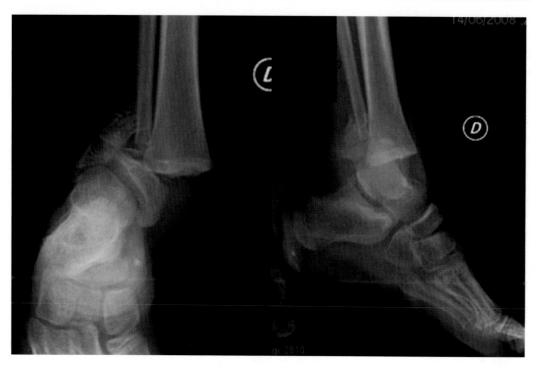

Fig. 5.3 Case 1: Basketball player showing a Salter–Harris type I fracture

posteriorly and laterally. The anterolateral portion of the growth plate is the last to ossify. Shear trauma causes an incomplete epiphyseal separation due to the different degree of maturation at the same level of the growth plate. An avulsed metaphyseal wedge occurs depending on the additional bending movement. The fractures planes lie in the epiphysis, the not mineralized part of the physis and the metaphysis. We can identified three types of transitional fractures: (1) pure two-plane fractures (e.g., Tillaux fracture) involve the epiphysis and a part of the growth plate; (2) type I triplane fractures have an additional metaphyseal component with the same epiphyseal pattern of the two-plane fractures; (3) type II triplane fractures have an additional Salter and Harris type IV to the two-plane component usually located in the medial region.

Some associated injuries, as distal fibular epiphysis, may occur. Important growth deformities are rare due to the age of the patients in which the transitional fractures occur. Articular surface gap, if not reduced, will lead to articular incongruence so to early arthrosis [16].

5.10 Apophyseal Fractures

The apophyseal fracture separates a projection (apophysis) of a bone from the main osseous tissue at a point of strong tendinous or ligamentous attachment. The apophyseal plate has the same morphological structure of the growth plate, but it is not involved in the longitudinal growth of the bone. They involve the epiphyseal side only in some cases: the distal part of the humerus (frequent the medial epicondyle) and the proximal tibia (the insertion of the cruciate ligament to the eminence of the tibia). They usually do not lead to growth disturbance. With respect to prognosis, we distinguish incomplete or not displaced fractures from completely displaced fractures [17].

In the proximal tibia, an apophyseal avulsion of the anterior tubercle is not rare in jumping sports. This fracture most often is an isolated

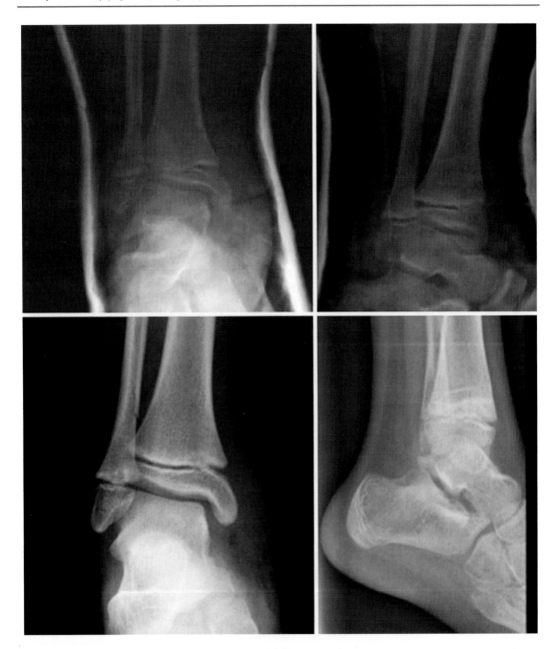

Fig. 5.4 Case 1: Conservative treatment with cast and follow-up results

injury related to push off or landing while jumping as the quadriceps eccentrically contracts to support the individual's weight. The fracture line is through the proximal tibial epiphysis and may extend into the anterior portion of the knee joint. The fracture pattern is dependent on the amount of physeal closure present at the time of injury because the physis of the proximal tibia closes from posterior to anterior. Open reduction and internal fixation are recommended, as reduction is difficult to maintain against the pull of the quadriceps muscle [18, 19].

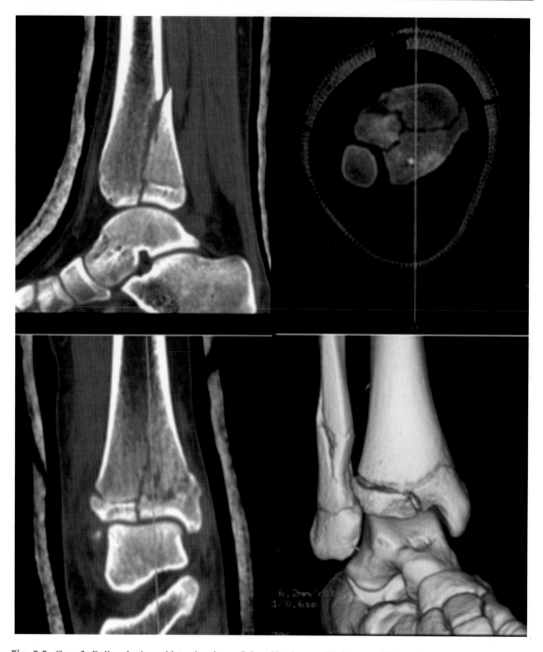

Fig. 5.5 Case 2: Roller skating athlete showing a Salter–Harris type IV fracture (CT scans)

5.11 Principles of Treatment

Salter and Harris types I and II injuries are usually managed by closed manipulation and plaster cast [20, 21]. Low-energy trauma SH I e SH II has minimal potential risk of growth damage (except for distal femur or proximal tibia) and has an excellent remodeling potential. The surgeon must gently manipulate in order to prevent an additional trauma to the physis. Sometimes an open reduction is required when a periosteal flap is located on the fracture gap (Figs. 5.3, 5.4).

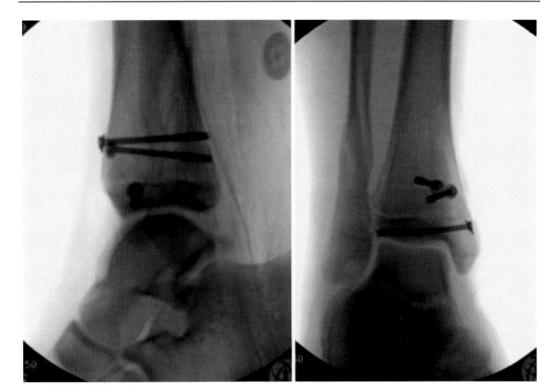

Fig. 5.6 Case 2: Surgical treatment with screws

Salter and Harris types III and IV injuries are intra-articular and need an anatomical reduction to obtain a normal articular surface and to prevent an epiphyseal–metaphyseal cross-union. Because they are often displaced, they often require open reduction and internal fixation. Computer tomography may help plan the procedure (Figs. 5.5, 5.6). The fixation device must be chosen carefully (Kirschner wires, screw, pins) and carefully placed in order to prevent bone bridges. It should not be plunged across the physis, or, at least, a small diameter device should be used.

5.12 Follow-up

Once the fracture heals, a long-term follow-up is usually necessary to monitor the child's recuperation and growth. Evaluation includes clinical examinations and X-rays of matching limbs at 6-month intervals for at least 2 years. Some

fractures can require periodic evaluations until the child's bones have finished growing. Sometimes a growth arrest line may appear as a marker of the injury in the metaphyseal bone (Fig. 5.7).

5.13 Prognosis

Growth plate injuries may heal with complications such as growth arrest and late angulation [22, 23] in high percentage (up to 50 %) of case.

The factors affecting the prognosis are as follows: severity of the trauma (vascular damage, exposed fracture), age of the patient (younger patients are expected to grow and the deformity will be greater), type of Salter and Harris fracture (types I and II rarely have growth problems, while types III and IV have a worse prognosis; type V should be suspected in most cases). It is very important to warn the parents of this possibility.

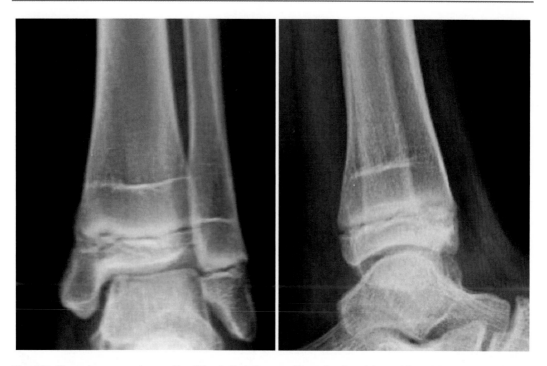

Fig. 5.7 X-ray shows growth arrest line (*Harris line*). Increased bone density of the position of the growth plate at the time of trauma

The occurrence of a growth disturbance depends more on the age at the time of injury than on the anatomical region involved. After trauma, the growth plate can increase or decrease function. The growth stimulation of the physeal plate depends on the extent and duration of the repair process. The treatment for the physeal fracture has a great influence on the duration of the repair process and consequently on the growth stimulation. Growth plate disturbances about the knee and the ankle have the worst prognosis. Angulation and leg length discrepancy can be corrected by osteotomy or epiphysiodesis or limb lengthening procedures.

References

1. Laer L (1991) Frakturen und Luxationen im Wachstumsalter. Thieme, Stuttgart
2. Mann DC, Rajmaira S (1990) Distribution of physeal and nonphyseal fractures in 2,650 long-bone fractures in children aged 0–16 years. J Pediatr Orthop 10:713–716
3. Pazzaglia UE, Zarattini G, Spagnuolo F, Superti G, Marchese M (2012) Growth and shape modeling of the rabbit tibia: study of the dynamics of developing skeleton. Anat Histol Embryol 41:217–226
4. Salter RB, Harris WR (1963) Injuries involving the epiphyseal plate. J Bone and Joint Surg Am 45(3): 587–622
5. Ogden JA (1981) Injury to the growth mechanism of the immature skeleton. Skeletal Radiol 6:237–253
6. Shapiro F (1982) Epiphyseal growth plate fracture-separations: a patho-physiologic approach. Orthopedics 5:720–736
7. Pozarny E, Kanat IO (1987) Epiphyseal growth plate fracture: Salter and Harris type V. J Foot Surg 26:204–209
8. Havranek P, Pesl T (2010) Salter (Rang) type 6 physeal injury. Eur J Pediatr Surg 20:174–177
9. Rogers LF, Poznanski AK (1994) Imaging of epiphyseal injuries. Radiology 191:297–308
10. Huckaby MC, Kruse D, Gibbs LH (2012) MRI findings of bilateral proximal radial physeal injury in a gymnast. Pediatr Radiol 42:1395–1400
11. Zionts LE, Harcke HT, Brooks KM, MacEwen GD (1987) Posttraumatic tibia valga: a case demonstrating asymmetric activity at the proximal growth plate on technetium bone scan. J Pediatr Orthop 7:458–462

12. Rosenbaum AJ, Dipreta JA, Uhl RL (2012) Review of distal epiphyseal transitional fractures. Orthopedics 35:1046–1049
13. Shapiro F (1982) Epiphyseal growth plate fracture-separations: a pathophysiologic approach. Orthopedics 5:720–736
14. Balckburn EW, Aronsoon DD, Rubright JH, Lisle JW (2012) Ankle fractures in children. J Bone Joint Surg Am 3:1234–1244
15. Podeszwa DA, Mubarak SJ (2012) Physeal fractures of the distal tibia and fibula (Salter-Harris type I, II, III and IV fractures). J Pediatr Orthop 32(Suppl 1):S62–S68
16. Crawford AH (2012) Triplane and Tillaux fractures: is a 2 mm residual gap acceptable? J Pediatr Orthop 32(Suppl 1):S69–S73
17. Kwon OS, Kamath AF, Kelly JD 4th (2012) Arthroscopic treatment of an anterior cruciate ligament avulsion fracture in a skeletally immature patient. Orthopedics 35:589–592
18. Pandya NK, Edmonds EW, Roocroft JH, Mubarak SJ (2012) Tibial tubercle fractures: complications, classification, and the need for intra-articular assessment. J Pediatr Orthop 32:749–759
19. Ogden JA (2000) Proximal tibial epiphyseal injuries. In: Ogden JA (ed) Skeletal injury in the child. Springer, New York, pp 1005–1010
20. Canale ST, Beaty JH (eds) (2008) Operative orthopedics, 11th edn. Mosby, St. Louis
21. Beaty JH, Kasser JR (eds) (2005) Rockwood and Wilkins' Fractures in children. Lippincott Williams and Wilkins, Philadelphia
22. Leary JT, Handling M, Talerico M, Young L, Bowe JA (2009) Physeal fractures of the distal tibia: predictive factors of premature physeal closure and growth arrest. J Pediatr Orthop 29:356–361
23. Basener CJ, Mehlman CT, DiPasquale TG (2009) Growth disturbance after distal femoral growth plate fractures in children: a meta-analysis. J Orthop Trauma 23:663–667

The Spine: Sports-Related Pathology

6

Pietro Bartolozzi and Guido Barneschi

Participation in sports by the pediatric population has increased over the years. Youth sports
participation carries an inherent risk of injury,
including overuse injuries. Acute injuries to the
spine in children are uncommon, accounting for
only 2–3 % of spinal injuries [1] and for 1 % of
pediatric fracture, but contribute to significant
morbidity in children. Acute injuries are the
same as those that occur in nonsporting accidents, whereas overuse or repetitive trauma
injuries are unique to sports medicine and represent approximately between 30 and 50 % of
all pediatric sports-related injuries. There are
substantial differences between children and
adults in the clinical presentation as well as
anatomy, diagnosis, treatment, complications,
and functional outcome for spine injuries,
especially for very young children.

6.1 Acute Injuries

6.1.1 Epidemiology

The incidence of spinal injuries among pediatric
patients is variable, depending on age and level
of activity. Injury rate and severity increase with
age: before puberty, boys and girls are equally
likely to sustain sports-related injuries; after
puberty, the incidence of injury is greater in
boys than in girls and boys tend to sustain more
severe injuries, possibly because they play
highest-risk games, but for certain sports, such
as horse riding, injuries are four times more
common in females. The most commonly
encountered lesions are soft tissue trauma and
include ligament sprains, muscle strains, and
soft tissue contusions; fractures and dislocations
are uncommon. Between 60 and 80 % of all
pediatric vertebral injuries are in the cervical
region and about 40 % of these are associated
with neurological involvement. This is in contrast to adults in whom cervical injuries constitute only 30–40 % of all vertebral injuries. Most
spinal injuries below the age of 12 years involve
the atlantoaxial or atlantooccipital joints,
although all levels are encountered. Thoracolumbar trauma is rare in children younger than
12 years of age, representing fewer than 8 %
[2]. Multilevel contiguous fractures are common, and between 6 and 12 % of patients

P. Bartolozzi
Director of Orthopedic Department, University of
Verona, Verona, Italy
e-mail: pietro.bartolozzi@gmail.com

G. Barneschi (✉)
Orthopedics, University of Florence, Florence, Italy
e-mail: g.barneschi@libero.it

V. Guzzanti (ed.), *Pediatric and Adolescent Sports Traumatology,*
DOI: 10.1007/978-88-470-5412-7_6, © Springer-Verlag Italia 2014

sustaining a spine injury had noncontiguous second fractures [3, 4].

Injury rates vary considerably among sports. The high-risk sports-related or recreation-related activities for acute spinal injuries are contact sports (American football, hockey, rugby , and wrestling), diving, winter sports (skiing, snowboarding, sledding, and tobogganing), horse riding, and gymnastic. A limited number of case reports of spinal trauma have been described in children or adolescents playing basketball or baseball, or following bicycle accidents.

American football is one of the most popular sports played by young athletes in USA. Spinal and axial skeleton injuries occur frequently in football and can result in significant time missed from practices and games. Cervical spine injuries are estimated to occur in 10–15 % of all football players, most commonly in linemen and defensive players. Injuries usually are secondary to high-velocity collisions between players and have a wide spectrum of severity. The burners and stingers syndrome is one of the most common injuries in American football. The cervical cord neurapraxia is a less common and more dangerous injury due to hyperextension, hyperflexion, or axial loading. Serious injuries (e.g., fractures, subluxations, dislocations) remain infrequent. Catastrophic cervical spine injuries with neurological sequelae in football are rare but tragic events. The mean incidence of neurological injury over the past 30 years has been approximately 0.5 per 100,000 participants at high school level and 1.5 per 100,000 at the collegiate level [5].

Cervical injuries in ice hockey are not rare. About half of major spinal injuries occur to players 16–20 years of age [6]. Impact of the head with the boards after being checked or pushed from behind is the most common mechanism of spinal injury. In rugby, cervical spine injuries are uncommon but have received growing attention owing to their often catastrophic nature. The majority of injuries occur after hyperflexion of the neck or after an axial compression mechanism and related "buckling" of the cervical spine [7].

Diving is the most common mechanism of spinal injury from recreational sport. Lesions occur almost exclusively in the cervical spine [8]. Diving accidents often strike young people, particularly children, who are more prone to take risks and fail to understand the consequences. The typical patient profile is of a teenager, athletic male, who suffered an injury to the cervical spine after diving into shallow water, usually during the summer months [9]. Injuries have a high tetraplegia rate, and the most commonly fractured vertebra is C5 [10].

Horseback riding has moderate to high risk of spinal injuries, and it is 20 times as dangerous as motor cycling [11]. In some countries, 70 % of all spine fractures caused by sports activities are sustained by equestrian activities. Other studies evidence that 7–10 % of all riders requiring hospital admission have a spinal injury [12]. As many as one-third of all horse riders are children. Female riders are more likely to be admitted with serious injury, but there are more women riding, and the number of accidents to female riders is probably in proportion to the total number of women riders [12]. Injuries are due to falls, and jumping is the most dangerous horse-riding activity. Lumbar and thoracic fractures are much more common than cervical fractures, the likelihood being that this is due to fall on the buttocks or being thrown against obstructions [13]. Most of the spine fractures occur at the thoracolumbar junction, and this is simply a reflection of the most common location of compression-type fractures.

Spinal injuries in snow sports are relatively rare but are on the increase with the development of acrobatic and high-speed activities on the mountains. Recreational alpine skiing and snowboarding may result in high-energy falls or collisions with other skiers, mountain equipment, or trees, resulting in significant trauma. Skiers usually suffer acute serious spinal injuries from falls or collisions at high speeds, whereas snowboarders are frequently injured from failing attempted jumps. Globally, the majority of severe spinal injuries are related to skiing, but rate of spinal injuries among snowboarders is fourfold that among skiers [14]. There is approximately one significant spinal injury every 100,000 skier-days. Snowboarders tend to fall backward, whereas skiers fall forward [15], so skiers tend to suffer from more cervical spine injuries related to falling forward, whereas those injured snowboarding had higher frequencies of injury to the lumbar spine. Concomitant injuries and multilevel fractures are common. The skiing injuries occurred to novices and top-class skiers alike, with one-third of those sustaining a fracture having associated spinal cord injury (SCI). Cervical spine trauma was associated with the highest likelihood of SCI. Nearly one-third of patients had fractures at more than one vertebral level: these injuries were often contiguous fractures of the vertebral body or transverse process fractures. The majority of thoracolumbar fractures are compression injuries with anterior column failures of less than 25 % vertebral body height [16].

6.2   Relevant Developmental Anatomy

There are certain anatomic and biomechanical differences between the immature spine of pediatric patients and adults. Children have hyperlaxity of ligamentous and capsular structures with hypermobility, poor development of musculature, incomplete ossification with the presence of epiphysis and synchondroses, unique features of the vertebral bony elements (e.g., flatter slope of the cervical facet joint and an immature uncinate process, wedge-shaped vertebral bodies). Younger children have disproportionately larger head than adults.

The subaxial cervical spine, as well as the thoracolumbar vertebrae, all follows a similar pattern of development with three ossification centers (Fig. 6.1): two in the neural arches and one in the centrum. At the puberty, secondary ossification centers appear in the tip of the spinous processes and transverse processes.

The formation of the atlas (C1) and the axis (C2) differs from the typical vertebral pattern. The atlas has three ossification centers

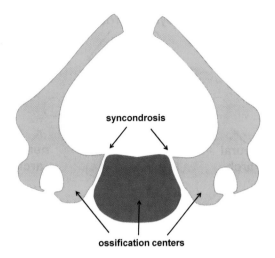

Fig. 6.1 Ossification of a subaxial cervical vertebra at 1 year of age

(Fig. 6.2), consisting of the body and two neural arches; synchondroses occur posteriorly and anteriorly on either side of central ossification center. The axis is formed from five primary ossification centers (Fig. 6.3): the centrum, the two neural arches, and two laterally situated centers that form the odontoid. The ossicle at the tip of the dens (os terminale) typically fuses by 12 years.

Growth of the vertebral bodies continues thoughtout childhood and adolescence and is completed between the ages of 18 and 25. In the immature spine, the intervertebral disk space is occupied by the nucleus pulposus, the annulus fibrosis, and the vertebral end plate. The child's disk has a high water content, is a better shock absorber than the adult, and is more resistant to injury than the vertebral bone. The end plate consists of a layer of hyaline cartilage that covers the surface of the disk and the physeal cartilage adjacent to the bony vertebral body. The physeal cartilage further consists in a physeal plate and a ring apophysis. In the immature spine, the cartilaginous end plate is attached to the ring apophysis and the annulus fibrosis. The ring apophysis develops between the ages of 6 and 8 years in girls and between the ages of 7 and 9 years in boys. At first, many foci of ossification coalesce to form a single rim, surrounding the upper and lower margins of the

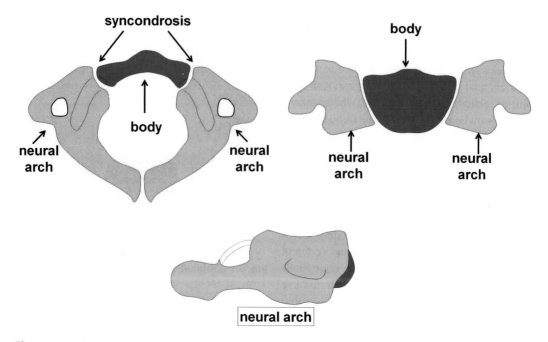

Fig. 6.2 Development of C1 at 1 year of age

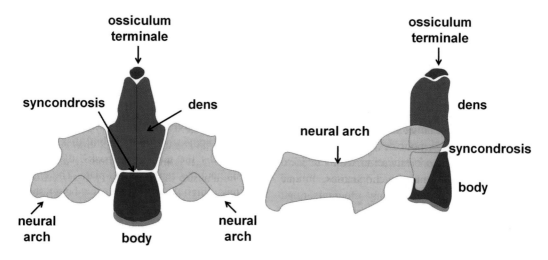

Fig. 6.3 Development of C2 at 1 year of age

vertebral body at the edges of the cartilaginous plate. By 12–15 years, the apophysis starts to ossify, forming the radiological ring. It usually fuses with vertebral body between the ages of 14 and 18 years. The ring apophysis does not specifically contribute to growth of vertebral body, but its fusion signals the cessation of longitudinal growth.

6.3   Cervical Trauma

Injury of the cervical spine in childhood and adolescence is relatively uncommon. There is a predominance of upper cervical lesions over lower cervical (the opposite of that seen in adults), due to increased head size. In children, sporting injury is the most common mechanism of cervical injury after motor vehicle-related accidents.

The most common mechanisms of injuries include athletic (American football, rugby, hockey, wrestling), recreational (skiing, snowboarding, horseback riding, mounting biking), and diving accidents. The most common sports-related injury of the neck is a ligament sprain or muscle strain. They are the result of a fall, impact, or contact with another person, object, or surface. In adolescent athletes, it is described as an equivalent of the clay-shoveler's fracture [17].

Anterior subluxation (hyperflexion sprain) [18] is a purely ligamentous injury associated with three column disruption, and it is the most unstable cervical spinal injury. Subluxation can be missed in plain radiograph because the initial radiological signs are subtle (in supine position), and even when recognized, the injury may not be considered significant. Additional studies, such as flexion–extension radiography and magnetic resonance imaging (MRI), are often used in the acute setting to assess injury status. Radiographically, anterior subluxation is characterized by a localized kyphotic angulation at the level of injury and anterior rotation or displacement of the subluxated vertebra; anterior narrowing and posterior widening of the disk space; widening of the space between the subluxated vertebral body and the subjacent articular masses; displacement of the inferior articulating facets of the subluxated vertebra with respect to their contiguous subjacent facets; and widening of the interspinous space. The treatment for such a kyphotic deformity may consist of surgical fixation of the lesion.

Disk herniations are often degenerative in nature, and such conditions should be considered chronic athletic injuries [19]. Disk herniation is sometimes associated with axial loading and hyperflexion (wrestling, diving, rugby, American football). Immature athletes tend to develop disk herniation at higher level than adults (C3–C4 or C4–C5).

Atlas fractures are extremely uncommon in children. Normal synchondroses should not be misinterpreted as a Jefferson fracture, but before age 7, fractures may occur through the neurocentral synchondroses. The computerized tomogram (CT) scan is the most sensitive tool for the diagnosis of these fractures. Normally, an immobilization with halo vest or halo cast is requested.

Odontoid fractures in young children always occur as an epiphyseal separation of the growth plate at the base of the dens. After the closure of the growth plate, fractures are extremely rare and they follow the patterns seen in adults. Neurological deficit is rare. The treatment for odontoid fractures traditionally has been halo stabilization for 8–12 weeks.

Subaxial cervical spine tends to be seen in the older child, and the injury patterns are similar to those seen in adults. Cervical end plate injury represents the only peculiar lesion. Injury to the physeal end plate is rare, frequently associated with neurological damage, and often unrecognized radiographically. In the subaxial spine, there is a wide variety of fracture types, ranging from simple linear fractures affecting the vertebral bodies or posterior portion of the spine, to complex fractures involving several elements of the spine or many vertebral levels. A fracture may or may not make the spinal column unstable, depending on its type and severity.

The decision to obtain radiographs can be made on the basis of the history and physical examination. Plain radiograph is typically the initial image test for the detection of cervical spinal injuries in traumatized children. In child who is alert, has no cervical tenderness, no painful distracting injuries, no neurological deficits, and is not intoxicated, X-rays are not necessary to exclude an injury.

The standard X-ray series consist in anteroposterior, lateral, and the open-mouth view. The latter is very difficult to obtain under age 8, and it is not useful for diagnosis. The most diagnostic view is the lateral film. Adequate lateral cervical radiograph visualizes the top of T1. Plain radiographs have a high sensitivity for cervical spine injury [21], but interpreting the cervical X-rays in skeletally immature patients is not always easy. Ossification centers may cause confusion as they appear and fuse at various ages.

Disturbance on alignment of the body may arouse concern about underlying occult injury. Special consideration includes the following (Fig. 6.4):

1. Pseudospread of C1 on C2: in open-mouth view, the ossification of the lateral mass of atlas may exceed that of the ossification of C2, simulating an atlas fracture.
2. Odontoid discontinuity (Fig. 6.4b): the synchondrosis in the waist of the dens can be mistaken for a fracture.
3. The atlantodental interval (ADI) in infants and young children can be wider than in adults, with up to 3–5 mm being considered normal (Fig. 6.4a).
4. Retropharyngeal swelling: prevertebral soft tissues are difficult to evaluate in infants and young children and can be up to 8 mm in width, especially when the child is crying (Fig. 6.4e).
5. Pseudosubluxation of the body of C2 on C3 and, less commonly, of C3 on C4: pseudosubluxation is the apparent anterior subluxation, commonly seen in normal pediatric population (Fig. 6.4c). A true ligamentous instability at the C2–C3 is extremely rare. The gliding of C2 on C3 depends on the relative horizontal plane of the articular process in the upper cervical spine but also on the hypermobility with ligamentous laxity. Finally, under age of 8 years, the C2–C3 articulation is the normal fulcrum of the cervical movement, in contrast to the normal fulcrum in adults which occurs at the C5–C6 level.
6. Anterior wedging of C3 (Fig. 6.4d) and C4 is often a normal finding and can be mistaken for compression fracture. Physiologic wedging gradually disappears as the child gets older.
7. Absence of cervical lordosis is a common normal finding seen in child (Fig. 6.4f).

If an upper cervical spine injury is suspected on standard X-rays, a CT scan should be obtained. If initial radiographs are normal and symptoms are continuing, flexion and extension lateral radiographs are needed after paraspinal muscle spasm has subsided. Radicular pain or

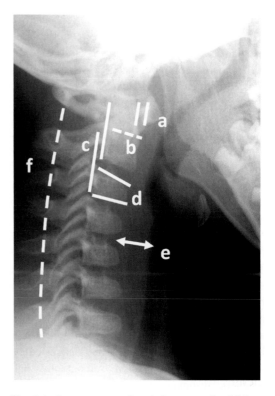

Fig. 6.4 Common normal variations seen in children: **a** widening of the atlantodental interval, **b** odontoid discontinuity, **c** pseudosubluxation of the body of C2 on C3, **d** anterior wedging of C3, **e** retropharyngeal swelling, **f** absence of cervical lordosis

neurological involvement prompts further evaluation with MRI. In the obtunded and high-risk pediatric trauma patient, high-resolution CT with sagittal and coronal reconstructions should be the basis for cervical spinal clearance, in combination with the interpretation of films by an expert radiologist [21]. Treatment for the cervical injuries depends on severity of diagnosed injury and can range from an individualized cervical spine rehabilitation program for cervical sprains to cervical spine decompression and fusion for more serious bony or ligamentous injury.

In pediatric cervical injuries, nonoperative treatment is more frequently employed than in adults and the overall prognosis is best in childhood. The current trend is represented by closed reduction and halo immobilization for instable injuries of the C1 and C2. For most patients treated in this manner, adequate bony healing occurs within 12 weeks of halo immobilization. Halo application is different in children: the size of the halo is smaller, the number of pins is higher, the location of pins is different, and less torque is used. Primary operative therapy is recommended for isolated ligamentous injuries of the cervical spine with associated deformity. The surgical procedures performed on children need to take not only their smaller size but also their unique biomechanics into consideration. Surgical dissection should be limited only to the involved levels. Spinal instrumentation is performed according to the type of lesion. The use of allograft bone should be avoided because it often results in poor fusion. Anterior or posterior fusion alone may be not appropriated in young children for the risk of rapidly progressive deformity.

Return-to-play decisions after a cervical injury are controversial [22]. Patients with minor injuries (i.e., spinous process fracture) or non-displaced subaxial fractures have no contraindication to return to sports after healing [19]. Absolute contraindications to return to play are atlantooccipital fusions, three or more levels of fusion, permanent instability of the spine, persistent neurological deficits, residual canal stenosis for fragments or trauma-induced sagittal malalignment. Return-to-play criteria for others conditions include the following: no pain, full range of motion, normal strength, normal neurological evaluation, ability to run and sustain contact without pain, no intake of pain medication, player education about preventive measures and future risks.

6.4 Burners and Stingers

Burners and stingers represent an upper cervical root injury (neurapraxia of a cervical nerve root or brachial plexus), due a traction, compression, or direct blow. Burners are most common in American football players but are also seen in those who participate in hockey, wrestling, and diving. The injury is named for the stinging or burning pain that spreads from the shoulder to the hand. Symptoms are usually transient and resolve quickly. The main treatment is rest until the symptoms disappear and muscle strength is regained. Return-to-play criteria after burners syndrome are resolution of pain and paresthesias, recovery of full range of motion and normal strength, negative brachial plexus stretch, and negative maneuver of axial compression.

6.5 Cervical Cord Neurapraxia

Neurapraxia is defined as transient post-traumatic paralysis of the motor and/or sensory tracts in the spinal cord. It has often been referred to as a "spinal cord concussion," or "transient quadriplegia." Although usually seen in athletes in traditional contact sports such as American football, wrestling, and ice hockey, neurapraxia may also be seen in other sport activities in which collisions occur, such as basketball, soccer, gymnastics, and baseball. Penning [23] postulated that an extreme movement can occur in high-velocity injuries, resulting in rapid compression of the spinal cord by the posterior–inferior cervical vertebral body and the subjacent spinal lamina ("pincers effect"). Return-to-play decisions after an episode of neurapraxia are controversial. Athletes with neurapraxia and documented ligamentous instability, MRI evidence of cord defects or swelling, neurological symptoms or signs for greater than 36 h, or more than one recurrence have an absolute contraindication [24]. It is also generally recommended that athletes with neurapraxia secondary to a herniated cervical disk, focal stenosis, or compressive osteophyte are not allowed to participate further in contact sports.

6.6 Thoracolumbar Trauma

The majority of pediatric thoracolumbar spine fractures occur in older children and adolescents [25]. The most common sport-related mechanism of injury is winter sports and horse riding.

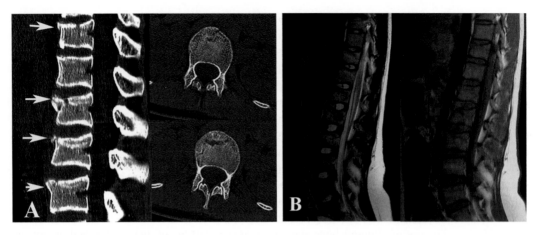

Fig. 6.5 Multiple thoracolumbar fractures in horse-riding child. Reprinted with permission [26]

The principal site of fracture is the thoracic spine, probably because the thorax is much more elastic in children than in adults, and the second most frequently affected site is the thoracolumbar junction. The most frequent fractures include compression fracture (wedge fracture) and fractures of posterior elements (transverse process, spinous process). Multiple contiguous fractures are more common in the child's spine than in the adult (Fig. 6.5). The incidence of neurological injuries in children is less than in adults, occurring between 14 and 35 % of spine fractures, and the prognosis is better. Children with permanent neurological lesions are at great risk of scoliosis formation. Deformities can also occur without neurological lesions when the growth zone of an end plate is affected, but significantly growth disturbance is rare.

There is no classification validated in children, and thoracolumbar fractures are typically described using adult classifications. The more commonly used classification in Europe is the AO/Magerl classification [27], based on the pathomorphological characteristics of the injury. Three mechanisms of injury, of which the effect is shown in the radiographs and CT scans, give name to the three main types: A = compression, B = distraction, and C = rotation fractures. A simple grid, the 3–3–3 scheme of the AO fracture classification, is used in grouping the injuries. Every type has three groups, each of which contains three subgroups with specifications.

Type A fractures represent the majority of thoracolumbar fractures in children. Over half of the Type A injuries are wedge fracture (A1) with the intact posterior wall of the vertebral body. These fractures are stable. Burst fractures (A3) are rare in young children [28], but in adolescents have almost the same incidence as in adults. The risk of neurological injury in burst fractures may be more closely related to the level of injury (thoracic) than the degree of spinal canal compromise, as in children the diameter of the canal is relatively larger and incidence of SCI is low despite significant retropulsion of bone fragments.

The diagnosis of thoracolumbar fracture in children may be difficult. The mechanism of the trauma, in combination with the complaints of the patient, generally gives rise to the suspicion of a spinal fracture. The patient's spine must be palpated using log roll to look for tenderness, swelling, bruising, or step off. The clinical examination had a good sensitivity and average specificity; however, missed injuries are common in pediatric patients [29], and clinical examination as a stand-alone screening tool for evaluation of the thoracolumbar spine is often inadequate. Most of spinal fractures in children are demonstrable in plain radiographs. Initial examination should include supine anteroposterior and lateral views of the thoracolumbar spine. Special attention should be given to look for additional levels of injury when a single-level spinal column injury has already been detected. In these patients, radiography showing at least 4 levels above and below the fracture should be performed [4]. Wedge vertebrae in Scheuermann's disease should not be misinterpreted as compression fracture. CT scan is sometimes necessary in suspected unstable fracture or in burst fracture to determine the degrees of canal compromise. MRI is useful in evaluating those patients with neurological injury, especially in cases that cannot be accounted for by osseous disruption on plain radiographs or CT scan. MRI can reveal the injury to the spinal cord, ligaments, annulus fibrosis, disk herniations, and epidural hematomas. Most spine injuries do not need operative treatment [25]. Compression fractures (wedge) in children usually require little treatment, with a good long-term outcome, particularly in those younger than 10 years of age (or Risser sign of 0 or 1). Fractures with less than 10 degrees of wedging require no treatment: after a few days of bed rest and analgesics, early mobilization can begin without a brace [30]. For fractures with a wedge angle greater than 10°, a brace should be prescribed. Most burst fractures and potentially unstable fractures can also be treated with bed rest, casting, and bracing for 8–12 weeks. Long-term studies lack to demonstrate improvement in kyphosis or clinical outcomes with surgical treatment in comparison with those treated conservatively. After rehabilitation, return to play is allowed if there is evidence of radiographic union, resolution of pain, and no neurological deficit. The main indication for surgical intervention is the presence of progressive neurological deterioration in documented spinal cord compression. Stabilization of the affected segment is required in case of unstable fractures. Early decompression and stabilization are indicated in children or adolescents with a partial deficit. Stabilization is also indicated in patients with complete neurological injury to prevent progression of deformity and facilitate nursing care. Prognosis for recovery of neurological injury is related to the severity of the initial damage. Under no circumstances should a laminectomy on its own be performed in patients with a neurological lesion as the risk of a severe post-traumatic kyphosis developing at a later date is great. Although the decision on when to return to play should be made on a case-by-case basis, patients who require a major surgical intervention with a spinal fusion and instrumental fixation may not able to return to participate in that specific sport.

6.7   Fracture of the Posterior Rim

Avulsion or fracture of posterior ring apophysis of lumbar vertebra is not a common clinical entity, and missed injuries are frequent. These fractures are typically seen in adolescents and young adults, because fusion in this area is not complete until the age of 18–25 years. Trauma resulting from strenuous sports activity has been reported as an important mechanism for this injury. Most of these lesions occur in lower lumbar spine. The cervical spine has also been reported as locations of these lesions.

Clinical signs usually imitate those of lumbar disk herniation: the most common symptoms are low-back pain and radicular pain due to nerve root irritation. Other symptoms and signs include paralumbar muscle spasm and tenderness, restricted back motion, tight hamstrings, limping (or a waddling gait with flexed knees), and neurological deficits caused by compressed nerve roots. Clinical signs may also be absent.

Based on the three-dimensional information that was obtained from computer tomography, Takata and colleagues [31] classified the fractures in three types: Type I is a simple separation of the entire arcuate posterior margin of the vertebra, and in this type there is no osseous defect in the posterior part of the vertebral body; Type II is an avulsion fracture of the posterior rim of the vertebral body, including a rim of bone; and Type III is a more localized fracture. Epstein and colleagues [32] added Type IV, a fracture of both cephalad and caudal end plates, which spans the full length of the posterior margin of vertebral body.

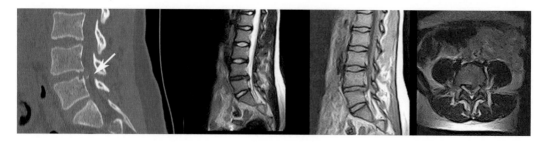

Fig. 6.6 CT scan and MR images of a 12-year-old boy with an avulsion fracture of the posterior rim of L5. The fragment is recognized only in computed tomography (*white arrow*)

For early detection of epiphyseal fracture, computerized tomography is recommended to show bony component of herniated material; posterior lumbar vertebral apophyseal ring fractures may be difficult to visualize on MRI imaging and MRI findings are less specific than CT signs. MRI can show prolapsed intervertebral disks (Fig. 6.6) and any associated nerve root compression useful for guiding surgical decision and intervention. Plain film radiographs of the lumbar spine show no abnormalities in many cases (but radiological signs of Scheuermann's disease are present in 50 % of the cases).

Treatment for this condition is not standardized. Conservative treatment such as rest, analgesics, modification of activity, and physical therapy should be used initially. The indication for surgical decompression is failure of conservative treatment, with persistent back pain adversely affecting the patient's ability to function, with or without neurological deficits. Usually, Type I fracture occurs in children less than 14 years and respond to conservative treatment well. Type II fracture occurs in somewhat older children between 14 and 18 years, and they also respond to conservative regimen with some potentiality for operative treatment. The most used surgical options are laminectomy with posterior discectomy and simultaneous excision of apophyseal fragments without spine fusion. Surgical outcomes are usually favorable, but recurrence requiring further surgery is seldom reported.

6.8 Spinal Cord Injuries

Spinal cord injuries constitute uncommon but nonetheless devastating occurrences to those participating in athletic events. The exact incidence of pediatric SCI is unknown, but reports vary from 1 to 10 % of all spinal cord injuries. These injuries happen primarily to athletes involved in the contact sports of American football, wrestling, and ice hockey, with football injuries constituting the largest number of cases. Spinal cord injuries can produce complete neurological loss or any of wide variety of incomplete patterns. Injury to the spinal cord in the cervical region, with associated loss of muscle strength in all 4 extremities, is termed tetraplegia (that replaces the term quadriplegia). Paraplegia is an injury in the spinal cord in the thoracic, lumbar, or sacral segments, including the cauda equina and conus medullaris.

SCI can be sustained through different mechanisms, with the following 3 common abnormalities leading to tissue damage: destruction from direct trauma; compression by retropulsed bone fragments into the canal, hematoma, or disk material; ischemia from damage or impingement on the spinal arteries.

The American Spinal Injury Association (ASIA) and the International Spinal Cord Society (ISCoS) published a system of tests used to define and describe the extent and severity of a patient's SCI, called the *International Standards for Neurological and Functional Classification of Spinal Cord Injury* (ISNCSCI), widely used to document sensory and motor impairments, following SCI. The standard classification can be used in subjects older than 6 years [33]. It is based on neurological responses, touch and pinprick sensations tested in each dermatome, and strength of ten key muscles on each side of the body. Traumatic SCI is classified into five categories on the ASIA Impairment Scale: A indicates a "complete" SCI where no motor or sensory function is preserved in the sacral segments S4–S5. Complete SCI usually does not recover. B indicates an "incomplete" SCI where sensory but not motor function is preserved below the neurological level and includes the sacral segments S4–S5. C indicates an "incomplete" SCI where motor function is preserved below the neurological level and more than half of key muscles below the neurological level have a muscle grade of less than 3, which indicates active movement with full range of motion against gravity. D indicates an "incomplete" SCI where motor function is preserved below the neurological level and at least half of the key muscles below the neurological level have a muscle grade of 3 or more. E indicates "normal" where motor and sensory scores are normal. The incomplete clinical syndromes are the *central cord syndrome* (incomplete loss of motor function with a disproportionate weakness of the upper extremities as compared with the lower extremities), the *anterior spinal cord syndrome* (complete loss of all motor function below the level of injury, in addition to loss of sensation of pain and temperature), the *Brown-Sequard syndrome* has been classically described as hemisection of the spinal cord with loss of ipsilateral motor function and contralateral spinothalamic (pain and temperature) modalities, the *posterior cord syndrome* (loss of proprioception and epicritic sensation below the level of injury with motor function, sense of pain, and sensitivity to light touch intact), the *conus midollaris syndrome* injury to the sacral cord and lumbar nerve roots leading to areflexic bladder, bowel, the *cauda equina syndrome* injury to the lumbosacral nerve roots in the spinal canal, leading to

areflexic bladder, bowel, with varying neurological involvement of the lower limbs. In children, incomplete SCI have high rate of neurological improvement.

The initial assessment of an injured player, who is suspected of having a vertebral column or SCI, begins by consideration of basic life support. The athlete should not be moved unless it is absolutely essential to maintain the airway, breathing, or circulation. The patients must be immediately immobilized and transported carefully to avoid neurological injury. When it becomes necessary to move the athlete, the head and trunk must be moved as one unit. Due to the difficulty in attaining a definitive exclusion regarding the possibility of spinal injury in an on-field setting, it is recommended that any athlete with significant neck or spine pain, diminished level of consciousness, or significant neurological deficits be transported, in an appropriate manner, to an emergency department, where a more formal neurological examination can be conducted and serial assessments can be completed with definitive diagnosis. In American football, neither the helmet nor the shoulder pads should be removed. Only the face mask, if present, should be removed, before transportation. At the hospital, the helmet is manually and carefully removed without moving the neck. Cervical spine injuries in children tend to displace on a standard spine board because of the relatively larger size of a child's head. There are special pediatric spine boards with head "cut out," or alternatively, the cervical spine flexion can be corrected by placing a folded towel or a bump under the patient's shoulders.

The principles involved in treatment for pediatric SCI are similar to those established in adults. Patients with severe spinal cord injuries diagnosed within 8 h of injury are usually administered a 24-h course of methylprednisolone based on the recommendation of the National Acute Spinal Cord Injury Study III , but the use of steroids in traumatic SCI in children is controversial [34]. Patients who have a demonstrable spinal cord compression and are having progressively worsening neurological deficits secondary to a fracture fragment impinging on the spinal cord, epidural hematoma, or extruded disk causing compression are candidates for early surgery. The main principles of treatment are correction of any spinal column deformity, decompression of the spinal cord if present, and recognition and management of unstable segments of the spine. The question of whether to allow an athlete to return to contact sports after a documented or suspected spinal injury has always been an issue. Any athlete who suffers a neurological injury to the spinal cord ordinarily should not be allowed to return.

6.9 SCIWORA

Spinal injury may also occur in the absence of a bony abnormality. This entity has been defined as SCIWORA, an acronyms that stands for spinal cord injury without radiological abnormalities. The estimated incidence of SCIWORA varies widely from 8 to 50 %, depending on the definition. The SCIWORA is usually defined as an SCI with no abnormality depicted on conventional radiography or CT scans. Younger patients account for 2/3 of all SCIWORA injuries and have a higher proportion of complete neurological injuries. Adolescents show a far less frequent incidence of complete SCI due to SCIWORA. This kind of SCI may occur in any location, but it is most common in the cervical spine.

SCI may be sustained as a result of lesser elasticity of the neural elements compared with that of the immature cervical spine structure in response to deforming stresses. The other suggested cause of SCIWORA is ischemia that results from direct vessel injury or hypoperfusion of the spinal cord parenchyma. Alternately, the pathology may be a radiographically inapparent fracture through vertebral cartilaginous end plate.

Profound or progressive paralysis occurs immediately or after a short latency period (usually within 48 h); transient symptoms can also occur, such as numbness, paresthesias, or paresis. This delay in diagnosis may be secondary to the development of spinal cord ischemia or spinal instability. The prognosis of SCIWORA depends on the degree of SCI. Once a SCIWORA injury is diagnosed, the child is at increased risk of recurrence of this episode. Recurrent injuries are typically more severe than initial injuries and may have permanent sequelae. Immobilization seems unnecessary in children with SCIWORA, but the data are conflicting and many centers maintain patients in external braces such as a stiff cervical collar for several months in order to prevent further injury.

6.10 Overuse Injuries

Spondylolysis and spondylolisthesis are the most common overuse injuries of the lower back in sport, especially in growing adolescents. The term of spondylolisthesis indicates a pathologic condition due to a forward slippage of one vertebra over the one below and can be considered one of the costs paid to the upright position. Spondylolisthesis can be secondary to a variety of causes, as well as differ sharply in terms of clinical characteristics and radiographic appearance. These considerations, together with factors such as severity, etiology, age, gender, and evolution, indicate the need for a case-by-case differentiation. Use of blanket term spondylolisthesis contributes little to the fulfillment of practical needs. Each case must be examined on its own merits, to ensure unerringly accurate diagnosis and to serve as the basis for correct treatment.

To achieve the most exact classification of spondylolisthesis is not only a scientific but, perhaps even more, a practical necessity. Classifications must be clear, simple, and comprehensive and based on totally unequivocal criteria. In 1997, Marchetti and Bartolozzi [35] proposed a new classification that has been internationally accepted and widely utilized. It distinguishes two main groups of spondylolisthesis: the developmental and the acquired with their subgroups (Table 6.1). Spondylolysis and spondylolisthesis in young athletes due to sport activities have to be classified as "acquired

Table 6.1 Marchetti and Bartolozzi classification system of spondylolisthesis [36]

Developmental
High dysplastic
• With lysis
• With elongation
Low dysplastic
• With lysis
• With elongation
Acquired
Traumatic
• Acute fracture
• Stress fracture
Post-surgery
• Direct surgery
• Indirect surgery
Pathological
• Local pathology
• Systemic pathology
Degenerative
• Primary
• Secondary

traumatic" even if it is not always possible to demonstrate that the lesion was not preexistent the beginning of the athletic training.

We distinguish two subgroups in the traumatic form: the ones due to an acute fracture and the others due to a stress fracture. In both cases, the fracture is the result of an efficient trauma in an essentially normal bone. When the trauma would be insufficient under normal conditions but results in fracture associated with congenital dysplasia, the spondylolisthesis is classified as developmental. The bony lesions characteristics of true acute traumatic spondylolisthesis occur not so much in the pars as in the articular masses. The injury is associated with fractures of the transverse processes and, frequently, with injuries to abdominal organs. These are generally cases of high-energy trauma. Traumatic spondylolysis caused by a true acute fracture of the pars rarely is observed with a mild slip; traumatic spondylolisthesis usually follows severe injury with various degrees of listhesis. Mild cases usually heal with a simple immobilization, whereas severe cases generally require surgical stabilization.

Stress fractures of the bony hook are an interesting form of spondylolisthesis and are common among those involved in competitive sports, such as gymnastics and weight lifting. The site of the lesion is usually the neural arch. Many authors have shown that athletes can have intact L4 and L5 vertebrae at the outset of their competitive careers but present a high incidence of isthmic spondylolysis or spondylolisthesis after some years. The pars is the weakest site on the bony hook and is the most subject to stress. The pars interarticularis of the posterior lumbar vertebral arch is a narrow bridge of cortical bone joining the lamina and inferior articular facet to the pedicle and superior facet. Repeated stress injury of the pars may lead to fatigue failure producing a fracture. Persistent motion through the fracture may result in the establishment of a pseudarthrosis. The aim of this chapter is the detection and treatment for this lesion.

The forces acting on the pars during flexion and extension of the spine are very strong. In flexion, resistance is applied to the spinous process; the lower part of the pars is subjected to forces of compression, and the upper portion is subjected to forces of traction. On the contrary, in extension of the spine, resistance is applied to the lower articular process. The forces acting on the lower portion of the pars are those of traction, whereas those acting on the upper part are those of compression. The frequency of lysis is not only of the isthmus, but also at the level of the pedicles and of the lamina so that more properly we define "isthmic" lysis, pedicle lysis or lamina lysis, often associated, is increased by the widespread of the CT scan (Fig. 6.7).

When the lysis occurs, the antisliding function of the arch is compromised. If the intervertebral disk, in association with the ligaments that are the structures absorbing the sliding forces, is whole, the lysis is not followed by the listhesis. Only after a progressive degeneration or an acute lesion of the disk, the listhesis could occur.

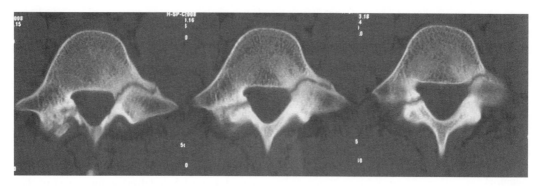

Fig. 6.7 A 17-year-old athlete presented with low-back pain: CT images reveled spondylolysis in the right pars interarticularis and lysis of the left pedicle of L5

People with these injuries typically present because of activity-related lumbar pain. Because spinal pain in the adolescent and young adult is a worrisome symptom, a careful evaluation is warranted when symptoms do not disappear. In the athletically active person particularly, the possibility of a pars interarticularis stress reaction or stress fracture should be considered. An acute injury resulting in a pars interarticularis fracture is unusual. Symptoms are gradual in onset, activity-related, and largely relieved with rest. Only when spondylolisthesis has occurred, neurological symptoms and associated hamstring muscle tightness are present and it is an exceptional situation. Although plain radiography, especially oblique views, may be revealing, they may not show a recent injury. In this respect, a pars interarticularis fracture is similar to a fatigue fracture of the metatarsus. If suspicion warrants a single-photon emission computed tomography (SPECT) scan is most useful in confirming the presence of a stress lesion. This kind of instrumental examination is not as specific as sensitive. For this reason, if positive, it should be followed by a CT scan of the suspect area. Whereas the SPECT scan may be indicative of metabolic activity, the CT scan will reveal whether actual fracture of the pars has occurred. Regardless of the treatment elected, the CT scan will be the most helpful study in determining the progress or lack thereof in healing of the pars.

Even if bracing of an established spondylolysis (or even spondylolisthesis) with clinical symptoms has been discussed, this lesion may have potential consequences: contralateral pedicle fracture, contralateral lamina fracture, spondylolisthesis, or subjacent disk degeneration. Thus, at least in the symptomatic person, treatment would appear to be indicated. Nonoperative treatment should provide satisfactory resolution of symptoms in the person with pain, a stress reaction but no established fracture. In this situation, the SPECT scan will reveal metabolic activity and the CT scan will show thickening of the pars. Avoidance of aggravating activity or the use of a brace has been effective treatments.

If a fracture has occurred and SPECT scan is positive, a trial of brace immobilization is warranted.

A period of 3 months is to be considered enough to understand whether or not this mode of treatment will be successful. Again, the CT is most helpful in reexamining the pars for evidence of healing. However, if a pseudarthrosis of the pars is clearly established, as evidenced by rounding of the fracture edges or inactivity on SPECT scan, then conservative treatment with a brace will have little prospect of obtaining union of the fracture. If the pain is resolved, the usual question is the follow: "May I take up the usual sport activity again?" The permission has to be carefully evaluated and only if the pain does not reappear. In these circumstances or if the pain compromises the daily activities, the surgical solution has to be considered.

In a symptomatic young patient with an established lesion of the neural arch, the surgical options are as follows: the direct repair or the stabilization of the motion segment. The direct repair has to follow the principles of treatment for a pseudarthrosis: debridement of the lesion and grafting with autologous bone, plus stabilization with different possibilities (Scot method with wire fixation or pedicle screw and sublaminar hooks). We must consider that this kind of surgery is not a minor one, that the risk of failure in the repair is high, and that a direct repair in case of listhesis ignores a certain degree of degeneration of the disk. The stabilization of the motion segment is a more aggressive procedure and modifies the normal anatomy, especially in young patients. The posterior fixation with screws and bars has to be completed with intersomatic cages (PLIF, TLIF, etc.) to avoid the risk of breakage of the instruments. The arthrodesis is posterolateral utilizing the laminar morselized bone. The surgical procedure is more delicate and demanding. After a surgical treatment, the young patient would have to be allowed to return to the previous sport activity.

References

1. Habelt S, Hasler CC, Steinbrück K, Majewski M (2011) Sport injuries in adolescents. Orthop Rev 6 3(2):e18
2. Dogan S, Safavi-Abbasi S, Theodore N, Chang SW, Horn EM, Mariwalla NR, Rekate HL, Sonntag VK (2007) J Neurosurg 106(6 Suppl):426–433
3. Mahan ST, Mooney DP, Karlin LI, Hresko MT (2009) Multiple level injuries in pediatric spinal trauma. J Trauma 67(3):537–542
4. Firth GB, Kingwell SP, Moroz PJ (2012) Pediatric noncontiguous spinal injuries: the 15-year experience at 1 pediatric trauma center. Spine (Phila Pa 1976) 37(10):E599
5. Rihn JA, Anderson DT, Lamb K, Deluca PF, Bata A, Marchetto PA, Neves N, Vaccaro AR (2009) Cervical spine injuries in American football. Sports Med 39(9):697–708

6. Tator CH, Provvidenza CF, Lapczak L, Carson J, Raymond D (2004) Spinal injuries in Canadian ice hockey: documentation of injuries sustained from 1943–1999. Can J Neurol Sci 31(4):460–466
7. Kuster D, Gibson A, Abboud R, Drew T (2012) Mechanisms of cervical spine injury in rugby union: a systematic review of the literature. Br J Sport Me 46(8):550–554
8. Aito S, D'Andrea M, Werhagen L (2005) Spinal cord injuries due to diving accidents. Spinal Cord 43(2):109–116
9. Korres DS, Benetos IS, Themistocleous GS, Mavrogenis AF, Nikolakakos L, Liantis PT (2006) Diving injuries of the cervical spine in amateur divers. Spine J 6(1):44–49
10. Amorim EC, Vetter H, Mascarenhas LB, Gomes EG, Carvalho JB, Gomes JF (2011) Spine trauma due to diving: main features and short-term neurological outcome. Spinal Cord 49(2):206–210
11. Firth JL (1985) Equestrian injuries. In: Schneider RC, Kennedy JC, Plant ML (eds) Sports injuries. Mechanisms, prevention, and treatment. Williams & Wilkins, Baltimore, pp 431–449
12. Siebenga J, Segers MJ, Elzinga MJ, Bakker FC, Haarman HJ, Patka P (2006) Spine fractures caused by horse riding. Eur Spine J 15(4):465–471
13. Silver JR (2002) Spinal injuries resulting from horse riding accidents. Spinal Cord 40:264–271
14. Tarazi F, Dvorak MF, Wing PC (1999) Spinal injuries in skiers and snowboarders. Am J Sports Med 27(2):177–180
15. Kary JM (2008) Acute spine injuries in skiers and snowboarders. Curr Sports Med Rep 7(1):35–38
16. Floyd T (2001) Alpine skiing, snowboarding, and spinal trauma. Arch Orthop Trauma Surg 121(8):433–436
17. Yamaguchi KT Jr, Myung KS, Alonso MA, Skaggs DL (2012) Clay-shoveler's fracture equivalent in children. Spine (Phila Pa 1976) 37(26):E1672–E1675
18. Green JD, Harle TS, Harris JH Jr (1981) Anterior subluxation of the cervical spine: hyperflexion sprain. AJNR Am J Neuroradiol 2(3):243–250
19. Kepler CK, Vaccaro AR (2012) Injuries and abnormalities of the cervical spine and return to play criteria. Clin Sports Med 31(3):499–508
20. Nigrovic LE, Rogers AJ, Adelgais KM, Olsen CS, Leonard JR, Jaffe DM, Leonard JC (2012) Utility of plain radiographs in detecting traumatic injuries of the cervical spine in children; Pediatric Emergency Care Applied Research Network (PECARN) Cervical Spine study group. Pediatr Emerg Care 28(5):426–432
21. Hutchings L, Atijosan O, Burgess C, Willett K (2009) Developing a spinal clearance protocol for unconscious pediatric trauma patients. J Trauma 67(4):681–686
22. Morganti C, Sweeney CA, Albanese SA, Burak C, Hosea T, Connolly PJ (2001) Return to play after

cervical spine injury. Spine (Phila Pa 1976) 26(10): 1131–1136

23. Penning L (1962) Some aspects of plain radiography of the cervical spine in chronic myelopathy. Neurology 12:513

24. Torg JS (2002) Cervical spinal stenosis with cord neurapraxia: evaluations and decisions regarding participation in athletics. Curr Sports Med Rep 1(1):43–46

25. Santiago R, Rafael MD, Guenther E, Carroll K, Junkins EP (2006) The clinical presentation of pediatric thoracolumbar fractures. J Trauma 60(1):187–192

26. Barneschi G (2007) Traumatologia vertebrale. Verduci Editore, Roma

27. Magerl F, Aebi M, Gertzbein SD, Harms J, Nazarian S (1994) A comprehensive classification of thoracic and lumbar injuries. Eur Spine J 3(4):184–201

28. Vander Have KL, Caird MS, Gross S, Farley FA, Graziano GA, Stauff M, Segal LS (2009) Burst fractures of the thoracic and lumbar spine in children and adolescents. J Pediatr Orthop 29(7):713–719

29. Junkins EP Jr, Stotts A, Santiago R, Guenther E (2008) The clinical presentation of pediatric thoracolumbar fractures: a prospective study. J Trauma 65(5):1066–1071

30. Pouliquen JC, Kassis B, Glorion C, Langlais J (1997) Vertebral growth after thoracic or lumbar fracture of the spine in children. J Pediatr Orthop 17:115–120

31. Takata K, Inoue S, Takahashi K, Ohtsuka Y (1988) Fracture of the posterior margin of a lumbar vertebral body. J Bone Joint Surg Am 70:589–594

32. Epstein NE, Epstein JA, Mauri T (1989) Treatment of fractures of the vertebral limbus and spinal stenosis in five adolescents and five adults. Neurosurgery 24(4):595–604

33. Chafetz RS, Gaughan JP, Vogel LC, Betz R, Mulcahey MJ (2009) The international standards for neurological classification of spinal cord injury: intra-rater agreement of total motor and sensory scores in the pediatric population. J Spinal Cord Med 32(2):157–161

34. Pettiford JN, Bikhchandani J, Ostlie DJ, Peter SD, Sharp RJ, Juang D (2012) A review: the role of high dose methylprednisolone in spinal cord trauma in children. Pediatr Surg Int 28(3):287–294

35. Marchetti PG, Bartolozzi P (1997) Classification of spondylolisthesis as a guideline for treatment. In: Bridwell K, de Wald R (eds) The textbook of spinal surgery 2. Lippincott-Raven, Philadelphia, pp 1211–1254

The Shoulder: Skeletal Injuries and Ligamentous Instability

7

Vincenzo Izzo and Carlo Fabbriciani

Shoulder injuries in the pediatric athletic population continue to increase with expanded participation and higher competitive levels of youth sports. Injury patterns are unique to the growing musculoskeletal system and specific to the demands of the sport involved. They could concern a direct contact from a collision or from a repetitive overhead motion. Both acute (sudden, traumatic) and chronic (long-term) injuries are common. Injuries requiring surgical intervention are even rarer. However, it is important for the practicing orthopedic surgeon to differentiate nonoperative injuries from the urgent and potentially operative injuries. Missing such an injury in the pediatric population could be potentially life threatening or lead to long-term disability. Open fractures or neurovascular-threatening fractures should be attended to immediately. Severely displaced proximal physeal humerus fractures in the older child often have a better long-term outcome after anatomic reduction. Finally, although glenohumeral dislocations, once reduced, are not life threatening or limb threatening, they do have a very high incidence of recurrence in adolescent patients. Posterior sternoclavicular dislocations should be differentiated from medial clavicular physeal injuries and promptly reduced. There is controversy regarding the appropriate treatment of these adolescent athletes—including debates on injury prevention, nonsurgical treatment versus surgical treatment, overuse injuries, and return to play after shoulder fractures, dislocations, and instability.

7.1 Anatomy and Development of the Shoulder

Understanding the anatomy in skeletally immature adolescents provides greater insight into typical pediatric and adolescent shoulder injuries. The major differences between the skeletally immature versus mature shoulder relate to the epiphyseal plates of the shoulder and collagen composition of the supporting ligaments and tendons. The proximal humeral epiphysis is responsible for 80 % of the humeral growth in length. The proximal humeral epiphyseal ossification, consisting in 3 different ossification centers, appears between the fourth and sixth months of life. The epiphyseal ossification core becomes radiologically evident in the first year of life. Between the second and third years of life, the second ossification core forming the greater tubercle and the third ossification core maturing to the lesser tubercle can be spotted radiologically. The tubercle core fuses with the core of the humeral head between the ages of 14

V. Izzo (✉) · C. Fabbriciani
Department of Orthopedics and Traumatology—"A. Gemelli" Hospital, Catholic University of Sacred Heart, l.go A. Gemelli, 8, 00168, Rome, Italy
e-mail: vincenzo.izzo@hotmail.it

C. Fabbriciani
e-mail: carlo.fabbriciani@rm.unicatt.it

V. Guzzanti (ed.), *Pediatric and Adolescent Sports Traumatology*,
DOI: 10.1007/978-88-470-5412-7_7, © Springer-Verlag Italia 2014

and 16. Around the age of 20, the entire humeral epiphysis shows fusion with the diaphysis [1, 2].

The presence of the physeal plates of the shoulder provides matrices of lesser strength than those provided by the adjacent capsules and ligaments or even in some cases by the periosteum. The physis has an age-related variability in strength. Apparently the physis and its perichondral ring weaken just prior to maturity. This fact is borne out clinically in the classic study by Peterson [3], who found that the physeal injuries occurred between 11 and 12 years in girls and between 13 and 14 years in boys.

The shoulder, like the hip, is a ball-and-socket joint, but with a great lack of restriction. Different capsuloligamentous and muscular stabilizers ensure stability of glenohumeral joint. Static stabilizers include capsule and labrum and the superior, middle, and inferior glenohumeral ligaments. Dynamic stabilizers include the rotator cuff, long head of the biceps, deltoid, and scapulothoracic muscles [2].

The combination of weaker epiphyseal plates, weaker muscle forces, and excessive laxity of the supporting structures in the setting of significant forces to the shoulder region during sport may predispose the young athlete to shoulder injury. Additionally, it is known that the amount of Type III collagen (the major protein of ligaments and tendons) produced in adolescents is significantly greater than in adults, potentially leading to excessive laxity in the shoulder capsule and ligaments.

7.2   Specific Sporting Events and Injuries

7.2.1   Macrotrauma

Football: Football and wrestling produced the greatest number of injuries overall, whereas swimming and tennis had the lowest injury rates. They rank only second after the knee in overall injuries sustained in football.

Most injuries to the shoulder sustained in football result in macrotrauma (i.e., fracture of the clavicle or glenohumeral dislocation) and

perhaps the outlawing of spearing, which brought a return of shoulder–body contact to tackling.

Wrestling: Twenty-nine percent of injuries occurring during high school wrestling season involve the upper extremity. Snook [4] found that almost 78 % involved the acromioclavicular (AC) joint. Such injuries are the result of a direct blow when the shoulder hits the mat. Since the object of wrestling is often to put leverage about the shoulder, one might expect. The incidence of glenohumeral dislocation, however, is quite low (less than 10 % of all shoulder injuries). This fact can probably be explained by the fact that the leverage forces applied to the shoulder are gradual and are strongly resisted by the muscular forces of the opponent.

Bicycling: Although bicycling is usually a recreational activity, it is becoming increasingly popular as an organized sport. Most bicycle injuries in the pediatric age group occur in children between 5 and 14 years old. In bicycle injuries, 85 % involve the upper extremity. One unique injury is the so-called "bicycle shoulder" (Fig. 7.1). This occurs when the cyclist is thrown over the front of the cycle when it is suddenly stopped. Failure to stay with the bicycle causes the cyclist to be thrown forward, landing directly on the shoulder. This forward propulsion over the wells produces a direct trauma to the Acromio-Clavicular (AC) area (fracture of distal clavicle or AC joint dislocation). A right teaching program explaining to the cyclist to maintain a tight grip on the handlebar and rolling with the cycle allows the body to absorb some forces of the fall, preventing shoulder injuries [5].

Skiing: During skiing, almost 30 % of the upper extremity injuries consist of shoulder dislocation or sprain. It was surmised that conditions that increased the speed of the skier, i.e., his ability and snow pack, increased the chances of sustaining an injury to the upper extremity [6].

Horseback riding: Two-thirds of the fractures sustained by young horseback riders occur in the upper extremities, after head and neck injuries. In Sweden, the major cause of fractures of the

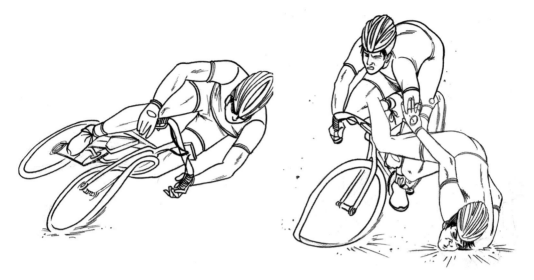

Fig. 7.1 Mechanism of trauma during cycling. Bicyclist lands directly on his shoulder after throwing forward over the handle bar. Falling in a proper and trained way leads a large distribution of force on the trunk preventing AC disruption or further shoulder major tears

proximal humerus in young girls is falling off the horse [7].

7.2.2 Microtrauma

Shoulder microtrauma and overuse syndrome can be divided into three categories: The first is *explosive* force such as that occurring in pitching a baseball; the second is *dynamic force*, sustaining a repetitive force for a longer period but without maximum forces such as in swimming; and the third is *static* in which isometric contractions are maintained across the shoulder for various periods of time.

Swimming: The most common orthopedic problem in competitive swimmers involves the shoulder and is almost exclusively seen in high-performance swimmers. In swimming, the athlete must pull the body over the arm. Athletes under the age of 10 rarely are affected by these injuries, but a dramatic increase is reported after that age. A unique aspect of swimming is the factor of upper extremity endurance. Competitive athletes may swim 10,000–14,000 m (6–8 miles) a day, 6 or 7 days a week. Distance swimmers may double that distance. This distance equates to 16,000 shoulder revolutions per week, or approximately 2,500 revolutions per day. Many of these revolutions are done in sequence, without any rest for the muscles to recover. It has been calculated that the average freestyle swimmer performs almost 400,000 strokes per arm per year, women 660,000 because they require more strokes to swim the same distance. Symptoms increased with the caliber of the athlete, were more common in the early and middle portions of the season, and were often exacerbated by the use of hand paddles during training.

The major cause of shoulder pain is an "impingement syndrome" between humeral head and rotator cuff on the coracoacromial arch. The sports medicine literature often refers to "swimmer's shoulder," an ill-defined condition that is widely synonymous with impingement syndrome and rotator cuff tendinitis (Fig. 7.2). Swimmer's shoulder pathology could involve a more complex pattern of lesions that follows repeated microtrauma and overuse strain of static and dynamic stabilizer of the shoulder. Diminished performance over a period of time (overuse) can sometimes lead to an acute injury, resulting in reduced ability or an inability to participate in the sport [2, 8].

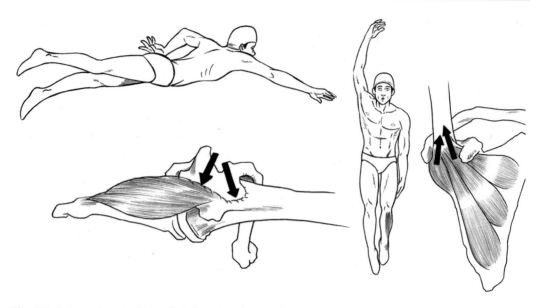

Fig. 7.2 Swimmer's shoulder. Pull-through phase: mechanism of impingement between humeral head and rotator cuff. In the backstroke, the initial phase of pull-through phase will be a tendency to place tension on the anterior part of glenohumeral capsule (*arrows*)

Gymnastic: Gymnastic events produce unique forces across the shoulder. Rather than performing motions repetitively, the gymnast often has to maintain one position for relatively prolonged period of time. In male gymnast who performs extensively on the rings, which produce a great deal of stress across the shoulder, a benign cortical hypertrophy often develops at the insertion of the pectoralis major muscle into the proximal humerus. This has been termed by Fulton the "ringman's shoulder lesion" [9]. In a study of female gymnast by Snook, the second most common injury was a supraspinatus tendinitis, which emphasized the great degree of tension and compressive forces about the shoulder that occur with gymnastics [10].

7.2.2.1 Baseball and Throwing Athlete

The act of throwing is one of the fastest and most violent maneuvers to which any joint in the body is subjected. For each pitch, the thrower must generate high levels of energy in the lower extremities and trunk to accelerate the ball to top velocity. The muscles and capsular structures of the shoulder must then dissipate this force after ball release and during arm deceleration. In elite pitchers, internal rotation of the humerus can reach velocities as great as 7,000 deg/s. To maximize the force that can be generated and transferred to the ball, the structures of the shoulder must strike a delicate balance between adequate laxity to achieve extreme range of motion and sufficient stability to inhibit subluxation and instability. This delicate equilibrium has been referred to as the "throwers paradox." At the extremes of motion, the forces generated and the speed with which this motion occurs, place the stabilizing structures of glenohumeral joint and scapula at risk [11].

Most studies demonstrated that at least 50 % of all players experienced shoulder pain at some point during the athletic season [12]. There are multiple causes of shoulder pain in overhead throwing athletes including Little League shoulder, rotator cuff injury, glenohumeral instability and glenohumeral internal rotation deficit (GIRD). Most shoulder injuries are due to chronic stress placed on the skeletally immature shoulder during repetitive throwing activities. These injuries occur in greatest frequency during the mid- to late teen years as the shoulder is subjected to progressively higher stresses with increasing muscular development.

The importance of core activation in initiating this kinetic chain of events has been advocated as an etiologic factor that leads to shoulder pain in more immature pitchers.

Children without injury throw with mechanics similar to adults but with several important differences. When comparing Little League to college and professional pitchers, the younger Little League pitchers generate slower trunk and hip rotation and shoulder external rotation velocities. In addition, their elbow may fall behind their body in the cocking phase and with overall poor synchronization of arm motion with body motion. These improper mechanics can lead to increased stress on the shoulder with a higher risk of injury [2, 12, 13].

Little League shoulder: Little League shoulder is an apophysitis caused by repetitive rotational stresses on the proximal humeral physis during overhead throwing activity. The injury is typically seen in baseball pitchers between 11 and 13 years of age when physeal growth is maximal.

Radiographs reveal widening of the proximal humeral physis, which may be subtle and require comparison views of the contralateral shoulder to detect. There may be associated fragmentation, sclerosis, demineralization, and cystic changes of the humeral physis. Since Little League shoulder is primarily a clinical diagnosis, magnetic resonance imaging (MRI) is rarely used to evaluate patients with suspected apophysitis. However, MRI may show widening and edema within and around the proximal humeral physis [14, 15].

The goal of therapy for the thrower who presents with shoulder pain is to develop a straightforward rehabilitation program. For an injured athlete, rest and recovery of range of motion is the first step. In an effort to decrease the number of youth overuse injuries, Little League Baseball and the American Sports Medicine Institute have recommended pitch count limits and appropriate number of rest days between pitching appearances. The days of rest required between appearances increases with player age and number of pitches thrown [2, 15]. The next goal is to improve muscular strength and endurance. Resistance is initially light with an emphasis on form. Volume is progressively increased. Once adequate endurance is obtained, the rehabilitation program focuses on strength and speed. It is important to train muscles to respond and contract at a speed that is consistent with performance speed. Once motion and strength with endurance is regained, the thrower begins a progressive throwing program.

The coordinated production and transfer of potential energy from the body to the upper extremity in the form of kinetic energy is required to propel the ball at top velocity. Continuative program of education of gesture with emphasis on proper throwing mechanics and control rather than speed is the key to lead to fewer future shoulder injuries. A coordinated approach among trainers, therapists and physicians is required for the comprehensive evaluation, diagnosis, and treatment of shoulder pain in the throwing athlete.

Finally, shoulder pain in young overhead athlete could be a consequence of the only referred glenohumeral pain even very rare in younger athletes. Repetitive stress may injure the AC and sternoclavicular joints (SCJs). Finally, less common causes of shoulder pain in the throwing athlete should be borne in mind. These include quadrilateral space syndrome, suprascapular nerve entrapment, axillary artery occlusion, axillary vein thrombosis, posterior capsule laxity, and glenoid spurs.

7.2.2.2 Glenohumeral Internal Rotation Deficit

Glenohumeral internal rotation deficit (GIRD) is defined as a condition resulting in the loss of internal rotation of the glenohumeral joint as compared to the contralateral side. Changes to the dynamic restraints of the glenohumeral joint caused by repetitive stress are found in most overhead athletes, especially younger ones; changes to the internal rotator cuff musculature have been documented in young swimmers and baseball and tennis players. A GIRD occurs primarily in overhead athletes often seen in baseball pitchers. A number of theories have been reported concerning a time line for developing GIRD, and the underlying etiology of these adaptations is controversial.

Glenohumeral internal rotation deficit occurs before any other motion adaptation and is sometimes followed by associated gains in ER. Contractures of the posterior capsule and tightening of the large anterior shoulder muscles are to blame for some of this change in motion. GIRD begins in the early years with a bony adaptation of the humerus. Higher humeral head retroversion, found in both Little League and college-age baseball players, have been attributed to the quick change in velocity during the late cocking-through-deceleration phases of the throwing motion [16]. IR alterations have also been documented in adult and college-age swimmers and adolescent tennis players as a consequence of soft tissue changes, static and dynamic stabilizers. If not detected, GIRD tends to worsen over time and ultimately alters normal scapular and shoulder biomechanics.

First line of treatment in younger athletes is rest from throwing and physical therapy for six months which include posterior capsule stretching (sleeper stretch) performed with internal rotation stretch at 90° of abduction with scapular stabilization, pectoralis minor stretching, subscapularis and serratus (anterior) strengthening. Although very uncommon in the adolescent population, operative treatment with posterior capsule release or anterior stabilization is required only if extensive physical therapy fails [17].

7.2.3 Capsuloligamentous Injuries

7.2.3.1 Glenohumeral Instability

Pediatric shoulder instability continues to be a significant clinical problem. It is a more commonly encountered shoulder problem in young overhead athletes. Traumatic dislocation of the shoulder in childhood is rare, accounting for only 0.01 % of all injuries in this age class.

Depending on age, joint injuries in children and adolescents far more commonly result in metaphyseal fractures than in injuries to the joint capsule, ligament disruptures, and dislocations.

More than 50 % of the dislocations occurred during sporting activities. Ninety-three percent of the casualties were aged over 10 years, and 62 % were female (Fig. 7.3). Only about 4 % of all dislocations of the shoulder affect patients in whom the growth plates are still open [18].

Glenohumeral instability is often characterized as traumatic or atraumatic. As in adults, 8 traumatic anterior dislocations account for 90 % of cases, usually following a fall onto the abducted, externally rotated arm; traumatic posterior dislocations are rare and reported only anecdotally [19].

Closed reduction under conscious sedation is often necessary and a post-reduction immobilization is mandatory. In the first time dislocation this could be a definitive choice of treatment unless there are some risk factors or complex articular joint tears that need an acute surgical treatment. The type of treatment by post-operative sling may be important. There has been growing interest in whether immobilizing the upper extremity in external rotation has an effect on treatment efficacy [20, 21].

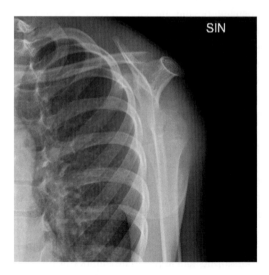

Fig. 7.3 Radiograph in an AP view shows first-time anterior dislocation of the glenohumeral joint

Despite a number of publications regarding this topic, there is a paucity of comparative studies to review as a basis for clinical decision-making. A Level II evidence exists to support the conclusion that post-reduction immobilization in external rotation may reduce recurrence, while Level I evidence suggests that immobilization in internal rotation does not reduce recurrence. A recent Cochrane review on this topic could only find one "flawed quasirandomized trial" comparing post-reduction immobilization in external rotation to immobilization in internal rotation [22]. No significant differences in terms of return to activity or recurrent instability or dislocation were found and similar numbers of patients discontinued their immobilization within 1 week of treatment in both treatment arms [20].

There is a paucity of literature regarding the outcome of skeletally immature patients who sustain a primary traumatic anterior shoulder dislocation [23]. Most published results focus on adolescents and young adults, using recurrent dislocation/instability as a determinant of outcome rather than a validated quality of life measurement tool. As early as 1956, Rowe [24] demonstrated a 100 % risk of recurrence if the patient sustained a primary dislocation before age 10 years. Another study by Marans et al. [25] also reported a 100 % rate of redislocation in 21 adolescent patients with open physis who sustained a traumatic anterior dislocation. However, these two studies did not report on the functional outcome of these patients.

Presently, isolated outcome data are limited regarding primary traumatic anterior shoulder dislocation in the skeletally immature pediatric population. Therefore, there is a lack of consensus for the ideal treatment of such a patient. Although an abundance of data exists on dislocation in a mixed population of adolescent and young adult patients, caution should be taken in extrapolating such data to the pediatric skeletally immature patient.

An important aspect to define is if dislocation occurs with a pathoanatomical tears of capsulolabral complex or only with their enlargement due to the congenital laxity or intrinsic characteristics of collagen. This lends credence to the idea that, regarding shoulder instability, children are not simply "little adults." The primary pediatric traumatic shoulder dislocation represents a distinct pathoanatomical entity. It has been hypothesized that the capsular structures of the pediatric shoulder have a much greater elasticity than their adult counterparts [26]. This finding, theoretically, would allow for a resilient shoulder that is resistant to structural damage. In addition, it is believed that a more laterally based capsular insertion on the glenoid in the pediatric skeletally immature patient would create a smaller anterior/inferior recess, as described by Rockwood and Matsen [22]. This would impart increased tension on the anterior capsule when healed, making recurrent instability less likely in the younger pediatric population. The high variable rate in recurrent dislocation after first-time dislocation reported in the literature is thus explained.

About the debate on conservative versus operative treatment of traumatic shoulder instability, there is a void in the data available, and it is unknown how patients present and how they respond to treatment. It is unclear whether children are similar to adult patients with the same diagnosis or whether they require different treatment, in the same way that certain pediatric fracture patients require different management than adult fractures at the same anatomic sites. The concerns with traumatic dislocations include the risk of recurrent instability and the right treatment of associated secondary injuries of the humeral head, articular cartilage, anterior and posterior capsule, glenohumeral ligaments and glenoid and biceps tendon.

The prevalence of dislocations in patients younger than 18 years is 19.7 in 10,000 for men and 5.01 in 10,000 for women. Age at the time of the initial dislocation is inversely related to the recurrence rate: Recurrent dislocation is higher in patients younger than 18 years old and in men. The presence of bony lesions has a dramatic impact on surgical outcome, as athletes participating in contact sports are at a higher risk of recurrence.

The arthroscopic treatment for traumatic shoulder instability in young athletes has recently become the best option for the majority of surgeons due to improvements in suture anchors and cosmesis as well as the possibility of identifying and treating additional intra-articular lesions such as HAGL, SLAP or posterior Bankart lesions. Studies comparing nonoperative treatment with immediate open or arthroscopic Bankart repair for initial traumatic anterior dislocations demonstrated a lower recurrence of dislocation after the surgical procedure with recurrence rates of 3–19 % [2, 27].

The major disadvantage of arthroscopic Bankart repair is still the rate of recurrence, even if recent studies have shown better outcome and lower recurrence rate [28].

Ligamentous laxity in young athletes can lead to atraumatic or multidirectional shoulder instability, especially in throwers, gymnasts, and swimmers. It results from chronic overload owing to excessive repetitive external rotation during overhead motion with high stresses on the anterior capsuloligament restraints. Patients with hyperlaxity often experience subluxation episodes with spontaneous reduction and reveal evidence of hyperlaxity of multiple joints. In contrast to surgery for traumatic dislocations, a specific rehabilitation program, often up to 6 months, is successful in more than 80 % of those with multidirectional instability [2, 28].

Since the introduction of arthroscopic techniques for refixation of the anterior labral complex using suture anchor systems, which are generally absorbable, this technique is the gold standard for surgical treatment of post-traumatic, recurrent, anterior shoulder instabilities, but arthroscopic labral refixation is suitable only for the small number of children and adolescents, suffering from post-traumatic shoulder instability (Fig. 7.4). The advantage of surgical treatment is not undisputed, and even current literature has nowadays no consensus about the right treatment revealing redislocation and instability rates of up to 20 % in longer follow-up periods of almost 100 months following arthroscopic surgical treatment. Five percent of redislocations are described even with

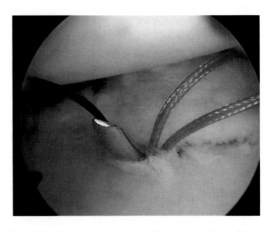

Fig. 7.4 Arthroscopic view. Traumatic labral injury with multidirectional instability in a 16-year-old high-performance basket player with labral refixation suitable only for the small number of young athletes, suffering from post-traumatic shoulder instability

immediate arthroscopic refixation of the labral complex after traumatic first dislocation [29].

The first rigorous differentiation must be made in this assessment regarding the laxness of the shoulder joint, which may vary greatly from one case to the next and regarding habitual shoulder joint instability, which is generally multidirectional. Early surgical stabilization has the advantage of a significantly lower recurrence rate for young active patients. However, early surgical intervention will result in some patients having unnecessary surgery, and further research is needed to establish prognostic factors that can stratify patient risk in order to identify individuals most likely to benefit from surgery. Patient age at first-time dislocation is clearly an important prognostic factor, but other issues, particularly patient activity level and specific sport participation, may provide further prognostic value to help determine which patients would benefit from early surgical intervention.

Arthroscopic labral refixation is a reliable, surgical treatment procedure, and it can be used successfully in children and young people prior to skeletal maturity. No alteration of the surgical procedure of Bankart repair in adults is necessary. Furthermore, arthroscopic stabilization using suture anchors appears to be comparable to open stabilization although, again, there may be certain subsets of patients, for example contact athletes, who would benefit from open stabilization.

7.2.3.2 SLAP Lesions

To understand the etiology of superior labral injuries, it is useful to first consider the two discretely different mechanisms of injury that have been proposed in the literature: superior compression and inferior traction. An acute traumatic superior compression force to the shoulder, usually due to a fall onto an outstretched arm with the shoulder positioned in an abducted and slightly forward-flexed position at the time of impact, was the most common mechanism of injury described. The throwing athlete appears to be prone to this mechanism. Both biomechanical and clinical explanations exist for the occurrence of SLAP lesions in overhead athletes. Large forces in the biceps tendon during the deceleration phase of the throwing motion may create SLAP lesions.

The diagnosis of SLAP tears can be difficult as they often coexist with other injuries. The clinical presentation of superior glenoid lesions is quite variable. A review of the literature does not identify a specific constellation of historical or physical findings that are pathognomonic for superior glenoid lesions.

Throwers may or may not relate a specific event to the onset of symptoms, and they will complain of an insidious onset of nonspecific shoulder pain, often occurring in the overhead position.

The value of imaging studies has been questioned in the orthopedic literature, in which detection of superior glenoid disease has been reported in only 9–38 % of cases. Plain radiographs cannot identify a SLAP lesion, but assessment of the acromial morphology and the AC joint is useful in considering associated disorders. The utility of MRI or computer tomography arthrograms for diagnosing this lesion is touted in the radiology literature. Recent data suggest that a 3T magnetic resonance arthrogram is the most sensitive study for the diagnosis of SLAP tears [2, 30]. Among the

four main types of SLAP tears, Type II is most common in throwers.

Most adolescents with a suspected superior labral lesion should undergo a period of conservative management, including rest, physical therapy, and rarely nonsteroidal anti-inflammatory drugs.

Despite the efforts to make the diagnosis preoperatively, most lesions are discovered and treated surgically at the time of arthroscopic diagnosis. Shoulder arthroscopy should be considered if symptoms do not improve after a correct rehabilitation program. Type I lesions require only debridement of the frayed labral edge. Type II lesions are most common and are best treated with suture anchor or biodegradable-tack fixation of the unstable biceps anchor. Type II lesions should be treated with debridement of the bucket-handle portion of the superior labrum. Finally, Type IV lesions may require debridement of the torn portion of labrum and biceps tendon, arthroscopic repair and stabilization, or biceps tenodesis, depending on the amount of biceps tendon involvement (Fig. 7.5). Controversial results regarding SLAP repairs are reported in the literature with different impairments of the return to their preinjury level. Oh et al. [31] published their results of 34 patients undergoing arthroscopic repair of isolated SLAP

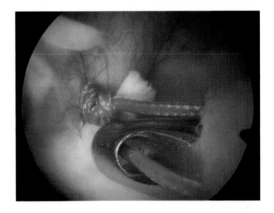

Fig. 7.5 Arthroscopic SLAP repair using suture anchor systems, which are generally absorbable. Labral debridement or repair depend on the type of tear found at surgery. Surgical technique is similar to that used in adults

tears using suture anchors [2]. At 33 months post-surgery only 22 % of those involved in overhead sports returned to their preinjury level without any limitations. This is in contrast to 63 % of those in nonoverhead sports activity.

7.2.3.3 Rotator Cuff Injuries

In the pediatric and adolescent population the overall incidence of rotator cuff injury is rare, with only small case series present in the literature. Although these injuries in children are relatively rare, their presence both in isolation and with other associated pathology must be recognized.

Furthermore, health care providers caring for adolescent athletes with shoulder pain must be able to identify the source of pain to prescribe the appropriate treatment. Frequently, these younger patients have a constellation of findings suggesting the diagnosis of internal impingement. First described by Walch et al. [32] in 1992, the concept of internal impingement has been well studied in adults. However, its presence in adolescents is not well characterized. Several theories exist as to the fundamental cause of the pathology, but the ultimate lesion often involves both posterior and posterosuperior glenoid labral tears and an articular-sided rotator cuff tear in an overhead athlete.

In addition, some authors suggest that anterior instability plays a significant role in the disease process, with increased anterior humeral head translation being the underlying process that leads to the posterior labral tears and P.A.S.T.A. (Partial Articular Sided Tendon Avulsion) lesions seen in these patients [33].

Furthermore, Eisner [34] reported a hypertrophic synovitis lesion in the posterosuperior region in addition to a P.A.S.T.A. lesion. Although this lesion has not been previously described, its presence may be within the spectrum of internal impingement in adolescents, representing a synovial response to increased contact between the humeral head and posterosuperior joint capsule and adjacent structures.

Treatment of rotator cuff pathology in adolescent patients generally begins, and is almost always conservative, with a course of physical therapy. If symptoms persist, surgical intervention may be warranted. Shoulder arthroscopy allows the treating surgeon to address the rotator cuff and associated capsulolabral, biceps or cartilaginous pathology, simultaneously. However, the outcomes of both conservative and surgical treatment of rotator cuff pathology in adolescent patients remain largely unknown [35, 36].

7.2.4 Upper Extremity Fractures and Joint Injuries in the Adolescent Athlete

7.2.4.1 Proximal Humerus Fractures

Most of proximal humerus fractures in adolescent are Salter Types I or II. Salter–Harris Type I physeal fractures occur primarily in neonates and children younger than 5 years old. Children aged between 5 and 11 primarily have metaphyseal fractures, whereas those older than 11 have Salter–Harris Type II injuries. Traditionally, pediatric proximal humerus fractures have been treated nonoperatively. This is because roughly 80 % of the longitudinal growth of the humerus occurs at the proximal humerus; therefore, there is great potential for remodeling at this site. Furthermore, the large arc of motion of this joint can compensate for a large degree of malunion and angulation. Accidentally, pathologic bone lesions such as unicameral bone cysts are found in up to 25 % of adolescents with proximal humerus fractures [2].

The correct treatment of fractures of the proximal humerus in children and adolescents depends on the fracture location, degree of displacement, and the child's age. Conservative treatment by a shoulder sling is the gold standard for no displaced or minimally displaced fractures. Because of the high potential of spontaneous correction due to the proximal humeral epiphysis the prognosis of proximal humerus fractures is good. Till the age of 12 years, a correction of 50–60° of shaft breaks in the frontal and sagittal planes is possible by a closed reduction. We recommend an immobilization for 3–4 weeks if the fracture is stable after closed reduction.

Beyond the age of 12 years the correction ability shrinks to half of the primary malposition, which can be tolerated to a maximum of 40 degrees of correction [2].

More frequent fractures that need a surgical fixation in adolescents are Salter–Harris Type II fractures, which entail a more proximal fracture line with a steeper angle compared with fractures in adults. This translates into a different pin configuration as well as a different reduction maneuver. There are a lot of many pin configurations, but it is important to emphasize that the goal with each of these pin patterns could be a perfect balance between fixation into the humeral shaft and humeral head, optimization of the biomechanical trajectory across the fracture line. No skeletal complications are rarely reported with injuries in this area. Transient axillary nerve paralysis has been described. Usually, however, these problems resolve by the time the athlete is ready to start the recovery or rehabilitation phase.

Brachial plexus paresis as well as complete disruption of the brachial artery is a very rare event and reported in the literature only as case reports.

7.2.4.2 Clavicle Fractures

Clavicle fractures are frequent injuries in young athletes due to its superficial location, its thin midshaft, the forces transmitted across it, but also the prominent use of the shoulder girdle during many athletic feats in different sports, like blocking and tackling in football as well as battering ram in hockey or rugby. Clavicle fractures comprise up to 15 % of all fractures in this population.

The anatomic site of the fracture is typically described using the Allman classification, which divides the clavicle into thirds: Group I (midshaft) fractures occur on the middle third of the clavicle, group II fractures on the lateral (distal) third, and group III fractures on the medial (proximal) third.

Midshaft fractures account for approximately 75–80 % of all clavicle fractures and typically occur in younger persons. Distal third fractures represent about 15–25 % of clavicle fractures. Medial third fractures are least common, accounting for less than 5 % of clavicle fractures.

The pediatric athlete usually has a distinct history of injury when a clavicular fracture is present. They typically hold the affected arm adducted close to the body, often supporting the affected side with the opposite hand. This position is most comfortable because it limits the pull from the weight of the arm on the fractured bone. Physical examination may reveal ecchymosis, edema, focal tenderness, and crepitation on palpation over the clavicle. The defect in the bone may be seen by visual inspection or localized by palpation. Despite the low incidence of complications, it is important to perform a neurovascular and lung examination, because the subclavicular vessels, brachial plexus, and lung apex can be injured in posteriorly displaced fractures.

Radiography should be performed on all patients with suspected clavicle fractures. Most fractures can be seen on a standard anteroposterior view of the clavicle; however, an anteroposterior view with 45° cephalic tilt minimizes the overlap of the ribs and scapula and allows for better assessment of displacement in the anterior and posterior plane [37]. Advanced imaging such as computer tomography is indicated only in rare cases of distal or proximal fracture to assess the extent of intra-articular involvement.

Consideration of anatomy within the area of the fracture is essential so that associated injuries can be diagnosed and appropriately treated. A standard sling or a "figure-of-8" brace, when the latter would not cause complications such as compression of axillary vessels and brachial plexopathy, is the gold standard treatment for nondisplaced or minimally displaced fractures in patients of all ages.

We would recommend that displaced fractures with or without compromised skin integrity, associated neurovascular injury, and floating shoulder must be performed by surgical approach. Open reduction internal fixation of significantly shortened or displaced fractures in skeletally immature adolescents or teenagers to improve time to union and decrease the incidence of symptomatic malunion [38]. Return to sporting activity is frequently quicker in such operatively treated patients. Patients usually can return to noncontact sports and full daily activities six weeks after injury. Contact and collision sports should be delayed for two to four months until solid bony union occurs. If surgery is performed, some surgeons recommend removal of hardware before returning to sports. However, plate removal may delay return to sports and is not recommended by other surgeons [2, 39].

7.2.4.3 Acromioclavicular Joint Injuries

Acromioclavicular joint injuries occur as a result of a direct force applied to the tip of the shoulder or due to indirect trauma such as a fall on the outstretched hand. These mechanisms lead to bone injuries in younger adolescents, while they lead to the AC sprain in the older ones.

Acromioclavicular joint dislocations range from a simple sprain of the acromioclavicular and coracoclavicular ligaments to widely displaced injuries with dislocations of the distal third of the clavicle.

Acromioclavicular dislocations are classified on the basis of the radiographic findings. X-ray includes a standard shoulder view or sometimes an additional "Zanca view," consisting of AP view with a 10° of superior tilt. Different classification systems are available, being that of Rockwood the most widely utilized. This classification takes into account not only the position of AC joint, but also the coracoclavicular ligament, the deltoid and trapezius muscles, and the direction of dislocation of the clavicle with respect to the acromion.

Type I injury is a partial tearing of the AC ligament but with the joint remaining intact. Type II injury is a complete disruption of the AC ligament, while the coracoclavicular ligaments are not completely disrupted. Type III injury results in a 25–100 % superior displacement of clavicle (a dislocation) as the AC and coracoclavicular ligaments are both completely disrupted. Rockwood then further delineated variations of the Type III as IV, V, and VI where the clavicle is captured by other soft tissues [40].

The majority of AC joint injuries are successfully treated nonoperatively with a period of sling immobilization followed by progressive physical therapy and shoulder range of motion exercises. Surgical management of AC joint injuries is indicated in Types IV, V, and VI injuries and in very selected cases, Type III. Many surgical techniques described in the literature involve the use of metallic implants for internal fixation or reconstruction of the CC (Coraco-Clavicular) ligament by transferring the AC ligament or using autograft or allograft tissues [2, 41].

7.2.4.4 Sternoclavicular Joint Injuries

Sternoclavicular joint (SCJ), like the AC joint, can suffer a spectrum of ligamentous injuries, even rare in the adolescent athlete. When it comes to dislocation, it can dislocate anteriorly or posteriorly, depending on the different mechanism of injury occurring during the sport event. The posterior structures are stronger than the anterior and this is why posterior SCJ dislocations are rarer than anterior dislocations. The key to diagnosis is a detailed patient history and physical examination, but in most cases occurs only a slight or none deformity. Nevertheless, before CT scan evaluation became possible, such injuries were often discovered very late.

Anterior dislocations are often successfully treated with closed reduction. Posterior dislocations have significant clinical implications because of the proximity of surrounding vessels and nerves, trachea, and esophagus. Any attempt at reduction in a posterior dislocation compressing the mediastinal structures requires the presence of a cardiothoracic surgeon. Patients with posterior dislocations are usually stable after reduction, and surgery is required only if a redislocation occurs or if there is symptomatic instability.

Many surgical procedures have been advocated for SCJ dislocation such as Kirschner wires or Steinmann pin fixation, polydioxane cords or custom-made plates. Arthrodesis of the SCJ is also contraindicated because of the marked restriction in shoulder movement which it produces. More recently, Bae reported satisfactory results with the use of a semitendinosus tendon graft in a figure-of-8 fashion through drill holes in the sternum and manubrium [42].

References

1. Chen FS, Diaz VA, Loebenberg M et al (2005) Shoulder and elbow injuries in the skeletally immature athlete. J Am Acad Orthop Surg 13: 172–185
2. Mariscalco MW (2005) Upper extremity injuries in the adolescent athlete. Sports Med Arthr Rev 19(1):17–26
3. Peterson CA, Peterson HA (1972) Analysis of the incidence of injuries to the epiphyseal growth plate. J Trauma 12:275–281
4. Snook GA (1982) Injuries in intercollegiate wrestling. A 5-year study. Am J Sports Med 10(3):142–144
5. Garrick JG, Requa RK (1978) Injuries in high school sports. Pediatrics 61(3):465–469
6. Carr D, Johnson RJ, Pope MH (1981) Upper extremity injuries in skiing. Am J Sports Med 9(6):378–83
7. Landin LA (1983) Fracture patterns in children. Analysis of 8,682 fractures with special reference to incidence, etiology and secular changes in a Swedish urban population 1950–1979. Acta Orthop Scand Suppl 202:1–109
8. Van de Velde A, De Mey K, Maenhout A, Calders P, Cools AM (2011) Scapular-muscle performance: two training programs in adolescent swimmers. J Athl Train Mar-Apr 46(2):160–167
9. Fulton MN, Albright JP, El-Khoury GY (1979) Cortical desmoid-like lesion of the proximal humerus and its occurrence in gymnasts (ringman's shoulder lesion). Am J Sports Med 7(1):57–61
10. Snook GA (1985) A review of women's collegiate gymnastics. Clin Sports Med 4(1):31–37
11. Sciascia A, Kibler WB (2006) The pediatric overhead athlete: what is the real problem? Clin J Sport Med 16:471–477
12. Putnam CA (1993) Sequential motions of body segments in striking and throwing skills: descriptions and explanations. J Biomech 26: 125–135
13. Lyman S, Fleisig GS, Andrews JR et al (2002) Effect of pitch type, pitch count, and pitching mechanics on risk of elbow and shoulder pain in youth baseball pitchers. Am J Sports Med 30:463–468
14. Adams JE (1966) Little league shoulder: osteochondrosis of the proximal humeral epiphysis in boy baseball pitchers. Calif Med 105:22–25
15. Kocher MS, Waters PM, Micheli LJ (2000) Upper extremity injuries in the pediatric athlete. Sports Med 30:117–135
16. Davis JT, Limpisvasti O, Fluhme D, Mohr KJ, Yocum LA, Elattrache NS, Jobe FW (2009) The effect of pitching biomechanics on the upper extremity in youth and adolescent baseball pitchers. Am J Sports Med 37(8):1484–1491
17. Yoneda M, Nakagawa S, Mizuno N et al (2006) Arthroscopic capsular release for painful throwing shoulder with posterior capsular tightness. Arthroscopy 7(801):e1–e5
18. Postacchini F, Gumina S, Cinotti G (2000) Anterior shoulder dislocations in adolescents. J Shoulder Elbow Surg 9:470–474
19. Von Laer L (2004) Pediatric fractures and dislocations. Thieme, Stuttgart
20. Deyle GD, Nagel KL (2007) Prolonged immobilization in abduction and neutral rotation for a first-episode anterior shoulder dislocation. J Orthop Sports Phys Ther 37:192–198
21. Itoi E, Sashi R, Minagawa H, Shimizu T, Wakabayashi I, Sato K (2001) Position of immobilization after dislocation of the glenohumeral joint. A study with use of magnetic resonance imaging. J Bone Joint Surg Am 83:661–667
22. Rockwood C, Matsen F (1990) The Shoulder. WB Saunders, Philadelphia
23. Handoll HHG, Hanchard NCA, Goodchild L, Feary J. (2006) Conservative management following closed reduction of traumatic anterior shoulder dislocation of the shoulder. Cochrane Database Syst Rev
24. Rowe C (1956) Prognosis in dislocations of the shoulder. J Bone Joint Surg Am 38(5):957–977
25. Marans H, Angel K, Schemitsch E, Wedge JH (1992) The fate of traumatic anterior dislocation of the shoulder in children. J Bone Joint Surg Am 74(8):1242–1244
26. Deitch J, Mehlman C, Foad S, Obbehat A, Mallory M (2003) Traumatic anterior shoulder dislocation in adolescents. Am J Sports Med 35(1):758–763
27. Cil A, Kocher MS (2010) Treatment of pediatric shoulder instability. J Pediatr Orthop 30:S3–S6
28. Jakobsen BW, Johannsen HV, Suder P et al (2007) Primary repair versus conservative treatment of first-time traumatic anterior dislocation of the shoulder: a randomized study with 10-year follow-up. Arthroscopy 23:118–123
29. Elmlund A, Kartus C, Sernert N, Hultenheim I, Ejerhed L (2008) A long-term clinical follow-up study after arthroscopic intraarticular Bankart repair

using absorbable tacks. Knee Surg Sports Traumatol Arthrosc 16:707–712

30. Magee T (2009) 3-T MRI of the shoulder: is MR arthrography necessary? AJR Am J Roentgenol 192:86–92

31. Oh JH, Kim SH, Kwak SH, Oh CH, Gong HS (2011) Results of concomitant rotator cuff and SLAP repair are not affected by unhealed SLAP lesion. J Shoulder Elbow Surg 20(1):138–145

32. Walch G, Boileau P, Noel E (1992) Impingement of the deep surface of the supraspinatus tendon on the posterosuperior glenoid rim: an arthroscopic study. J Shoulder Elbow Surg 1:238–245

33. Heyworth BE, Williams RJ III (2009) Internal impingement of the shoulder. Am J Sports Med 37:1024–1037

34. Eisner EA, Roocroft JHM, Moor MA, Edmonds EW (2013) J Pediatr Orthop 33(1)

35. Kibler WB, Sciascia A (2010) Current concepts: scapular dyskinesis. Br J Sports Med 44:300–305

36. Taylor DC, Krasinski KL (2009) Adolescent shoulder injuries: consensus and controversies. J Bone Joint Surg Am 91:461–473

37. Johnson TR, Steinbach LS (2003) Fracture of the clavicle. In: Rosemont Ill (ed) Essentials of musculoskeletal imaging. American Academy of Orthopaedic Surgeons, pp 180–1

38. Sarwark JF, King EC, Luhmann SJ (2006) Proximal humerus, scapula, and clavicle. In: Beaty JA, Kasser JR (eds) Rockwood and Wilkin's fractures in children, 6th edn. Lippincott-Raven, Philadelphia, pp 704–771

39. Vander Have KL, Perdue AM, Caird MS (2010) Operative versus nonoperative treatment of midshaft clavicle fractures in adolescents. J Pediatr Orthop 30(307–312):18

40. Rockwood CA (1982) Fractures of outer clavicle in children and adults. J Bone Joint Surg Br 64:642–649

41. Shah RR, Kinder J, Peelman J (2010) Pediatric clavicle and acromioclavicular injuries. J Pediatr Orthop 30:S69–S72

42. Bae DS, Kocher MS (2006) Chronic recurrent anterior sternoclavicular joint instability: results of surgical management. J Pediatr Orthop 26:71–74

The Elbow: Ligamentous and Skeletal Injuries

8

Filippo M. Sénès, Nunzio Catena and Silvio Boero

During the stages of child growth, the elbow is frequently a site of injury. Many peculiarities arise, depending on the age of the child and the mechanism of the injury.

In order to fully understand the different types of trauma in the varying phases of growth, knowledge of elbow anatomy is necessary, in addition to expertise in relation to how primary and secondary ossification nuclei appear and fuse.

From the time of birth up to the first year of life, the elbow is predominantly cartilaginous. Only between the first year and second year of life does the first nucleus of secondary ossification appear. This is represented by the capitulum humeri and is followed in succession by

- The radial head (caput radii): at the age of 3 years
- The medial epicondyle (epicondylus medialis humeri): at the age of 5 years
- The humeral trochlea (trochlea humeri): at the age of 7 years
- Olecranon: at the age of 9 years

- The lateral epicondyle (epicondylus lateralis humeri): at the age of 10 years in a girl and 11 years in a boy (Fig. 8.1).

The mnemonic acronym CITROE may be helpful to remember the order in which the secondary nuclei appear [1]. It stands for the following:

C = Capitellum
R = Radial head
I = Internal (medial) epicondyle
T = Trochlea
O = Olecranon
E = External (lateral) epicondyle

All secondary ossification nuclei are intra-articular with the exception of the medial and lateral epicondyles. Their fusion takes place in a sequential and progressive manner, with an order which differs depending on appearance and age ranges. This timeline can be summed up by the following [2]:

- Capitulum, trochlea, and olecranon: at the age of 14 years
- Medial epicondyle: at the age of 15 years
- Lateral epicondyle and the radial head: at the age of 16 years.

The elbow allows for flexion and extension movements, by means of the ulnar–humeral component and pronosupination, thanks to the proximal radioulnar joint.

The majority of joint stability, both static and dynamic, is because of the structural characteristics of the skeletal component, particularly at the level of articulation between the distal humerus and olecranon.

F. M. Sénès (✉) · N. Catena · S. Boero
Microsurgery and Hand Surgery Unit, Orthopedics and Traumatology Unit, Istituto G. Gaslini, Largo G.Gaslini 5, 16147, Genoa, GE, Italy
e-mail: filipposenes@fastwebnet.it

N. Catena
e-mail: nunziocatena@gmail.com

S. Boero
e-mail: silvioboero@ospedale-gaslini.ge.it

V. Guzzanti (ed.), *Pediatric and Adolescent Sports Traumatology*,
DOI: 10.1007/978-88-470-5412-7_8, © Springer-Verlag Italia 2014

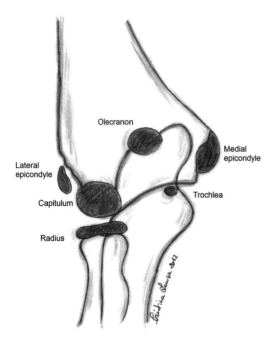

Fig. 8.1 Elbow anatomy featuring the cartilaginous components that are commonly fractured during child growth

The ligament complex and the origin of the muscles in the medial and lateral regions allow for joint stabilization techniques, especially in relation to the pressure exerted in varus and valgus.

The ulnar collateral ligament is located in a medial position and it is composed of three bundles (anterior, posterior, and oblique), which represent the principle stabilizers against valgus stress. Theses bundles are further assisted by the common tendon of origin to the flexor–pronator muscles (pronator teres, flexor carpi radialis, the palmar gracile muscle, and the flexor carpi ulnaris muscle) [3].

On the other hand, on the lateral side, you can find the radial collateral ligament system, which represents the main obstacle to rotations and subluxation of the humeral–ulnar joints. With the aid of the originating tendon for extensor–supinator muscles, it provides for maintaining the lateral stability of the elbow [4].

8.1 General Aspects of Sports Injuries to the Elbow

During school-going age and adolescence, there is a steady commitment to gymnastic sport activities. In general, this age group marks a consequent increase in skeletal disorder and ligamentous trauma to the axial skeleton, but more particularly to the elbow area, since the latter is often involved in traumatic events because of its anatomical peculiarities, to the detriment of the skeleton. The anatomical area comprised of the elbow, forearm, and wrist is involved in about twenty-five percent of traumatic lesions, which occur during sports practice. Dislocations and damage to cartilage growth account for 75 % of all elbow injuries [5].

Isolate traumatic ligament injuries are somewhat rare in the stages of child growth. On the other hand, traumatic ligament lesions associated with other types of fracture can be found. The pathology of overuse is much more frequent, for example medial epicondylar apophysitis, olecranon apophyseal injury, Panner's disease, and osteochondritis dissecans, which will be discussed at the later stage in the book [6].

Certain sporting disciplines are linked to a significant incidence and percentage of elbow trauma, with a greater risk of injury due to contact or fall:

- American football: 2–6 %
- Rugby: 2.6 %
- Skating: 11 %
- Ice hockey: 2–6 %
- Snowboarding: 2–5 %
- Skiing: 1.5–3 %
- Gymnastics: 3.7–8.5 %.

On the contrary, other disciplines such as baseball, tennis, and javelin are characterized by a higher occurrence of repeated microtrauma diseases, which may give rise to other types of overuse symptoms in a skeleton, which is not fully developed. This depends on the type of repetitive movement which takes place, be it a throw, push, or pull [7].

The most common type of skeletal lesions is as follows:

- Supracondylar fractures of the humerus
- Medial epicondyle fractures
- Dislocation of the elbow
- Radial head fractures.

One lesion, which is often present and not to be underestimated, is the Monteggia dislocation fracture. Both the classic form of the injury and the Monteggia-like form are more typical during the stages of child growth. In children, it is rare to come across olecranon fractures as they are typically more common in adults, while fractures of the humeral condyle are more frequent in children under the age of six. Although these latter types of fractures are not so rare, they can be seen due to the fact that children are beginning to participate in sporting activities at an earlier age.

We must consider the type of sport being practiced in order to determine the various types of lesions. It is important to take into account whether or not it is a contact sport, as well as considering how the elbow functions in the different sporting disciplines. Supracondylar fractures, dislocations, and fractures of the radial head are often a result of injury due to a fall on a flexed or extended elbow, while other fractures, such as a fracture of the medial epicondyle, are due to abnormal strain during traction, which the medial compartment of the elbow is frequently subjected to, in order to counteract movements with a strong valgus deformity [8].

Traction forces in the lateral compartment are rarer, where instead you can frequently find strain during compression, possibly brought on by the overuse symptom. One last thing to consider is that often, traumatic events in the elbow region can have a negative outcome, with varying degrees of disability in adulthood.

8.1.1 Supracondylar Fractures of the Humerus

In developmental age, supracondylar fractures of the humerus are the most frequent type of lesions to the elbow joint, which are caused by a reduced anterior–posterior diameter in the humerus at that level. This creates a so-called locus minoris resistentiae in the event of trauma to the upper limb [9]. The average age of the individuals concerned is 5–7 years, although recently you can note an increase in such fractures at an older age with degrees of displaced fractures and complications with long-term effects. This is in antithesis of what happens at a younger age [10].

The production mechanism for this type of lesion, that is, falling on the palm of the hand with the elbow extended, causes fractures from overextension (98 %), which are more frequent than those resulting from flexion (2 %). Dislocations of the distal stump may occur at varying levels of severity. A great number of anatomical pathology classifications exist for this type of lesion, depending on whether it is a major or minor displacement. You may recall the proposal by Lagrange and Rigault, which is useful for obtaining direct results during the treatment.

- Grade I: Compound fracture
- Grade II: Slightly displaced
- Grade III: Displaced but with contact between the stumps
- Grade IV: No contact between the stumps.

Anglo-Saxon authors prefer classifications deriving from Gartland, which, in practice, merge Phase II and III into one [11].

The clinical presentation of these lesions varies depending on the severity of the injury. Even in the case of compound fractures, a distinct swelling of the elbow, with limited functionality, is evident. With displaced fractures, you can observe an important bayonet deformity in the region, with diffused ecchymotic swelling (Fig. 8.2). The skin bends inward and is subject to traction by the bone stumps, while exposure is rare. Nerve deficits are habitually present, which may frequently affect the radial nerve as well as the median and ulnar nerves which are often connected to apraxia and have a tendency to resolve themselves spontaneously in the months following the fracture reduction.

Particular attention should be paid to the vascular system of the limb, before, during, and post-treatment for this fracture. Ischemia as a result of the humeral artery being pinched or even just a reflex spasm of the artery due to trauma (Fig. 8.3) can be the cause of Volkmann's syndrome, that is, ischemic paralysis of the muscles in the forearm and hand, a condition which requires immediate surgical exploration of the artery [12].

This syndrome is accompanied by a mnemonic sign ("the 4 p's") as referred to by the Anglo-Saxon authors: pain, paleness, paralysis,

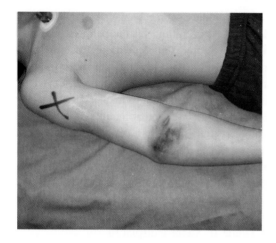

Fig. 8.2 The clinical appearance of fractured elbow presenting with bruising, swelling, and angular deformity

that approximately 10–20 % of patients with displaced supracondylar fractures present with a diminished or an absent pulse. A diminished or absent pulse (the difference can be obtained by Doppler sonography) does not indicate a complete ischemic syndrome if the hand is warm, as collateral circulation may keep the limb well perfused.

The treatment for Grade I fractures only provides for the application of a plaster cast to the upper limb, while in the event of a Grade II fracture, a closed reduction is necessary, which is obtained by flexing the fracture site as much as possible. If the reduction seems somewhat unstable, it is advisable to have an X-ray under the plaster after a week.

and absence of pulse. A delay in surgical intervention in these cases involves paralysis and therefore irreversible tissue necrosis and retraction of the muscles in the forearm, resulting in the loss of hand function. It must be underlined

In Grades III and IV fractures, the treatment allows for two different methods; the first involves the application of a traction using transolecranon wire for 3–5 days while assessing the limb's vascular system in the meantime, followed by reduction under general anesthetic

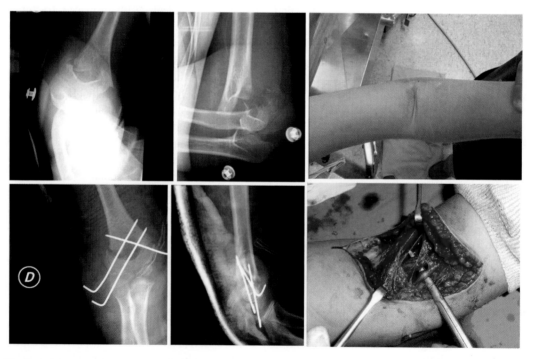

Fig. 8.3 Severe deformity and diffuse ecchymotic swelling in "Grade IV "supracondylar fracture. Ischemia of hand and forearm was lasting during closed reduction and pinning and therefore the condition required the surgical exploration of the artery. The vasculonervous bundle appeared to be compress at the fracture site

and stabilization by osteosynthesis with a minimum of two Kirschner wires (crossed by lateral and medial insertion or parallel/diverging with only one lateral insertion) and a plaster cast for a four-week period. With the second methodology, you proceed to immediate reduction under anesthetic, always performing minimum synthesis with wires and a plaster cast. The traction period in bed should diminish the occurrence of neurovascular complications, while the extemporaneous reduction in fractures would reduce the hospitalization period and it would be better tolerated by a child, who is not forced to spend days in bed; the topic is still controversial. The quality of the obtained result is evaluated directly by X-ray in the operating room, with restoration of the normal angle formed by the physeal cartilage of the humeral condyle with the humeral shaft. Good reduction in the frontal plane helps to minimize complications such as cubitus varus and cubitus valgus deformities of the elbow, deformities which worsen with the growth of the humeral segment in the child, especially nullifying cubitus varus, resulting in a deformity of the humerus in the medial concavity, which may require consequent surgical correction. Supracondylar humeral osteotomy is best performed toward the end of growth to avoid subsequent recurrence of the deformity [13].

Incomplete reduction in the sagittal plane and the residual rotational deficit are better tolerated because they are gradually corrected over time.

The advantages of percutaneous osteosynthesis are represented by an adequately stable fixation under the plaster, with good control of the distal fragment. The literature is not unanimous as to which type of osteosynthesis is more appropriate. In fact, some authors claim that the use of cross-pinning offers greater stability to the reduction, although the risk of iatrogenic injury to the ulnar nerve, while the medial wire is being introduced should be considered [14]. For this reason, some authors prefer to use lateral pinning with Kirschner wires [15].

In comparison with lateral pinning, the cross-pinning methodology seems to provide better stability, primarily for the rotational component of the fracture as per Types III and IV, even if some authors in a perspective random study did not find substantial differences in the outcome between the two types of osteosynthesis [16].

Complications are rare, and they are represented by the possibility of infection at the wire entry points and the migration of the same. Nerve lesions pertain to the radial (Fig. 8.4) and median nerve, while there are less occurrences of damage to the ulnar nerve, which is frequently iatrogenic (for traction purposes when in bed or for cross-pinning) [17].

The indications for open reduction are exceptional and in practice are limited to exposed fractures, which require thorough cleaning and washing with antiseptic and as already mentioned, and in the event of vascular lesions, an examination of the humeral artery is necessary.

On removing the plaster cast and percutaneous wires, clinical examination and X-ray demonstrate the consolidation of the fracture, which is followed by the gradual recovery of movement in the elbow. The child is stimulated to recover autonomous movement with monthly out-patient visits, reserving the use of conservative rehabilitation therapy for cases with distinct stiffness. Any residual nerve deficit is controlled by electrophysiological techniques (motor and sensory nerve conduction velocities) until they have been resolved. A surgical reduction would only be carried out if full recovery has not been made 6 months after the injury [18]. Growth disturbance must be always considered after any treatment as a consequence of primary physeal injury.

8.1.2 Fractures of the Epicondyle and Medial Epicondyle

Both the epicondyle and the medial epicondyles are apophyses and therefore do not participate in the growth in the length of the humerus. This single type of fracture and detachment from the epicondyle are rare.

Medial epicondyle fractures are more frequent and result in the apophyseal cartilage, detaching itself due to the traction exerted by the

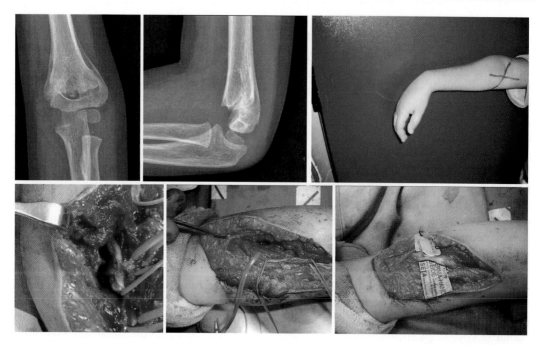

Fig. 8.4 Radial nerve entrapment in the fibrocartilaginous bone during the bone healing phase consequent to a supracondylar fracture

muscles, which insert themselves there. This may be associated with a lateral dislocation of the elbow [19].

Four stages can be identified, depending on the type of displaced fracture. In the first stage, if it displaces "in situ" of the medial epicondyle. In the second stage, it has a minimum displacement of the nucleus as a result of the epicondyle muscles. In the third stage, the apophyseal fragment is dislocated at the level of the humeroulnar joint. In the fourth stage, the apophysis is trapped inside the elbow joint, which is the consequence of a dislocation which occurred at the time of injury and which reduced spontaneously.

The clinical presentation of these lesions is linked to pain and local swelling and to any signs of instability and loss of movement in the elbow. The treatment is more frequently conservative, with a plaster cast for injuries, which present as a displaced fracture less than 5 mm.

With regard to surgical treatment, the signs that reduction and osteosynthesis are needed, both in the case of percutaneous repair and in the case of open repair, are represented by

- Displaced fractures and rotation greater than 5 mm/1 cm (since no reduction could lead to the flexor–pronator muscles weakening, as well as a significant cosmetic deformity of the elbow)
- Persistence of intra-articular fragment after the reduction in the elbow dislocation.
- Acute injury to the ulnar nerve
- Valgus instability in the elbow (Fig. 8.5).

The reduction is carried out through a medial approach to the elbow, and osteosynthesis can be executed both with a cannulated screw and with a Kirschner wire (Fig 8.6). Some authors advise the possible reconstruction of the ulnar collateral ligament, in the event of the associated lesion being verified [20]. However, certain authors do not agree with a surgical approach. This single

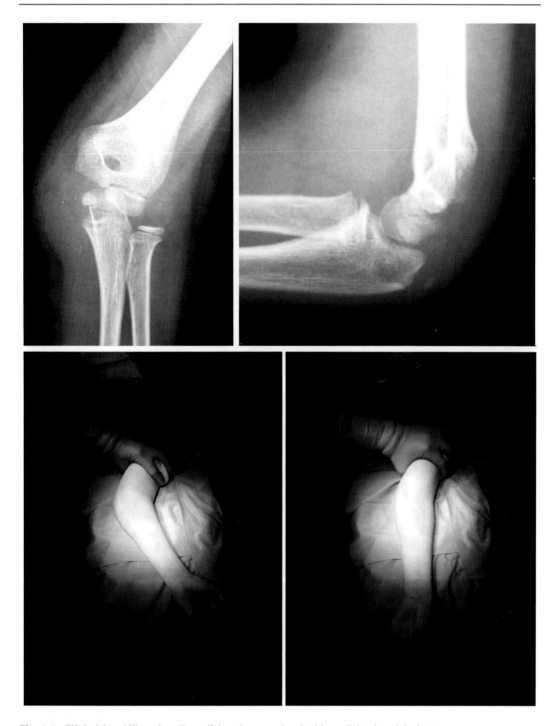

Fig. 8.5 Clinical instability *after* elbow dislocation associated with medial epicondyle fracture

type of fracture, even in the case of displaced fractures, is between 5 and 15 mm. In terms of how much authors support claims that complications do not exist further on and in the occurrence of non-union, the literature attests to the formation of a fibrous bridge that guarantees

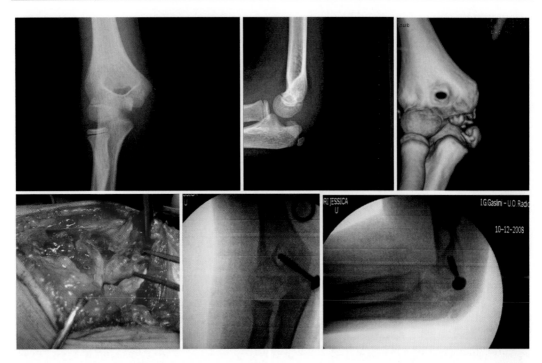

Fig. 8.6 Open reduction and osteosynthesis executed with a cannulated screw in a medial epicondyle fracture

correct stability of the medial epicondyle [21]. However, if left untreated, it is reported that ulnar nerve entrapment occurs further down the line.

8.1.3 Humeral Condyle Fractures

It always deals with particular fractures with the involvement of articular cartilage and the one connected to growth. In addition to the ossification nucleus of the humeral condyle, the fractured fragment comprises of a metaphyseal fragment, thus constituting on the whole, a Type IV epiphyseal detachment [22].

The muscles attached to the epicondyle are responsible for frequently displaced fractures. The fracture occurs as displaced and separated, and the condyle goes around the horizontal and sagittal axes.

The clinical presentation may be poor, highlighting only local pain and even, relatively modest swelling; no injuries associated with the neurovascular are present.

The X-ray assessment in the two standard views can fool the untrained eye; the anteroposterior view due to an overlap of the stumps because of rotation often leads to and underestimation of the displaced fracture, which is usually more evident in lateral view (Fig. 8.7). Different classifications exist for humeral condyle fractures, which categorize the dislocation of the solid condylar. Jakob and his collaborators provide for three types of classification. In the first type, the rim of the fracture affects the condyle, but does not reach the articular surface. In the second type, it interrupts the articular surface with minimal displacement and separation, and in the type three, the solid condylar is dislocated and rotated around its axis [23]. The treatment requires an adequate reduction, in order to reestablish a physiological articular surface and with a view to minimizing the eventual consequences of the physeal cartilage and thus to the subsequent growth of the humerus [24]. The growth disturbances secondary to the primary injury of growth cartilage are described.

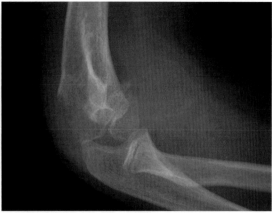

Fig. 8.7 A displaced lateral condyle fracture

Compound fractures with maximum displacement and separation of 2 mm of the rim of the fracture can be immobilized using a plaster cast, by carrying out an X-ray directly under the cast after the space of a week and by advising the child's parents of the possibility of surgical intervention in the case of secondary displacement fractures. With displaced fractures, surgical intervention is imperative; it is possible to attempt it with external maneuvers, but if this does not guarantee an anatomical relocation of the condyle, surgical intervention is indicated. This should be gentle to avoid the detachment of dislocated fragment from the muscular insertions, which ensure the blood supply and thus survival of the vascular system. The joint capsule should still be opened by controlling the reconstruction of the articular surface. In the event of a reduced fracture, osteosynthesis is carried out in each case using a cannulated screw, which offers stability to the structure. The plaster cast is kept on for 4 weeks post-surgery. If consolidation occurs, surgical removal of the screw is programmed for 1–2 months later.

There are complications frequently, even following correct treatment, the worst of these being ischemic necrosis, followed by post-traumatic osteoarthritis [25].

A bone formation linking the metaphyseal bone and the epiphysis through the physeal cartilage can determine the development of cubitus valgus, while an unsatisfactory reduction and unstable osteosynthesis are often caused by cubitus varus and pseudarthrosis, that is, the failure of the fracture to heal.

8.1.4   Elbow Dislocations

Dislocated elbows are rare, but they do not exhibit distinct characteristics in developmental age in comparison with those in adulthood [26]. Depending on the type of dislocation of the forearm, they are distinguished as posterior, lateral, medial, anterior, and divergent, posterior being the most frequent. The fractures habitually associated with this are fractures of the medial epicondyle, although fractures of the lateral condyle and osteochondral fractures of the olecranon have been reported as being less common [27, 28].

Nerve damage to the ulnar nerve, median nerve, and rarely to the radial nerve, in addition to associated vascular problems, are seldom described but still possible and treacherous [29, 30]. The clinical presentation is explanatory, even if a differential diagnosis of the supracondylar fracture needs to be applied. However, X-rays always resolve the situation.

Reduction is achieved by cautious traction and flexion maneuvers, often with no need to resort to general anesthetic with immediate relief for the suffering patient (Fig. 8.8). The plaster cast of the upper limb, which is kept on for

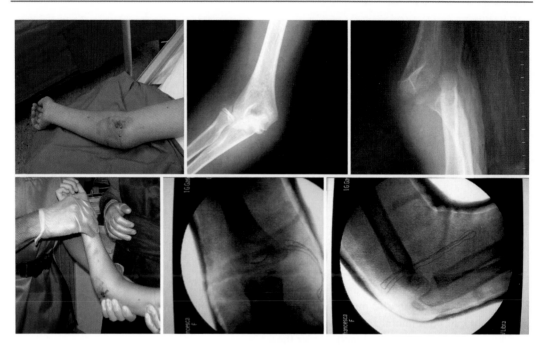

Fig. 8.8 Clinical and radiographic aspects of elbow dislocation. Manual reduction and plaster casting

20 days, is done with a little padding to minimize the risk of possible redislocation under the plaster. The prognosis is always good with rapid recovery of movement. With time, the results highlight the particular calcification, that is, X-ray evidence that is not usually associated with clinically evident limitations. Cases of fractures associated with the medial epicondyle, with or without incarcerated fragmentation present, may require osteosynthesis as aforementioned.

8.1.5　Olecranon Fractures

Olecranon fractures are rare at developmental age, and X-ray images are frequently difficult to interpret due to the presence of physeal cartilage at the base of the olecranon process. These are the results of direct trauma or a sudden contraction of the triceps. Clinically, it shows local pain and swelling, which is more pronounced and associated with signs of an unstable elbow in the event of associated dislocation.

Treatment depends on the displacement of the fragment. If it is inferior to 5 mm, it is sufficient to make a plaster cast; if it is greater than

5 mm, it is necessary to carry out an open or closed reduction performed by means of osteosynthesis with screws or with two Kirschner wire pins and metal cerclage wire or nonabsorbable wire. This is then followed by a plaster cast for 4 weeks [31].

The results of the treatment are invariably good, and a few cases of complications further to the treatment have been reported. A rare but serious complication is the entrapment of the ulnar nerve due to changes in the epitrochlear–olecranon canal, once the fracture has been healed [32].

8.1.6　Radial Head Fractures

In the majority of cases, it has to do with the epiphyseal separation of Types I and II, which recognizes falling on the palm of one's hand as a traumatic mechanism [33]. The clinical presentation is characterized by the local pain and swelling proportionate to the severity of the displaced fracture. This varies from absent (displaced "in situ") to noticeable, with the radial epiphysis rotated to 90° and supported from a posterior angle and laterally on the diaphysis of the radius. The magnitude of the angle can be measured based on the epiphysis–diaphyseal angle. Depending on age, angles between 45 and 60° can be tolerated. If the angle exceeds 60°, a closed reduction under general anesthetic is required. It is possible to achieve a complete reduction even in the event of more grave displaced fractures using traction maneuvers with a flexed elbow, associated pronation, and supination of the forearm with direct pressure on the displaced fragment. Synthesis of the fragment is reached from the reverse side using Kirschner wire, which is introduced at the extreme distal and pushed toward the proximal epiphysis of the radius (Fig. 8.9) [34].

After 4 weeks, the wire is removed at the same time as the plaster cast. With this procedure, complications are rare; they are limited to temporary joint stiffness. Surgical reduction and transarticular synthesis of the radial head are often associated with persistent joint stiffness, proximal radioulnar joint synostosis, infection, and necrosis of the radial head. Likewise, the resection of the fractured radial head should not be performed in pediatric age for the possible outcome of cubitus valgus.

8.1.7 The Monteggia Dislocation

The Monteggia dislocation represents a relatively common injury in the stages of child growth. It is characterized by a diaphyseal

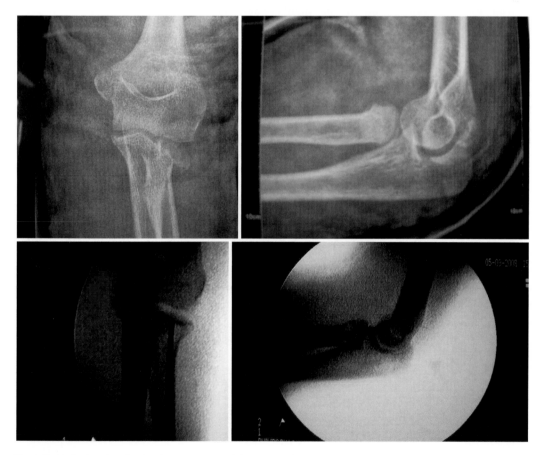

Fig. 8.9 A displaced radial head fracture treated by means of Kirschner wire which was introduced at the extreme distal and pushed toward in order to repair the proximal emphasizes of the radius

fracture of the ulna, involving dislocation of the radial head.

Today, the classification is done according to what was proposed by Bado, which subdivides the Monteggia lesion into 4 types: [35]

- Type 1 (60 %): Ulnar fracture of the middle-third with front angles associated with anterior dislocation of the radial head.
- Type 2 (15 %): Ulnar fracture of the middle-third proximal with posterior angles associated with posterior dislocation of the radial head (often with associated fracture).
- Type 3 (20 %): Ulnar fracture scarcely proximal to the coronoid process, with lateral dislocation of the radial head.
- Type 4 (5 %): Ulnar fracture of the middle-third proximal with anterior dislocation of the radial head, with its fracture lying below the bicipital tuberosity.

With trauma types 1 and 4, the injury mechanism allows for a fall on an extended elbow with a pronated forearm, which involves a compressive force determining the ulnar fracture and traction by the biceps tendon, which dislocates the front of the head. In trauma type 2, the fall occurs on a flexed elbow with a pronated forearm, while in type 3, there is a traumatic force direct from the medial to lateral side.

During the stages of child growth, the detection of Monteggia-like lesions is possible. It is extremely important for this to be discovered in order to receive the proper treatment; the principal forms are as follows:

- Plastic deformation of the ulnar bone with anterior dislocation of the radial head
- Diaphyseal ulnar fractures associated with radial head fractures
- Diaphyseal ulnar and olecranon fractures associated with anterior dislocation of the radial head
- Posterior dislocation of the elbow and diaphyseal fracture of the ulnar bone, with or without the proximal radius.

The clinical presentation is characterized by pain, by functional weakness, and by the position of the forearm being in fixed pronation. In order to make this diagnosis, a proper X-ray examination, which includes the elbow, forearm, and wrist, is essential to be able to exclude injuries associated with distal humerus (fractures of the distal humeral part, which can provoke floating elbow) and the distal radioulnar joint (associated with Galeazzi injury) (Fig. 8.10).

In high-level trauma, it is possible to have both immediate complications, which involve the soft parts, as well as the radial, median, and

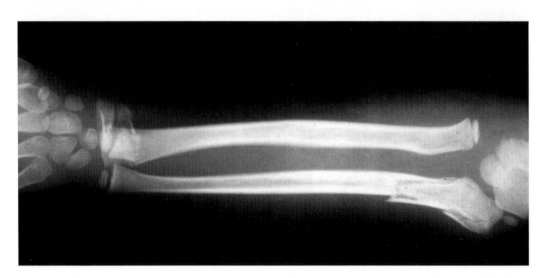

Fig. 8.10 A Monteggia lesion showing the lateral dislocation of the radial head and the third proximal fracture of the ulnar bone

ulnar nerves, connected to the typology and extent of dislocation of the radial head [36].

The importance of a sharp diagnosis and proper treatment may prevent the onset of complications with time. Such a loss of joint movement in the elbow when the forearm is flexed in pronation and supination is mainly caused by an abnormal growth of the radial head with secondary cubitus valgus, which is unstable and has a compressed pathology involving the posterior interosseous nerve.

The treatment for the Monteggia injury is based on the reduction in ulnar fractures with possible osteosynthesis, usually by means of an intra-medullary pin. This procedure normally leads to a spontaneous reduction in the radial head. If the head is unstable after the reduction, it is possible to proceed to temporary radiohumeral arthrodesis, which allows for good joint stabilization in the majority of cases [37].

Some authors propose the use of surgical reduction with the annular ligament reconstruction procedure, which in our opinion can also be performed as a secondary surgery in the event of dislocation recurring [38]. No matter which treatment is executed, it will be followed by the immobilization of the upper limb in a plaster cast for a period of 4 weeks [39].

References

1. Benjamin HJ, Briner WW Jr (2005) Little league elbow. Clin J Sport Med 15:37–40
2. Bradley JP (1994) Upper extremity: elbow injuries in children and adolescents. In: Stanitski CL, De Lee JC, Drez D (eds) Pediatric and adolescent sports medicine. Orthopedic sport medicine: principles and practice, vol 3. WB Saunders, Philadelpia, pp 242–261
3. Callaway GH, Field LD, Deng XH et al (1997) Biomechanical evaluation of medial collateral ligament of the elbow. J Bone Joint Surg Am 79:1223–1231
4. Regan WD, Korinek SL, Morrey BF et al (1991) Biomechanical study of ligaments around the elbow joint. Clin Orthop Relat Res 271:170–179
5. Maffulli N (1995) Children in sport: questions and controversies. In: Maffuli N (ed) Colour atlas and texts of sport medicine in childhood and adolescence. Mosby-Wolfe, London, pp 7–14
6. Rudzki JR, Paletta GA Jr (2004) Juvenile and adolescent elbow injuries in sports. Clin Sports Med 23:581–608
7. Magra M, Caine D, Maffulli N (2007) A review of epidemiology of paediatric elbow injuries in sports. Sports Med 37(8):717–735
8. Sabick MB, Torry MR, Lawton RL et al (2004) Valgus torque in youth baseball pitchers: a biomechanical study. J Shoulder Elbow Surg 13:349–355
9. Maylahn DJ, Fahey JJ (1958) Fractures of the elbow in children; review of three hundred consecutive cases. Am Med Assoc 166(3):220–228
10. Fletcher ND, Schiller JR, Garg S, Weller A, Larson AN, Kwon M, Browne R, Copley L, Ho C (2012) Increased severity of type III supracondylar humerus fractures in the preteen population. J Pediatr Orthop 32(6):567–572
11. Heras J, Duran D, de la Cerda J, Romanillos O, Martinez-Miranda J, Rodriguez-Merchan EC (2005) Supracondylar Fractures of the Humerus in Children. Clin Orthop Relat Res 432:57–64
12. Clement DA (1990) Assessment of a treatment plan for managing acute vascular complications associated with supracondylar fractures of the humerus in children. J Ped Orthop 10:97–100
13. Wilkins KE (1990) Residual of elbow trauma in children. Orthop Clin North Am 21:291–314
14. Brauer CA, Lee BM, Bae DS, Waters PM, Kocher MS (2007) A systematic review of medial and lateral entry pinning versus lateral entry pinning for supracondylar fractures of the humerus. J Pediatr Orthop 27(2):181–186
15. Mulpuri K, Wilkins K (2012) The treatment of displaced supracondylar humerus fractures: evidence-based guideline. J Pediatr Orthop 32(Suppl 2):S143–S152
16. Gaston RG, Cates TB, Devito D, Schmitz M, Schrader T, Busch M, Fabregas J, Rosenberg E, Blanco J (2010) Medial and lateral pin versus lateral-entry pin fixation for Type 3 supracondylar fractures in children: a prospective, surgeon-randomized study. J Pediatr Orthop 30(8):799–806
17. Franchin F, Sénès FM, Asquasciati G, Andaloro A, Pinelli G (1998) Complicanze ed esiti delle fratture del gomito nell'età pediatrica. Minerva Ortop Traumatol 49:241–246
18. Senes FM, Campus R, Becchetti F, Catena N (2009) Upper limb nerve injuries in developmental age. Microsurgery 29(7):529–535
19. Rasool MN (2004) Dislocations of the elbow in children. J Bone Joint Surg Br 86(7):1050–1058
20. Lieber J, Zundel SM, Luithle T, Fuchs J, Kirschner HJ (2012) Acute traumatic posterior elbow dislocation in children. J Pediatr Orthop B 21(5):474–481
21. Farsetti P, Potenza V, Caterini R, Ippolito E (2001) Long—term results of treatment of fractures of the medial humeral epicondyle in children. J Bone Joint Surg Am 83(9):1299–1305

22. Jakob R, Fowles JV, Rang M, Kassab MT (1975) Observations concerning fractures of the lateral humeral condyle in children. J Bone Joint Surg Br 57(4):430–436

23. Mirsky EC, Karas EH, Weiner LS (1997) Lateral condyle fractures in children: evaluation of classification and treatment. J Orthop Trauma 11(2):117–120

24. Badelon O, Bensahel H, Mazda K, Vie P (1988) Lateral humerus condylar fractures in children: a report of 47 cases. J Ped Orthop 8:31–34

25. Flynn JC (1989) Nonunion of slightly displaced fractures of the lateral humeral condyle in children: an update. J Ped Orthop 9:691–696

26. Frongia G, Günther P, Romero P, Kessler M, Holland-Cunz S (2012) Elbow dislocation in childhood. Long-term observational study. Unfallchirurg 115(2):125–133

27. Kirkos JM, Beslikas TA, Papavasiliou VA (2003) Posteromedial dislocation of the elbow with lateral condyle fracture in children. Clin Orthop Relat Res 408:232–236

28. Song KS, Jeon SH (2003) Osteochondral flap fracture of the olecranon with dislocation of the elbow in a child: a case report. J Orthop Trauma 17(3):229–231

29. Reed MW, Reed DN (2012) Acute ulnar nerve entrapment after closed reduction of a posterior fracture dislocation of the elbow: a case report. Pediatr Emerg Care 28(6):570–572

30. Simon D, Masquijo JJ, Duncan MJ, Kontio K (2010) Intra-articular median nerve incarceration after spontaneous reduction of a pediatric elbow dislocation: case report and review of the literature. J Pediatr Orthop 30(2):125–129

31. Dormans JP, Rang M (1990) Fractures of the olecranon and radial neck in children. Orthop Clin North Am 21:257–268

32. Ertem K (2009) An unusual complication of ulnar nerve entrapment in a pediatric olecranon fracture: a case report. J Pediatr Orthop B 18(3):135–137

33. D'souza S, Vaishya R, Klenerman L (1993) Management of radial neck fractures in children: a retrospective analysis of one hundred patients. J Ped Orthop 13:232–238

34. Métaizeau JP (2005) Reduction and osteosynthesis of radial neck fractures in children by centromedullary pinning. Injury 36(Suppl 1):A75–A77

35. Bado SL (1967) The Monteggia lesion. Clin Orthop 50:71–86

36. Güven M, Eren A, Kadioğlu B, Yavuz U, Kilinçoğlu V, Ozkan K (2008) The results of treatment in pediatric Monteggia equivalent lesions. Acta Orthop Traumatol Turc 42(2):90–96

37. Pesl T, Havránek P (2010) Monteggia lesions in the growing skeleton: principles of therapy. Acta Chir Orthop Traumatol Cech 77(1):32–38

38. Speed JS, Boyd HB (1940) Treatment of fractures of the ulna with dislocation of head of the radius (Monteggia fracture). JAMA 115:1900–1940

39. Beutel BG (2012) Monteggia fractures in pediatric and adult populations. Orthopedics 35(2):138–144

Wrist and Hand: Ligamentous and Skeletal Injuries

9

Antonio Tulli, Antonio Pagliei, Guiseppe Taccardo,
Francesco Catalano and Francesco Fanfani

In most sports, the hand and wrist are exposed, causing them to have a 30 % of incidence of injury [1].

The literature reports studies concerning the relation between a type of fracture and specific sport activities or between different types of fractures and general sport activities [2–5].

The experience of the authors, conversely, is that traumatic lesions of hand and wrist linked to a specific sport activity in children and adolescents are not as much recorded as they are in adults.

This is true except for horseback riding. Due to possible high-energy traumas involving arms, it is possible to observe a high incidence of elbow fractures and dislocations. Other typical lesions are fractures (or epiphyseal separations) of the base of distal and middle phalanx in basketball. The treatment of skeletal lesions in the course of growth is characterized by closed reduction and percutaneous fixation, especially intramedullary. In this case, it should try to save physis (epiphyseal cartilage) where possible, fixing fractures when strictly necessary with few, smooth, and small-sized wires.

A. Tulli (✉) · A. Pagliei · G. Taccardo · F. Catalano
· F. Fanfani
Department of Geriatrics, Neurosciences and
Orthopedics, Orthopedic Clinic, Orthopedics and
Hand Surgery Division, Complesso Integrato
Columbus, Università Cattolica del Sacro Cuore,
Via G.Moscati 31/33, 00168, Rome, Italy
e-mail: tulli.antonio@libero.it

A. Pagliei
e-mail: paglieiantonio@yahoo.it

This approach generally does not lead growth deficiency, or axial deviation secondary to an epiphysiodesis or physeal lesions.

Concerning ligamentous lesions, except for elbow lesions often associated with fractures due to high-energy injuries, no surgical reconstruction appears necessary. These lesions were mainly proximal interphalangeal sprains which only require a conservative treatment, as well as the mallet finger.

Crush injuries of the distal phalanx involving nails are extremely frequent in children, but rarely related to sport activities.

9.1 Anatomy

The refined function of the hand requires a very complex and delicate framework which include numerous bones and multifaced small joints. The interphalangeal and metacarpophalangeal joints are bound together by a particular arrangement of ligaments. The wrist consists of multiple joints and contains multiple (eight) growing carpals bones arranged in two row. There is a midcarpal joint between the two rows, as well as intercarpal joints between individual bones in each row. The distal row articulates with the five metacarpal bones. The first carpometacarpal joint has a saddle-shaped surface that allows it to move in all directions. This gives the thumb its freedom of motion. In addition, the thumb is characterized by the opposability. In

V. Guzzanti (ed.), *Pediatric and Adolescent Sports Traumatology*,
DOI: 10.1007/978-88-470-5412-7_9, © Springer-Verlag Italia 2014

contrast to the first metacarpal, the other rays of the hand have limited mobility.

The proximal row of the carpal bones articulates with the two bones of the forearm forming the radiocarpal and radioulnocarpal joints. The distal radius and ulna articulate with each other, forming the distal radioulnar joint that allows the pronation and supination of the forearm. The movements of the other wrist joints are complex; together they produce the wrist movements of flexion, extension, radial deviation, and ulnar deviation.

The distal end of the radius has a styloid process, which forms part of the radiocarpal joint surface. The distal end of the ulna has also a styloid process which articulates directly with the carpus by interposition of a disc of fibrocartilage. The radiocarpal and ulnocarpal joints together form a single continuous joint cavity and are sometimes considered as one radiocarpal joint.

The joints of the wrist are enclosed by a fibrous joint capsule and are further bound together by multiple ligaments which blend with the capsule. The radial and ulnar sides of the wrist, respectively, are the 11 radial and ulnar collateral 11 ligaments. The volar radiocarpal ligaments support the palmar aspect of the wrist, and the dorsal radiocarpal ligaments support the dorsal aspect of the wrist. The collateral, volar, and dorsal ligaments are outside the joint capsule, while the intercarpal ligaments (connecting the individual carpal bones) are inside the capsule.

The ulnar side of the wrist is bound together by a group of structures known as the triangular fibrocartilage complex. The perfect mobility of the hand and wrist depends from the integrated and perfect function between the flexors and extensors muscles and tendons, the intrinsic muscles (the interosseous muscles that abduct and adduct the fingers), the lumbrical muscles (that make fine adjustments in the positions of the fingers), and the nerves. The integrity of the carpal tunnel and of the Guyon's canal is crucial for function as the long flexor tendons pass together through a carpal tunnel along with median nerve and the ulnar nerve passes through a Guyon's canal. The radial nerve sensitive branch crosses over the radial styloid (on the

radial side of the wrist) to reach the dorsum of the hand.

9.2 Treatment

As derived from complex, functional anatomy is easy to understand that surgery of the hand, wrist, and forearm requires a particular approach whether treating fracture as this whole region works as a single unit, and the dysfunction of a single part needs consideration of the whole. That is particularly true and delicate in case of skeletally immature patients as due to the presence of the growth plates and the fact that each interruption, either temporarily or permanently, of the function can determine a limitation, temporary, or permanent, of learning functions so delicate and so refined.

9.2.1 Phalanges

9.2.1.1 Distal Phalanx

Distal phalanx, as mentioned above, is rarely involved in sports injuries. In case of crush trauma with nail avulsion and fracture of the apical tuft, the nail avulsion can be treated by suturing the nail bed wound, too often misunderstood and always present when the nail plate comes out of the nail fold, and by repositioning the nail plate fixing it with a bridge suture. Fractures of the apical tuft only do not need to be treated. In cases of type II (Salter–Harris) fractures, no internal fixation is required (Fig. 9.1b). Type II radiographs may show the "Werenskiold" sign, consisting in the shadow of the layer of calcified metaphyseal cartilage that remains attached to the metaphysis [6]. Generally, the cases of epiphyseal separation (Fig. 9.1a) of the distal phalanx are not in connection with sports injuries. Cases of Segond fractures can be observed in adolescents with a complete physis fusion; such lesions, typically related to volleyball or basketball, can be treated surgically because immobilization with only a Zimmer splint is often inefficient (Fig. 9.1c). Sometimes treatment with splint causes

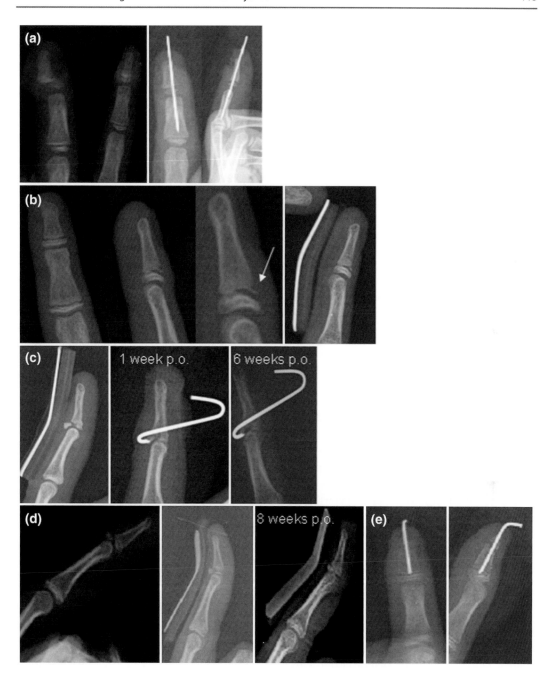

◄ **Fig. 9.1** **a** An 8-year-old patient. Physis separation of the second finger six days after injury; treated by closed reduction and retrograde percutaneous osteosynthesis. K-wire removed after 30 days. **b** A 14-year-old patient. Type II (Salter) physis fracture of the distal phalanx of the fourth finger (the pointer indicates the Werenskiold sign). Treated by immobilization with a short volar splint, removed 30 days after injury. **c** A 15-year-old patient. Segond fracture: insertional detachment of a large articular fragment from the distal phalanx base, without subluxation of the volar phalanx. Splint treatment does not ensure a satisfactory reduction, which may otherwise be obtained by closed reduction and application of a percutaneous dorsal–volar K-wire hooking and reducing the fragment ("umbrella handle technique").

The wire is tensioned by means of a button fixed on the volar side of the fingertip working as a pull-out. The wire is maintained up to 5 weeks after the surgical procedure. **d** A 12-year-old patient. Segond fracture: distal phalanx base fracture, with no volar subluxation of phalanx. Splint treatment allows a quite satisfactory reduction. An X-ray control 50 days after trauma still shows a nonunion of the fracture. By removing the splint, the recovery in the finger extension appears satisfactory (10 % deficit in the extension). **e** A 9-year-old patient. Distal phalanx apex fracture of the thumb (trauma by crushing), with nail plate avulsion and nail bed injury. The necessity for treating soft tissue injury requires a retrograde percutaneous osteosynthesis

complete recovery of the extension, but no consolidation of the fracture (Fig. 9.1d). Another type of lesion due to crush of the distal phalanx can produce a middle third distal fracture which require an osteosynthesis (Fig. 9.1e).

9.2.1.2 Middle Phalanx

Most middle phalanx fractures are of type II (Salter–Harris). Transverse diaphysis fractures are infrequent, and distal epiphysis or articular fractures are rare (Fig. 9.2a). Every physis fracture can be treated by closed reduction and percutaneous fixation even for small displacements (Fig. 9.2b). The diaphysis fractures can be treated or by fixing with percutaneous interfragmentary Kirschner wires, or using lately percutaneous fixation from the apex of the distal phalanx through the distal interphalangeal (DIP) joint up to the middle phalanx, associated with an interfragmentary anti-rotation K-wire.

9.2.1.3 Proximal Phalanx

Proximal phalanx fractures are frequent in sports injuries; most are of type II (Salter–Harris), with a dorsal displacement of diaphysis. After 10 days, these fractures could be very difficult to reduce because an altered consolidation has already occurred (Fig. 9.3a]. In case of a small displacement, a conservative treatment is possible. However, the treatment usually consists in a closed reduction under fluoroscopy and a fixation with an interfragmentary (possibly anterograde) K-wire

(Fig. 9.3d) passing first through the epiphysis, then through the metaphysis and fixed in the diaphysis compact bone. By entering the epiphysis on the side of the metaphyseal fragment, which is characteristic of type II fractures, the grip of the K-wire is improved and the application simplified. In distal metaphyseal fractures, where the fracture line passes through a spongy bone, should be preferred a percutaneous fixation with two K-wires placed crosswise and should be one of the two wires only pass through the periosteum of a fragment, the stabilizing action would be nonetheless guaranteed (Fig. 9.3b).

Epiphyseal fractures, very infrequent, can be treated by closed percutaneous reduction with interfragmentary fixation (Fig. 9.3c) or, in the presence of a small distal fragment hardly fixable, by means of a cantilever percutaneous fixation (Fig. 9.3e).

9.2.1.4 Metacarpals

Metacarpal fractures, which are uncommon, are usually due to epiphyseal separation (Fig. 9.4a): Distal diaphyseal fractures are more infrequent and midshaft fractures even more (Fig. 9.4b). All of these fractures are very often subject to secondary displacements. They were mainly treated surgically by means of a closed reduction and an intramedullary anterograde percutaneous fixation by applying manually an appropriately modeled K-wire, under fluoroscopy (Fig. 9.4c). The wire passing through the physis never produced any growth disturbance, given its small diameter

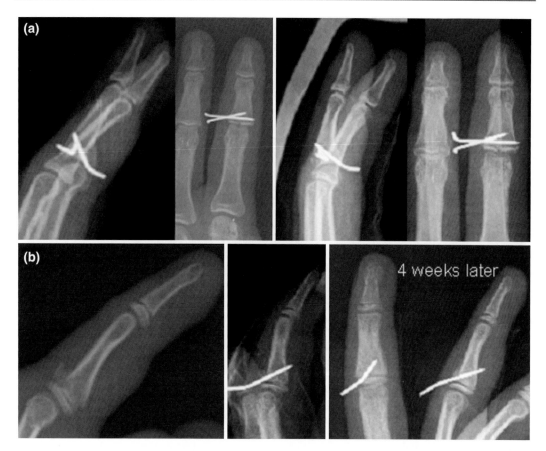

Fig. 9.2 a A 14-year-old patient. Middle phalanx base articular fracture, second finger, treated by closed reduction and percutaneous fixation six days after trauma. Post-operative control 35 days after trauma. **b** An 11-year-old patient. Physeal fracture of the middle phalanx base, fourth finger. Fracture reduction facilitated by the lever effect of a percutaneous K-wire which allowed osteosynthesis. Control performed 30 days after surgery (37 days after trauma). Consolidation of the fracture with an excellent functional outcome: no extension deficit in the PIP joint

(max 1.5 mm). The treatment is simpler in metaphyseal fractures during the phase of physeal closure, typical of boxing traumas (Fig. 9.5a, b). Cases treated conservatively were closely followed by radiographs in order to promptly identify displacements. There are no specific radiographic images of lesions in the phalanges of first finger, whereas the metacarpal is characterized by a high incidence of physis fractures, thus behaving as a proximal phalanx as far as skeletal growth is concerned (Fig. 9.5c). As for phalanges, the treatment consists in a closed reduction, only rarely in an open reduction, and a percutaneous interfragmentary fixation.

9.2.1.5 Carpus

The carpus is only exceptionally involved in pediatric fractures associated with sports activities since injuries usually cause a radius physis separation. Rarely, it can be observed a compound fracture of the distal third of the scaphoid. When the fracture is located in the middle third, it is necessary to fix with a screw, especially if exists a third fragment (Fig. 9.6a).

Alternatively, a middle third scaphoid fracture can be fixed with a memory staple (Fig. 9.6b): This technique has proved to be simpler and faster compared to screw osteosynthesis, which presents difficulties in the reduc-

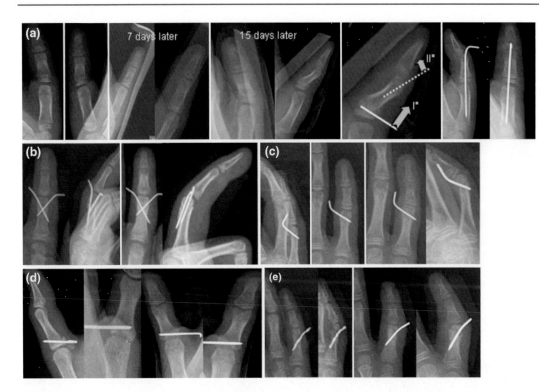

Fig. 9.3 a A 9-year-old patient. Proximal phalanx physeal fracture, first finger, not clearly evident during X-ray control in emergency. Nonoperatively treated, with radiographic evidence of proper alignment, after 7 days. During the following control (15 days after), a serious displacement detected requiring surgery. This difficult reduction achieved by using a percutaneous intrafocal K-wire applied with a lever effect (*arrow I*), followed by stabilization by means of an axial retrograde percutaneous transarticular wire (*arrow II*). **b** A 12-year-old patient. Distal metaphyseal fracture, potentially unstable, treated by osteosynthesis with two percutaneous crossed K-wires. In the lateral radiograph, one of the wires is found to be definitely subperiosteal. The reduction remains stable, as evidenced by a following control (35 days after trauma).

The periosteal callus, incorporating the subperiosteal wire on the proximal fragment, is relevant and evident. **c** A 9-year-old patient. The small size of the cephalic fragment requires a percutaneous intrafocal osteosynthesis ("cantilever style"). During control (35 days after injury), a satisfactory consolidation noticed. No residual stiffness was recorded. **d** A 13-year-old patient. Physeal fracture in first finger base, treated by closed reduction and anterograde osteosynthesis. Post-operative control and control after healing. **e** A 7-year-old patient. The cephalic fragment is potentially unstable and partially deformed. Although the reduction is not anatomical (also because of the deformation), the final control (after 37 days) shows a satisfactory reconstruction of the meta-epiphysis. No remnants of functional deficit

tion in the fracture and the retrograde percutaneous screw fixation. Intercarpal and radioulnocarpal ligament injuries, quite common in adults, are generally not observed in children.

9.2.1.6 Radius and Ulna

Distal radius and ulna fractures are the most common among fractures of the upper limb. A common problem to the treatment of these fractures it that must be considered the relationship between the possible deviations of the axis and the ability of the remodeling due to growth.

Metadiaphyseal and diaphyseal greenstick fractures must be followed with great attention as are subject to secondary displacement. If promptly treated, they must be corrected and stabilized whenever possible by closed reduction and percutaneous osteosynthesis, even at the risk of leaving a slight deformity of the axis. When this deformity corresponds to the anatomical

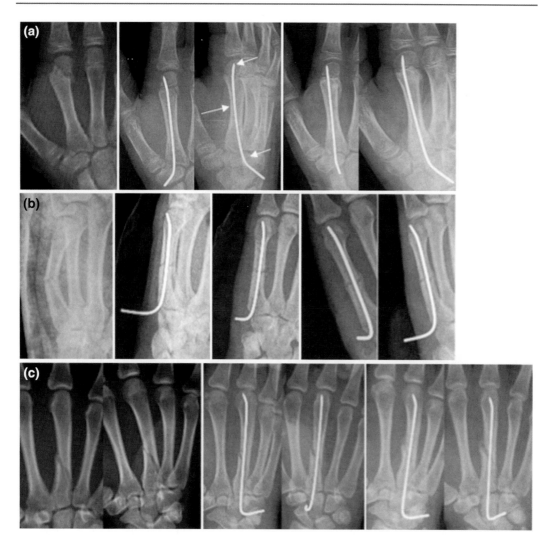

Fig. 9.4 a An 11-year-old patient. Physeal fracture of the second metacarpal treated by closed reduction and percutaneous anterograde fixation. The diameter of the wire (1.5 mm) provides the necessary passage through the growth plate without sequelae. Control 36 days after trauma shows a satisfactory consolidation. The *arrows* show the three gripping points of the wire, according to the principles of elastic osteosynthesis. **b** A 16-year-old patient. Displaced diaphyseal fracture observed 15 days after trauma. Treated by closed reduction and percutaneous anterograde fixation. Control after 60 days shows fracture consolidation. **c** A 15-year-old patient. Proximal metadiaphyseal oblique fracture of the third metacarpal. Treated by closed reduction and percutaneous anterograde fixation. Control after 37 days shows a satisfactory fracture consolidation

morphology achieved by the end of growth, it is considered acceptable. It must therefore be kept in mind that the final orientation of the radius articular surface (about 15° in a proper lateral wrist projection) is obtained gradually. In males, up to about 14 years old and in females up to about 13 years old, the radius articular surface is perpendicular to the radius longitudinal axis.

The incidence of complete isolated metaphyseal fractures of the radius is very high, and epiphyseal displacement is usually dorsal. Moreover, a great number of diaphyseal and metaphyseal fractures of the forearm are observed (single or double bone) which are associated with contact sports and result from crushing or trampling (Fig. 9.7a, b).The possibility of a secondary

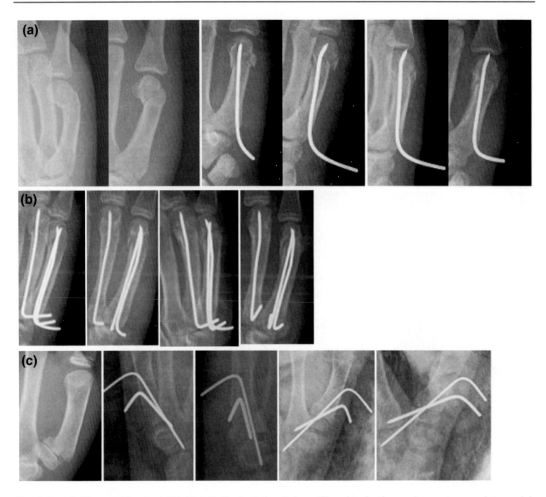

Fig. 9.5 **a** A 15-year-old patient. Distal metadiaphyseal fracture of the 5th metacarpal after 30 days. Difficult closed reduction and osteosynthesis. Control 30 days after osteosynthesis. **b** A 14-year-old patient. Distal metadiaphyseal fractures of 4th and 5th metacarpal after 8 days. Closed reduction and percutaneous intramedullary osteosynthesis. Control 36 days after trauma. **c** A 13-year-old patient. Physeal fracture of the first metacarpal with severe displacement in adduction. Closed reduction and percutaneous fixation with two K-wires

displacement is high both in metaphyseal and in diaphyseal fractures, even after a successful closed reduction and cast immobilization. This requires a strict radiographic control every 5–7 days during the first two weeks in order to correct any displacement that might occur [possibly with a closed or at least minimally invasive reduction (Fig. 9.7c)]. Any even slight displacement means that the fracture is not stable and will inexorably evolve toward a greater displacement notwithstanding cast immobilization. The first radiograph after injury shows the state of the two stumps not at the moment of maximum lesion impact, but when the stumps are already closer due to tissue elasticity, which makes it difficult to evaluate soft tissue tear (periosteum, muscle insertion, and retinacular septa). It would thus be misleading to evaluate stability by considering the number of fragments, the morphology of stumps, and the initial displacement. Only subsequent radiographs may show a possible displacement trend: An "ad axim" displacement in particular might indicate a progressive reduction loss. This type of displacement implies an imbalance in muscle forces applied and the presence of a displacement

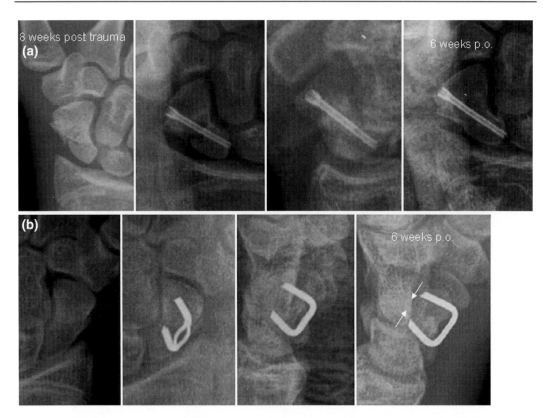

Fig. 9.6 a A 16-year-old patient. Carpal scaphoid fracture of the middle third, 50 days after trauma. Given the fracture site and time elapsed after trauma, a distal-proximal screw osteosynthesis was performed. **b** A 15-year-old patient. Carpal scaphoid fracture 15 days after trauma. The fracture site and the young age of the patient recommended fixation with a memory staple. Control 50 days after fracture clearly shows the compression effect (*arrows*) exerted by the staple and fracture consolidation

torque (Fig. 9.8), while an "ad latus" displacement, even if not anatomically corrected, is well compensated by skeletal growth. It can therefore be said that it is preferable to obtain an imperfect reduction by closed fixation than a perfect anatomical by open reduction (Fig. 9.9a). The treatment of metaphyseal fractures benefits from closed reduction under fluoroscopy, which is almost always possible. Fixation is always performed by entering the fracture line dorsally and percutaneously from the displacement side, using the wire inserted in the diaphyseal canal and deformed like a crossbow by the contact with the volar cortex to promote reduction and impede displacement. According to the stability assessed intraoperatively, an additional percutaneous wire may be applied from the radius distal

fragment, with an oblique course, by transfixing the epiphyseal cartilage if necessary, with an intramedullary application or passing through the opposite cortex. Can be used "canon tip" wires (Fig. 9.9b) with a blunt tip suited to sliding on the cortex of the intramedullary canal. The steels used must have good elasticity and shape memory; when properly applied, they are able to counteract displacement forces whose direction must be studied before and during surgery. By reducing radius displacement, it is also possible to reduce an ulnar displacement when present. Poor reliability of young patients almost always requires maintaining a forearm–metacarpal plaster cast until wire removal in order to avoid reduction loss, but mainly to prevent percutaneous wire contamination.

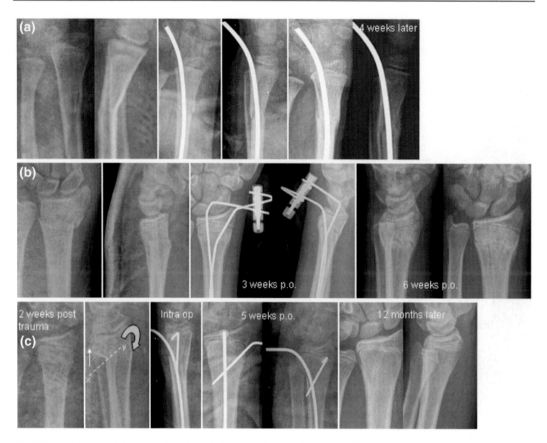

Fig. 9.7 a A 7-year-old patient. Diaphyseal fracture of radius 8 days after trauma, clearly unstable with volar displacement. Treatment by percutaneous retrograde osteosynthesis, without passing through the physis. The use of a single intramedullary wire dorsally inserted in a fracture tending toward a volar displacement recommends a greater extension prebending of the wire. Control 40 days after injury. **b** A 15-year-old patient. Metaphyseal fracture of the distal radius. Fracture site and skeletal age of the patient required a closed reduction and a percutaneous retrograde intramedullary osteosynthesis with two wires externally fixed on a plate and crossbow tensioned. The radial wire passing through the styloid necessarily transfixes the physis without causing any secondary growth disturbance. Control shows consolidation. **c** An 11-year-old patient. Radius physeal fracture observed more than 15 days after trauma. The initial consolidation of the fracture required the application of an intrafocal wire with a lever reducing effect introduced percutaneously along the x–y direction, favoring closed reduction. The same wire, proceeding in the anterograde direction and with an intramedullary course, exerted a crossbow stabilization effect; the osteosynthesis was completed by applying a percutaneous bicortical K-wire. Control 12 months after surgery shows the absence of fracture and surgery aftermath

Usually 35 days after injury, the X-ray control performed once the cast is removed shows healing of the fracture, thus allowing the wires to be removed in sedoanalgesia. Not normally is found any post-traumatic stiffness, nor any clinical or radiographic evidence of deformity, nor any wire site infection, but is possible to occur only a slight inflammatory reaction around percutaneous holes, which recedes after removal. There is a risk of a keloid reaction on wire sites. The surgical treatment of fractures is never performed in emergency so that limb swelling may recede. This procedure allows better fracture reduction, reducing the incidence

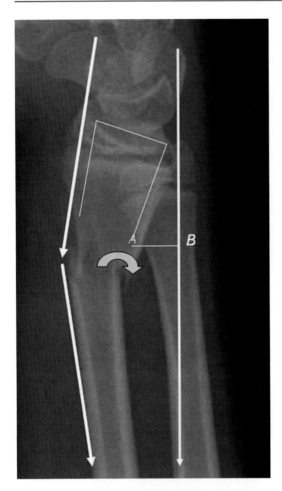

Fig. 9.8 Diagram shows the change in balance between flexor and extensor muscles in an extension deformity of a wrist metaphyseal fracture represented by a *curved arrow*. This condition results in a torque, i.e., a force in rotation, proportionate to the length of the AB segment; this torque tends to progressively increase the extension deformity

of skin disorders on wire sites and of postoperative pain. Ultimately, distal metaphyseal fractures are suitable for closed reduction and interfragmentary percutaneous fixation (Fig. 9.9c) or, in adolescents, for intramedullary retrograde percutaneous fixation (Figs. 9.9d–9.10a) or a mixed technique (Fig. 9.10b).

In the presence of very distal double-bone fractures in which the fracture line mainly involves the cancellous bone, an

interfragmentary fixation is more reliable than an intramedullary fixation (Fig. 9.10c). Whenever possible, closed reduction with intramedullary osteosynthesis is to be preferred (Fig. 9.11a, b). Sometimes, the ulna may be difficult to infibulate due to canal narrowness: In such cases, the ulnar fracture can be fixed by means of an interfragmentary osteosynthesis. Single- or double-bone diaphyseal fractures, in addition to problems mentioned above concerning distal fractures, present practical difficulties in reducing because, as mentioned before, the displacement at the time of trauma may have been greater, thereby allowing the interposition of soft tissues. Since a closed reduction during surgery is not easy to achieve, further traumatic actions and often futile attempts to reduce the fracture are not advisable. It would be better to choose a less biological, but more reliable open reduction. However, an intramedullary fixation with percutaneous wires forming intersecting arches, as in metadiaphyseal distal fractures, or with Rush nails does not require too large exposure of the fracture site, nor a real deperiostation, thus ensuring a greater respect for fracture biology which thereby favors a faster and safer healing. Proximal diaphyseal fractures can also benefit from an intramedullary osteosynthesis (Fig. 9.11e).

9.3   Ligament Injuries

The most common ligament injury is the detachment of the volar plate from the proximal interphalangeal (PIP) joint, typical of volleyball, basketball, and football (goalkeepers) injuries. It consists in the tearing of the volar plate of the PIP joint, almost always with a bone plug or a small type III (Salter) physeal fracture involving the base of the middle phalanx. These injuries are treated by immobilization with a Zimmer splint maintaining the PIP joint in extension or slightly in flexion for not more than one week, given the risk of a scarring retraction of the volar plate with a PIP

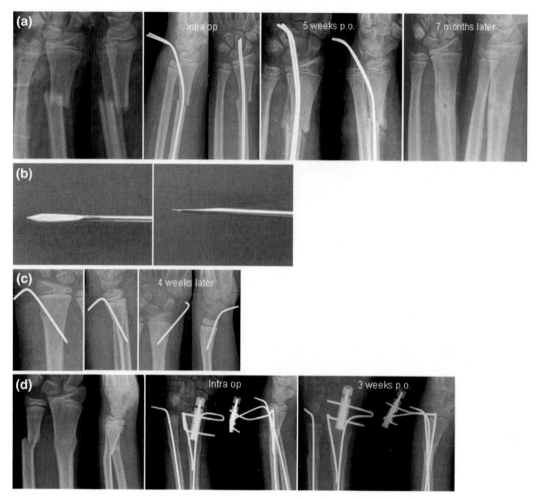

Fig. 9.9 a A 10-year-old patient. Diaphyseal fracture closed, reduced, and fixed with percutaneous intramedullary wires. Displacement "ad latus" is offset by growth, as shown by X-ray control after 7 months. **b** Canon tip—see text. **c** A 8-year-old patient. Metadiaphyseal fracture of the distal radius treated by closed reduction and percutaneous interfragmentary osteosynthesis. **d** An 11-year-old patient. Metadiaphyseal double-bone fracture of distal forearm. Closed reduction and percutaneous retrograde intramedullary fixation with three wires: two for the radius and one for the ulna. X-ray control shows consolidation

joint secondary flexion stiffness impossible to correct. Flexion and extension mobilization of the finger, both passive and active, 10 days after the injury (including bone avulsions) never resulted in bone and joint deformities nor stiffness (Fig. 9.12a).

9.4   Tendon Injuries

A complete lesion of the extensor apparatus at the DIP joint (the so-called mallet finger) with apparently no bone injury can be observed,

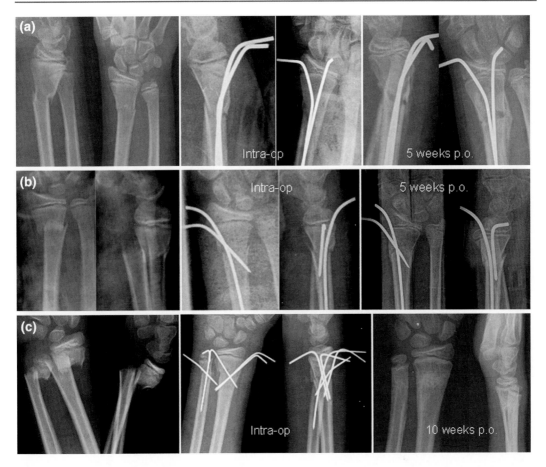

Fig. 9.10 a A 12-year-old patient. Metadiaphyseal fracture of the distal radius. Closed reduction and fixation with two percutaneous intramedullary retrograde wires. X-ray control 40 days after fracture. **b** A 12-year-old patient. Metaphyseal fracture of distal radius treated by combined internal fixation (percutaneous intramedullary retrograde wire and interfragmentary wire). **c** A 12-year-old patient. Double-bone fracture of metaphyseal distal forearm. The fracture site and the age of the patient suggest that the medullary canal is not well developed. Interfragmentary osteosynthesis is preferred, except for the ulna

especially in a basketball trauma. The lesion, also if is proved to be a Segond fracture, can be treated by immobilization with a short splint and a DIP joint hyperextension for 40 days, which resulted normally in a complete recovery of finger extension (Fig. 9.12b).

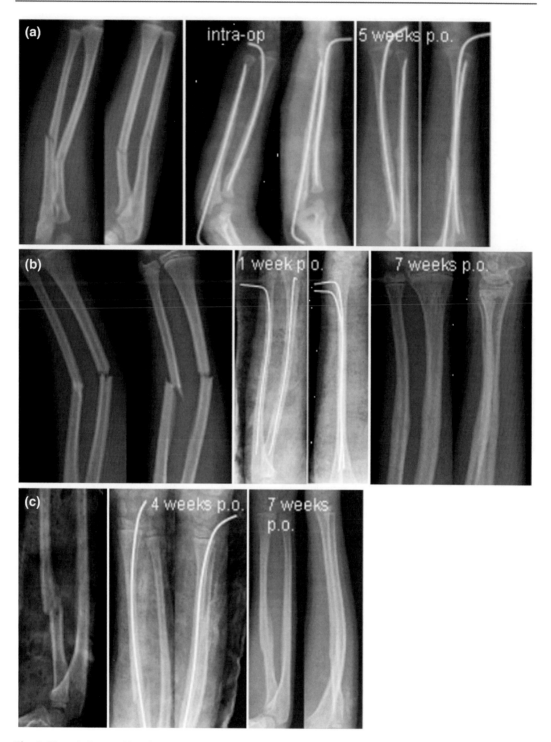

Fig. 9.11 **a** A 5-year-old patient. Double-bone diaphy-seal fracture of the forearm. Closed reduction and percutaneous intramedullary osteosynthesis. X-ray control 40 days after injury. The application of an ulnar wire, through the olecranon ossification nucleus, did not result in skeletal growth damage, given the size of the wire (2 mm diameter). This technique is also simpler and quicker. Alternatively, both percutaneous intramedullary wires can be applied in a retrograde direction (**b**). **c** A 7-year-old patient. Proximal radial diaphyseal fracture treated by closed reduction and percutaneous intramedullary retrograde fixation

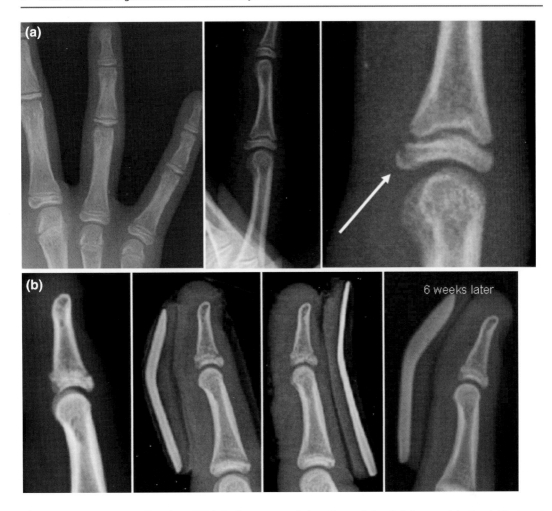

Fig. 9.12 a An 11-year-old patient. PIP joint hyperextension injury of the 4th finger with marginal epiphyseal fracture by avulsion of the distal volar plate insertion. The radiographic diagnosis of this lesion requires a strictly lateral X-ray projection of the finger involved. **b** A 13-year-old patient. Segond fracture of the distal phalanx base of the 3rd finger, *right hand*. Treatment with an hyperextension splint maintained for 40 days. It is safer in such cases to switch the splint from volar to dorsal side every 10–15 days. The dorsal splint, much more suitable to contain the fracture, may cause a dorsal decubitus

References

1. Zaricznyj B, Shattuck LJ, Mast TA, Robertson RV, D'Elia G (1980) Sports-related injuries in school-aged children. Am J Sports Med 8(5):318–324
2. Kraus R, Szalay G, Meyer C, Kilian O, Schnetter R (2007) Distal radius fracture-a goalkeepers' injury in children and adolescents. Sportveletz Sportschaden 21(4):177–179
3. Badia A, Stennett C (2006) Sports-related injuries of the elbow. J Hand Ther 19(2):206–226
4. Mitts KG, Hennrikus WL (1996) In-line skating fractures in children. J Pediatr Orthop 16(5):640–643
5. Curtin J, Kay NR (1976) Hand injuries due to soccer. Hand 8(1):93–95
6. Costard P (1990) Les fractures de la main chez l'enfant Cahier d'enseignement de la Société Française de Chirurgie de la Main -2, Expansion Scientifique Française

The Hip: Femoro-Acetabular Impingement

10

Luca M. Pierannunzii and Marco d'Imporzano

Femoro-acetabular impingement (FAI) is a common source of hip joint degenerative changes. It is more and more frequently recognized in the adult and young adult population, thank to the wider circulation of its knowledge among orthopedists and radiologists.

Although it may be referred to as a "disease," the term defines more properly a pathomechanism, while diseases are its possible consequences: labral injuries, chondral damage, and lastly degenerative joint disease (DJD).

In 1936, Smith-Petersen introduced the concept of the impingement of the femoral neck on the anterior acetabular margin [1] and anticipated the recent development on FAI surgery [2].

In 1986, Harris stated that 90 % of cases of so-called primary hip osteoarthritis are somehow characterized by subtle anatomical abnormalities, mostly represented by mild acetabular dysplasia and pistol grip deformity of the proximal femur [3]. Few years later Ganz and coworkers suggested a classification of FAI [4] based on different abnormal contact between the femoral neck and the acetabular rim.

10.1 Pathophysiological Classification

From a pathophysiological point of view, FAI may be divided into two mechanisms, the pincer-type and the cam-type (Fig. 10.1) [5]. The FAI is defined mixed if both mechanisms occur.

10.1.1 Pincer-Type FAI

The pincer-type FAI depends on excessive acetabular coverage that reduces the range of motion between neutral position and rim–neck contact (Fig. 10.1b). Since the joint congruency is intact and both articular surfaces are perfectly round, no significant strain is put on the cartilage; the labrum is the main victim, being pinched between the bony rim and neck.

In long-lasting pincer-type FAI, some chondral damages may develop because of recurrent head subluxations due to lever effect. Interestingly, while labral damages are mostly antero-lateral, chondral damages—if any—mainly occur in the postero-lateral quadrant of the socket. This topographical pattern of injuries is consistent with the hypothesized lever mechanism.

L. M. Pierannunzii (✉)
Sports Traumatology Unit, Gaetano Pini Orthopedic Institute, Piazza Cardinal Ferrari 1, 20122, Milan, Italy
e-mail: lmcpierannunzii@hotmail.com

M. d'Imporzano
Orthopedics, Istituto Auxologico Italiano, Via Mercalli 30, 20122, Milan, Italy
e-mail: dimpomarco@live.it

V. Guzzanti (ed.), *Pediatric and Adolescent Sports Traumatology*,
DOI: 10.1007/978-88-470-5412-7_10, © Springer-Verlag Italia 2014

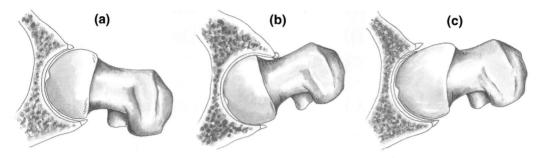

Fig. 10.1 Cross section of a normal hip, a pincer-FAI and a cam-FAI. **a** In the normal hip, the head is perfectly round and a large rim–neck clearance guarantees wide range of motion without impingement. **b** In pincer-FAI, the prominent rim determines early rim–neck contact, with antero-superior labral crushing and postero-inferior chondral countercoup lesion. **c** In cam-FAI, the out-of-round extension of the head (bump) everts the antero-superior labrum and causes delamination of the adjacent acetabular cartilage

Overcoverage may affect the whole acetabulum, leading to a global pincer-FAI, or just the antero-lateral sector of the socket, leading to a focal pincer-FAI.

Global pincer-FAI, already known as coxa profunda and protrusio acetabuli (according to deformity severity), was recognized as a weak cause of secondary hip osteoarthritis long time before FAI concept was born. However, little is known about the etiology of such a condition. Recently, the location of the acetabular fossa relatively to the ilioischial line was demonstrated to be unrelated to true overcoverage [6], and the center-edge angle has become the most predictive indicator of global pincer-type impingement.

Focal pincer-FAI is also named "retroverted acetabulum," as the antero-lateral focal overcoverage makes the superior pole of the socket retroverted [7]. Since the inferior pole of the socket is still anteverted, the helitorsion of the acetabular rim generates a special roentgenographic feature named cross-over sign (Fig. 10.2). This subtle developmental abnormality of the socket is considered a peculiar variant of the acetabular dysplasia, whose most common variant shows excessive anteversion and reduced lateral coverage.

Isolated pincer-FAI was rarely addressed in pediatric and adolescent patients, as this pathomechanism does not cause early articular damages and is usually diagnosed in adulthood.

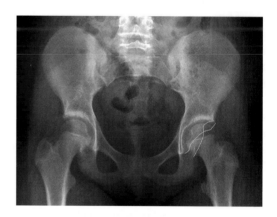

Fig. 10.2 Incidental finding of acetabular retroversion in an 11-year-old child. The cross-over sign is clearly visible on both sides, although the acetabular growth is still ongoing and the acetabular morphology after skeletal maturity is unpredictable

10.1.2 Cam-Type FAI

Cam-FAI is an out-of-round deformity of the proximal femur (Fig. 10.1c) [8]. In mechanics, a cam is a device that transforms rotation into linear translation and vice versa. Similarly, the cam deformity of the proximal femur transforms the rotation of the head into compression/abrasion of the acetabular cartilage.

The first chapter that considered an out-of-round shape of the femoral epiphysis as a possible cause of DJD was written by Murray back in 1965 [9]. At the time, the deformity was considered a subclinical (but potentially

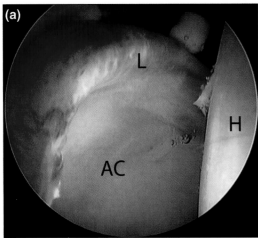
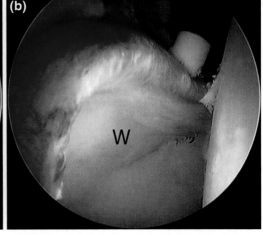

Fig. 10.3 Cartilage delamination in the right hip of 17-year-old female dancer affected by cam-FAI. If the labrum (L) is pushed inward with the probe, the adjacent acetabular cartilage (AC) bulges (wave sign, W), demonstrating that the chondral flap is detached from the bony acetabulum. H: femoral head. **a** Before probing. **b** While probing

dangerous) form of slipped capital femoral epiphysis (SCFE) and named "tilt deformity." Later, it was re-named pistol grip deformity for its resemblance with the handle of an old gun [10].

The knowledge of the cam mechanism has recently elucidated why the pistol grip deformity is strongly related to early DJD: the cam deformity everts the labrum and abrades the cartilage, resulting in chondral delamination and chondro-labral strain (Fig. 10.3). The chondro-labral junction lastly fails, the labrum dislocates peripherally and the acetabular cartilage margin is left unbound and unprotected. The cartilage flap is quickly disrupted and the subchondral bone is exposed.

The location of the so-called "bump," usually antero-lateral, is strongly related to the location of articular secondary damages that involve mainly the antero-lateral quadrant of the acetabulum.

As for the etiology, two kinds of cam deformity exist: primary and secondary. The secondary cam, in young patients, is commonly due to SCFE (Figs. 10.4, 10.5), Legg-Calvè-Perthes disease, neoplasms, less commonly to post-traumatic deformities after neck fracture. The primary cam, by far the commonest, is referred to as "idiopathic lack of head–neck offset," and its origin is still debated (Fig. 10.6).

Although Murray's tilt hypothesis might explain a few cases of primary cam deformity as outcome of subclinical SCFE, most patients would not fit this explanation. Some Authors believe that repetitive functional rim–neck abutments due to high range-of-motion sports activity might lead to secondary cam development [11], but this theory is far from being demonstrated. More likely, excessive loads transferred through the joint in adolescents practicing contact sports might induce the femoral physis to remodel abnormally. The physeal plates in lower limbs are aligned perpendicularly to the direction of compressive forces, so that the shear stress is minimum [12]. Their slope is known to change over the growth [13], with a theoretical self-adaptation to forces orientation. If this theory is true, the epiphyseal plate is perpendicular to the neck axis due to the tension band effect of the abductor mechanism (glutei and tensor fasciae latae muscles), transforming the traction forces running along the lateral aspect of the neck into compressive forces [14]. Impact load might change stress distribution through the physis, thus inducing an adaptive, horizontal re-orientation of the antero-lateral

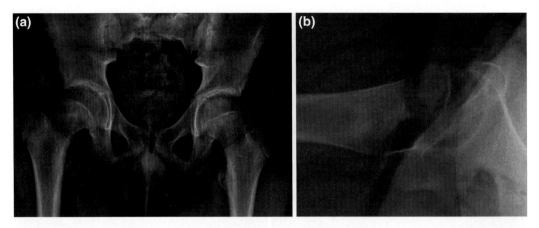

Fig. 10.4 Secondary right hip cam-FAI in a 15-year-old male who had a SCFE pinned in situ with resorbable hardware 5 months before. The posterior tilt of the head makes the anterior metaphysis prominent and virtually cancels the anterior head–neck offset. **a** Antero-posterior view. **b** Axial view. (courtesy of Dr. Antonio Memeo, Gaetano Pini Orthopaedic Institute, Milan)

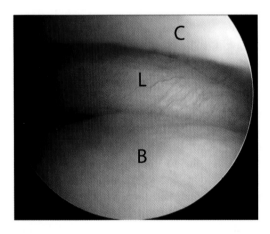

Fig. 10.5 Arthroscopic visualization of the cam-impingement mechanism due to post-SCFE deformity of the proximal femur in a 18-year-old soccer player. The hip is flexed at 70° and internally rotated. The bump (*B*) slides below the labrum (*L*) and everts it. *C* capsule

side of the plate [15]. So far the direction of such a remodeling process cannot be explained but temptatively, as if the balance between traction forces (due to vertical load of an oblique femoral neck) and tension band-related counter-forces was somehow impaired in favor of traction forces. A recent epidemiological investigation among male preprofessional soccer players aged 12–19 years found a cam deformity in 26 % of them versus 17 % in an age-matched non-athletic control population [16]. The abnormal head–neck junction was identifiable from the age of 13 years.

10.2 Clinical Presentation

The hip pain shows up in a similar fashion regardless of the underlying pathology [17]. The patient usually complains about a groin, buttock, or peritrochanteric pain, frequently pointing at all of these locations spreading his hand around the hip, with the thumb on the buttock and the other fingers in the groin or vice versa. Being the hand cupped like a "C" around the hip, this presentation is known as C-sign.

The observation of limp, lower limb malrotation, leg length discrepancy, together with age at presentation and familiar medical history, is of paramount importance to suspect developmental dysplasia of the hip (DDH), SCFE, or Legg-Calvè-Perthes disease.

The main tests performed in hip examination do not allow precise diagnosis, as positivity may be related to FAI, but also to any other cause of hip pain [18].

The most useful test is known as FADDIR (Fig. 10.7), from Flexion, ADDuction, and Internal Rotation. It is considered positive when

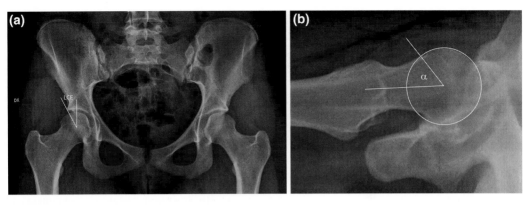

Fig. 10.6 Primary right hip cam-FAI in a 16-year-old female gymnast. **a** The pelvis antero-posterior view shows a *lateral center-edge angle* close to the lower limit of the normal range (28°) and a good spherical shape of the epiphysis. **b** The cross-table axial view of the *right hip* shows limited ventral cam deformity (alpha angle = 56°)

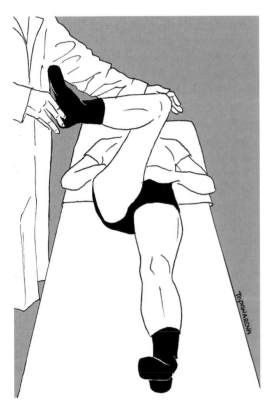

Fig. 10.7 FADDIR test

it elicits pain. Since it brings the antero-lateral head–neck junction below the corresponding acetabular rim, this maneuver is also known as "impingement test." However, the low specificity makes that definition quite inaccurate.

Another commonly performed test is known as FABER or Patrick's test (Fig. 10.8), from Flexion, ABduction, and External Rotation. The positivity may depend on pain and/or on restriction: the distance between the table and the knee is augmented in the painful hip (and is recorded as FABER distance).

Tenderness over the greater trochanter might be considered a sign of extra-articular pathology: unfortunately a positive sign does not rule out intra-articular injuries, although the relationship between trochanteric pain and joint disease is still obscure.

Several other tests may be added to augment completeness and accuracy of the physical examination (log-roll test, resisted straight leg raise test, etc.), but in no case, they will lead to the ultimate diagnosis that relies essentially on an adequate imaging.

10.3 Imaging

Imaging of FAI may be divided in three levels. The first level is usually sufficient to make the diagnosis, while the second one is needed to confirm it and to rule out other causes of pain.

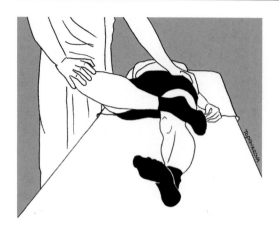

Fig. 10.8 FABER test

The third level is seldom resorted to for preoperative planning.

10.3.1 First Level: Conventional X-Rays

The standard antero-posterior view of the pelvis, together with the axial view of the affected hip, represents the most useful exam for FAI diagnosis [19].

The adequateness of the AP view is dictated by no lateral rotation (i.e., the vertical axis of the sacrum and coccyx points at the pubic symphysis) and normal pelvic tilt (i.e., in late-adolescents and adults, the distance between the sacrococcygeal joint and the upper border of the pubic symphysis is about 3 cm in males and 5 cm in females; unfortunately, this measure might be unreliable for younger patients).

On standard AP view, several angles and landmark should be noticed. These are the most useful for FAI assessment:

- LCE = lateral center-edge angle (Fig. 10.6a). It measures the acetabular coverage in the frontal plane and should range between 25 and 39°. When the upper limit is exceeded, the acetabulum is deeper (coxa profunda) and may determine a global pincer-type FAI.
- Alpha angle [20]. It measures the angle formed in the hip center of the rotation by the neck axis and the point of beginning asphericity of the head–neck junction. It is usually

lower than 50°. When higher than 55°, it is considered pathological and suggestive of cam-type FAI.

- Anterior and posterior walls. If the acetabular anatomy is normal, the walls diverge from the top to the bottom of the socket, with no intersections. If the acetabulum is retroverted, anterior and posterior walls cross each other at the level at which the socket changes its version from posterior to anterior. This sign is known as cross-over sign (Fig. 10.2). In case of positive cross-over sign, it is mandatory to verify that the hip center of rotation lies on the posterior wall profile (i.e., the retroversion is simply due to a prominent anterior wall). If the center is lateral, the retroversion is likely due to a deficient posterior wall and this is a relevant issue as for the surgical treatment.

On the axial view (either cross-table or frog-leg), the anterior profile is investigated. This allows to measure the alpha angle on the sagittal plane (Fig. 10.6b). Since the cam deformity may be located anywhere from postero-lateral to anterior, viewing the head–neck junction both on the frontal and on the sagittal plane is fundamental not to miss the deformity.

Some surgeons ask also for other views, the false profile view (that measures the anterior coverage through the anterior center-edge angle (ACE) and the Dunn view (that visualizes the antero-lateral profile of the neck, allowing to measure the alpha angle in an intermediate position between the lateral contour demonstrated by the AP view and the anterior contour demonstrated by the axial view).

10.3.2 Second Level: Magnetic Resonance

Since the FAI-associated radiographic abnormalities may be retrieved in asymptomatic subjects [21, 22], the magnetic resonance imaging (MRI) allows to rule out most of the confounding causes of hip pain [23] that might coexist with the aforementioned radiographic signs like

- osteoid osteoma;

- synovitis, that may be the early appearance of a juvenile rheumatoid arthritis or of a septic arthritis;
- avascular necrosis, that sometimes involves very young subjects, especially when secondary to sickle cell anemia or to steroid treatment;
- Malignancies.

If the clinical presentation is consistent with true hip pain, X-rays show impingement-associated signs, and MRI finds no other plausible causes for patient's symptoms, the diagnostic work-up may be considered concluded.

MRI allows precise spatial definition of the deformity, giving the surgeon the possibility to measure the alpha angle on all the radial planes passing through the head–neck axis. This may be useful in preoperative planning. Moreover, it allows to measure the acetabular version with good reliability.

A little information might be obtained about labral and chondral injuries, although the accuracy is much lower than for contrast-enhanced MRI.

10.3.3 Third Level: MR Arthrography

Direct MR arthrography (MRA) is the golden standard in hip chondro-labral evaluation [24]. This imaging technique is extremely useful in adults' FAI, where an accurate assessment of degenerative changes and irreparable injuries is needed to make a rational decision between conservative and prosthetic surgery. It is rarely useful in the very young patients, where such an advanced damage is not expected, and joint replacement is never an option.

Since direct MRA is based on intra-articular injection of gadolinium, it might be also unfeasible or scarcely accepted in young patients. Indirect MRA, obtained with intra-venous contrast administration, has been advocated as a viable option at least to increase the sensitivity versus labral injuries [25] and early synovitis [26]. The diffusion of 3T magnets might reduce the actual need for MRA, since those powerful

scanners generate more detailed images even without contrast enhancement [27].

10.4 Treatment

Given the large prevalence of FAI-related radiological signs in the young, healthy, asymptomatic population [28, 22], care should be taken not to overtreat this condition. Thus, an adequate attempt to relieve the symptoms should include sports activity modification [29] and core stability exercise to avoid excessive anterior pelvic tilt.

This approach is feasible in most children and adolescent practicing recreational sport. A temporary transition toward activities that do not include deep flexion (to keep the joint far from the end range) nor load impact (not to induce further bump formation, if the physis is still open) might be safe and effective.

Little is known about the chance of hip osteoarthritis development in patients showing FAI-related abnormalities. What is known for sure is that FAI is a potential cause of secondary osteoarthritis [30], while the true risk likely depends on several cofactors, such as lifestyle, level of activity, body weight. Careful monitoring is mandatory for all the children and adolescents who developed a temporary painful FAI, since future relapse might suggest the need for surgical treatment before degenerative changes occur. Same solution is recommended if unacceptable limitations are requested to keep the hip asymptomatic, or if the conservative approach fails immediately.

The timing of surgical correction is still debated. From a theoretical point of view, engaging the growth plates might be potentially dangerous and lead to abnormal development of the acetabulum (in case of rim trimming) and growth arrest of the proximal femur or acute SCFE due to perichondral ring violation (in case of head–neck junction osteochondroplasty) [31]. Fortunately, FAI diagnosis is mostly done in late adolescence, when the physis is closed or closing. If the patient was symptomatic earlier and

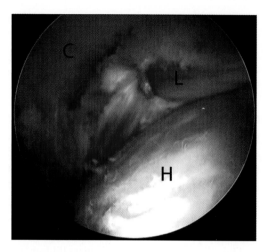

Fig. 10.9 Labral refixation after antero-superior rim trimming for acetabular retroversion. The refixed labrum (*L*) lies over the head (*H*) with adequate restoration of its sealing effect. *C* capsule

no relief could be obtained by conservative management, some series report adequate safety of the corrective surgery even in very young subjects. Rebello and coworkers [32] did not report any physeal disturbance in a 58-case series of surgical dislocation due to severe FAI-related hip deformities (SCFE, Perthes, osteonecroses, DDH, exostoses). Four cases developed avascular necrosis, but all of them

underwent a neck or intertrochanteric associated osteotomy that might be responsible for this severe complication. Unfortunately, the authors did not specify how many patients had open physes, but they might be a few, since the mean age of their sample was as high as 16 years. Philippon and coworkers recently published the 2-to 5-year results of arthroscopic de-impingement procedure in a population aged between 11 and 16 years. [33]. The authors wrote that the cam lesion was addressed only if non-communicating with the open physis, otherwise a delayed surgery would have been recommended. With this strategy, they did not have any growth disturbances among their patients. However, out of 60 patients, only six had open growth plates and eleven partially open plates. In conclusion, there is a very limited evidence in favor of early surgical correction of FAI in hips with open physis . Whenever possible, a conservative management up to radiological closure is recommended.

FAI correction may be performed with a surgical dislocation [5] or with hip arthroscopy [34]. The principles of the procedure (resection osteoplasty) are identical, whichever surgical technique is employed: the protruding rim is resected, possibly sparing the labrum that should

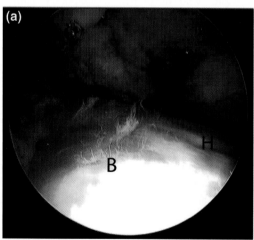

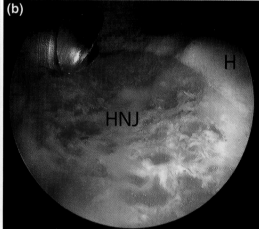

Fig. 10.10 Arthroscopic osteochondroplasty in a 19-year-old soccer player affected by left hip idiopathic cam-FAI. **a** The antero-lateral bump (*B*) is visualized, close to the head (*H*) and the labrum (*L*). The overlying abraded cartilage demonstrates the impinging area. **b** The arthroscopic burr is used to restore the proper concavity of the head–neck junction (*HNJ*)

be detached and subsequently refixed to the trimmed acetabular wall (Fig. 10.9); the aspherical extension of the head is removed, restoring the natural concave contour of the head–neck junction. All the associated injuries, like labral tears and chondral damages, are addressed as well.

Some recent reviews demonstrated that hip arthroscopy is better tolerated than surgical dislocation and mini-open surgery, is associated with less morbidity, and gains at least the same therapeutic result [35, 36]. The minimally invasive feature of arthroscopy makes it the actual best option for most FAI cases, especially in athletic patients aiming to return quickly to their preinjury level. Obviously severe deformities (secondary FAI) still require surgical dislocation, as it allows extensive corrections and associated procedures like relative femoral neck lengthening, intertrochanteric osteotomy, neck osteotomy, SCFE reduction. [32].

Lastly, in very selected cases of acetabular retroversion associated with posterior wall deficiency, the resection of the antero-superior rim might determine a significant reduction of the load-bearing surface. In this atypical dysplastic condition, the periacetabular osteotomy (PAO)—originally conceived to correct excessive anteversion and shallowness of conventional dysplastic sockets—may be indicated to correct the retroversion. This procedure is named reverse PAO [37] (Fig. 10.10).

References

1. Smith-Petersen MN (1936) Treatment of malum coxae senilis, old slipped upper femoral epiphysis, intrapelvic protrusion of the acetabulum, and coxa plana by means of acetabuloplasty. J Bone Surg Am 18:869–880
2. Rachbauer F, Kain MS, Leunig M (2009) The history of the anterior approach to the hip. Orthop Clin North Am 40(3):311–320
3. Harris WH (1986) Etiology of osteoarthritis of the hip. Clin Orthop Relat Res 213:20–33
4. Beck M, Kalhor M, Leunig M, Ganz R (2005) Hip morphology influences the pattern of damage to the acetabular cartilage: femoroacetabular impingement as a cause of early osteoarthritis of the hip. J Bone Joint Surg Br 87:1012–1018
5. Lavigne M, Parvizi J, Beck M, Siebenrock KA, Ganz R, Leunig M (2004) Anterior femoroacetabular impingement: part I. Techniques of joint preserving surgery. Clin Orthop Relat Res 418:61–66
6. Anderson LA, Kapron AL, Aoki SK, Peters CL (2012) Coxa Profunda: is the deep acetabulum overcovered? Clin Orthop Relat Res 2012 Aug 17. [Epub ahead of print]
7. Reynolds D, Lucas J, Klaue K (1999) Retroversion of the acetabulum. A cause of hip pain. J Bone Joint Surg Br 81(2):281–288
8. Siebenrock KA, Wahab KH, Werlen S, Kalhor M, Leunig M, Ganz R (2004) Abnormal extension of the femoral head epiphysis as a cause of cam impingement. Clin Orthop Relat Res 418:54–60
9. Murray RO (1965) The aetiology of primary osteoarthritis of the hip. Br J Radiol 38:810–824
10. Harris WH (1986) Etiology of osteoarthritis of the hip. Clin Orthop Relat Res 213:20–33
11. Hogervorst T, Bourma HW, de Vos J (2009) Evolution of the hip and pelvis. Acta Orthop Suppl 80:1–39
12. Smith JW (1962) The relationship of epiphysial plates to stress in some bones of the lower limb. J Anat 96:58–78
13. Mirkopulos N, Weiner DS, Askew M (1988) The evolving slope of the proximal femoral growth plate relationship to slipped capital femoral epiphysis. J Pediatr Orthop 8:268–273
14. Fetto J, Leali A, Moroz A (2002) Evolution of the Koch model of the biomechanics of the hip: clinical perspective. J Orthop Sci 7(6):724–730
15. Ng VY, Ellis TJ (2011) More than just a bump: Cam-type femoroacetabular impingement and the evolution of the femoral neck. Hip Int 21(01):001–008
16. Agricola R, Bessems JH, Ginai AZ, Heijboer MP, van der Heijden RA, Verhaar JA, Weinans H, Waarsing JH (2012) The development of Cam-type deformity in adolescent and young male soccer players. Am J Sports Med 40(5):1099–1106
17. Byrd JW (2007) Evaluation of the hip: history and physical examination. N Am J Sports Phys Ther 2(4):231–240
18. Martin RL, Irrgang JJ, Sekiya JK (2008) The diagnostic accuracy of a clinical examination in determining intra-articular hip pain for potential hip arthroscopy candidates. Arthroscopy 24(9):1013–1018
19. Tannast M, Siebenrock KA, Anderson SE (2007) Femoroacetabular impingement: radiographic diagnosis–what the radiologist should know. AJR Am J Roentgenol 188(6):1540–1552
20. Nötzli HP, Wyss TF, Stöcklin CH, Schmid MR, Treiber K, Hodler J (2002) The contour of the

femoral head–neck junction as a predictor for the risk of anterior impingement. J Bone Joint Surg Br 84:556–560

21. Hack K, Di Primio G, Rakhra K, Beaulé PE (2010) Prevalence of cam-type femoroacetabular impingement morphology in asymptomatic volunteers. J Bone Joint Surg Am 92(14):2436–2444

22. Kapron AL, Anderson AE, Aoki SK, Phillips LG, Petron DJ, Toth R, Peters CL (2011) Radiographic prevalence of femoroacetabular impingement in collegiate football players: AAOS exhibit selection. J Bone Joint Surg Am. 93(19):e111(1–10)

23. Carpineta L, Faingold R, Albuquerque PA, Morales Ramos DA (2007) Magnetic resonance imaging of pelvis and hips in infants, children, and adolescents: a pictorial review. Curr Probl Diagn Radiol 36(4):143–152

24. Kassarjian A (2006) Hip MR arthrography and femoroacetabular impingement. Semin Musculoskelet Radiol 10(3):208–219

25. Zlatkin MB, Pevsner D, Sanders TG, Hancock CR, Ceballos CE, Herrera MF (2010) Acetabular labral tears and cartilage lesions of the hip: indirect MR arthrographic correlation with arthroscopy–a preliminary study. AJR Am J Roentgenol 194(3):709–714

26. McQueen FM (2000) Magnetic resonance imaging in early inflammatory arthritis: what is its role? Rheumatology 39:700–706

27. Robinson P (2012) Conventional 3-T MRI and 1.5-T MR arthrography of femoroacetabular impingement. AJR Am J Roentgenol 199(3):509–515

28. Hack K, Di Primio G, Rakhra K, Beaulé PE (2010) Prevalence of cam-type femoroacetabular impingement morphology in asymptomatic volunteers. J Bone Joint Surg Am 92(14):2436–2444

29. Emara K, Samir W, el Motasem H, Ghafar KA (2011) Conservative treatment for mild femoroacetabular impingement. J Orthop Surg 19(1):41–45 (Hong Kong)

30. Ganz R, Leunig M, Leunig-Ganz K, Harris WH (2008) The etiology of osteoarthritis of the hip: an integrated mechanical concept. Clin Orthop Relat Res 466(2):264–272

31. Wenger DR, Kishan S, Pring ME (2006) Impingement and childhood hip disease. J Pediatric Orthopaedics B 15:233–243

32. Rebello G, Spencer S, Millis MB, Kim YJ (2009) Surgical dislocation in the management of pediatric and adolescent hip deformity. Clin Orthop Relat Res 467(3):724–731

33. Philippon MJ, Ejnisman L, Ellis HB, Briggs KK (2012) Outcomes 2 to 5 years following hip arthroscopy for femoroacetabular impingement in the patient aged 11 to 16 years. Arthroscopy 28(9):1255–1261

34. Bare AA, Guanche CA (2005) Hip impingement: the role of arthroscopy. Orthopedics 28:266–273

35. Matsuda DK, Carlisle JC, Arthurs SC, Wierks CH, Philippon MJ (2011) Comparative systematic review of the open dislocation, mini-open, and arthroscopic surgeries for femoroacetabular impingement. Arthroscopy 27(2):252–269

36. Botser IB, Smith TW Jr, Nasser R, Domb BG (2011) Open surgical dislocation versus arthroscopy for femoroacetabular impingement: a comparison of clinical outcomes. Arthroscopy 27(2):270–278

37. Siebenrock KA, Schoeniger R, Ganz R (2003) Anterior femoro-acetabular impingement due to acetabular retroversion. Treatment with periacetabular osteotomy. J Bone Joint Surg Am 85(2):278–286

Erratum to—The Hip: Avulsion Fractures

Luca M. Pierannunzii, Marco d'Imporzano and Antonio Memeo

Erratum to:
Chapter 11 in: V. Guzzanti (ed.),
Pediatric and Adolescent Sports
Traumatology,
DOI 10.1007/978-88-470-5412-7_11

In the original version of this chapter, one of the authors "Antonio Memeo" was missing.

Below are the authors with their affiliations who have contributed to Chap. 11:

L. M Pierannunzii
  SC Traumatologia Sportiva, Gaetano Pini Orthopaedic Institute, Piazza Cardinal Ferrari, 1, 20122 Milan, Italy
  e-mail: lmcpierannunzii@hotmail.com

M. d'Imporzano
  UO Ortopedia, Istituto Auxologico Italiano, Via Mercalli, 30, 20122 Milan, Italy

A. Memeo
  UO Ortopedia Infantile, Gaetano Pini Orthopaedic Institute, Piazza Cardinal Ferrari, 1, 20122 Milan, Italy

The online version of the original chapter can be found under DOI 10.1007/978-88-470-5412-7_11

L. M. Pierannunzii (✉)
SC Traumatologia Sportiva, Gaetano Pini
Orthopaedic Institute, Piazza Cardinal Ferrari, 1,
20122 Milan, Italy
e-mail: lmcpierannunzii@hotmail.com

M. d'Imporzano
UO Ortopedia, Istituto Auxologico Italiano,
Via Mercalli, 30, 20122 Milan, Italy

A. Memeo
UO Ortopedia Infantile, Gaetano Pini Orthopaedic
Institute, Piazza Cardinal Ferrari, 1, 20122 Milan,
Italy

The Hip: Avulsion Fractures

11

Luca M. Pierannunzii and Marco d'Imporzano

11.1 Introduction

Avulsion fractures of the pelvis are common injuries among sporting youngsters. A powerful, sudden, eccentric muscle contraction is the primary cause of these indirect injuries [1]. Most of them occur between the puberty and the middle of the third decade [2]. Their incidence is estimated to be increasing as the participation of adolescents in competitive sports is becoming more and more extensive.

In the adulthood, the muscle–tendon–bone complex usually fails at the muscle–tendon junction; on the contrary, before skeletal maturity, the weak junction is within the bony attachment. The physeal plate interposed between the tendon insertion (ossification center) and the rest of the bone is prone to distraction injuries when the applied force overcomes the ultimate tensile strength of the cartilage [3]. Some of these lesions, occurring in the late adolescence, seem to involve completely fused apophyses: in those cases, the radiologic fusion is supposed to conceal a persistently weak connection.

L. M. Pierannunzii (✉)
SC Traumatologia Sportiva, Gaetano Pini
Orthopaedic Institute, P.zza Cardinal Ferrari, 1,
20122, Milan, Italy
e-mail: lmcpierannunzii@hotmail.com

M. d'Imporzano
UO Ortopedia, Istituto Auxologico Italiano, Via
Mercalli, 30, 20122, Milan, Italy

The most commonly involved anatomical sites are the ischial tuberosity (IT) and the anterior inferior iliac spine (AIIS), followed by the anterior superior iliac spine (ASIS), the superior corner of the pubic symphysis (SCPS), the iliac crest (IC), the lesser trochanter (LT), and the greater trochanter (GT) [2, 4].

11.2 Clinical Presentation and Imaging

The patients who sustain an acute avulsion injury of the pelvis complain about a sudden, acute pain arisen from a forceful muscular contraction. Usually, the subject falls and keeps the limb and/or the trunk in an antalgic position suitable to relax the corresponding muscle.

Soft tissues above the apophysis are tender, usually swollen, sometimes ecchymosed. If the anamnestic data (young age, sport, indirect mechanism) are crossed with an elementary physical examination that reveals significant pain whenever the involved muscle–tendon unit is voluntarily contracted or passively stretched, the diagnosis is easily suspected.

The standard anteroposterior view of the pelvis is sometimes sufficient to confirm the diagnosis Oblique views of the pelvis and/or an axial view of the hip are often added. The hip anteroposterior view is inappropriate, given the scarcely predictable radiologic appearance of ossification centers. The comparison between the affected side and the contralateral healthy

V. Guzzanti (ed.), *Pediatric and Adolescent Sports Traumatology*,
DOI: 10.1007/978-88-470-5412-7_11, © Springer-Verlag Italia 2014

side is fundamental not to misdiagnose a simply unfused apophysis as an injury or vice versa [5].

In doubtful situations, the CT scan may solve the diagnostic dilemma, although the relatively higher radiation dose discourages from routine use. The magnetic resonance imaging (MRI) is an accurate, but also expensive technique we should save for very young patients, where the apophyses are still unossified [6]. Ultrasound scan might be as effective as MRI in experienced hands, without the risk of relevant motion artifacts in noncompliant children [7]. Lastly, if the traumatic history is not clear, late presentations of pelvic avulsions may be misdiagnosed as bone tumors: An adequate MRI may allow an accurate differential diagnosis [8].

11.3 Site-Specific Features

11.3.1 Ischial Tuberosity

A powerful contraction of the hamstrings is responsible for IT detachment. Soccer, sprinting, fencing, tennis, and gymnastics are the most commonly involved sports. Pain is located posteriorly, in the buttock. The hip is kept extended and the knee flexed, to relax the hamstrings. Due to the proximity to the ischiadic nerve, a few cases of secondary nerve irritation were described [9–11].

11.3.2 Anterior Inferior Iliac Spine

The direct tendon of the rectus femoris originates from the AIIS and may determine its avulsion (Fig. 11.1). A violent kick, either hitting the ball or missing it, is the commonest mechanism of injury among young soccer players. Tennis players, track and field athletes, and gymnasts may develop the same injury, although rarely, with explosive flexions of the hip associated with knee extension. The pain is

located in the groin, and the hip and knee are flexed to relieve the tension.

When the AIIS heals back in an elongated fashion, it may determine a peculiar type of extra-articular femoroacetabular impingement, limiting flexion and abduction [12]. An arthroscopic spinoplasty was proposed to treat this rare complication.

11.3.3 Anterior Superior Iliac Spine

Sartorius and tensor fasciae latae insert onto the ASIS. Since both these muscles take part in hip flexion, together with abduction and external rotation, their proximal avulsion strikes the same sports listed above for AIIS lesions. The pain, more lateral in the groin, has a similar presentation.

11.3.4 Superior Corner of the Pubic Symphysis

The SCPS is the insertion of the rectus abdominis. A violent contraction, as it might occur in soccer, gymnastics, or fencing, may determine this rare injury. The pain is located over the pubis, and the patient avoids deep breathing, coughing, and laughing.

11.3.5 Iliac Crest

The same sports responsible for SCPS avulsions are involved in IC avulsions (Fig. 11.2). In this case, the oblique abdominal muscles may detach the IC as a consequence of a sudden twist of the trunk. A similar injury may be determined by blunt trauma to the pelvis in various kinds of accident (car accidents, knocking down, etc.). The tenderness located over the IC is associated with the same antalgic behavior described above.

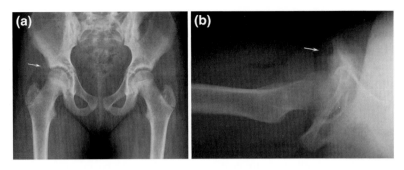

Fig. 11.1 Right AIIS type II avulsion fracture (*arrow*) in a 14-year-old female soccer player. **a** Anteroposterior view of the pelvis. **b** Axial view of the hip

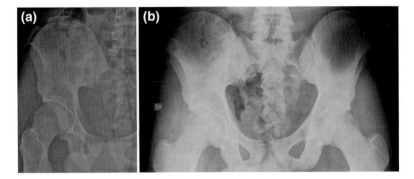

Fig. 11.2 Right type III combined avulsion fracture of IC and ASIS in a 17-year-old high-end male soccer player. Given the large size of the fragment and the patient's high level of activity, a surgical repair was offered. **a** Iliac view of the right pelvic bone at the time of injury. **b** Anteroposterior view of the pelvis 1 month after open reduction and internal fixation with multiple resorbable screws. The anatomy of the iliac wing is perfectly restored, when compared with the contralateral unaffected side

11.3.6 Lesser Trochanter

The LT is the distal insertion site of the iliopsoas tendon that flexes and rotates laterally the hip. This uncommon avulsion (Fig. 11.3) affects mostly track and field athletes and gymnasts, and the pain is radiated along the medial side of the proximal thigh. Hip extension and internal rotation are painful and consequently avoided.

11.3.7 Greater Trochanter

Glutei medius and minimus insert onto the GT. An abrupt abduction against resistance may determine GT avulsion. Being an extremely rare lesion, it is not possible to determine a sport-specific epidemiology [13, 14].

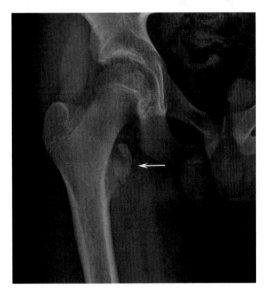

Fig. 11.3 Right type II LT avulsion fracture (*arrow*) in a 14-year-old male gymnast

Differently from most pelvic avulsions that have excellent prognosis, the rare GT avulsion was seldom associated with a severe complication, the femoral head osteonecrosis, regardless of the treatment—surgical or conservative [15].

11.4 Classification

The displacement is the most relevant prognostic factor, since large dislocations may determine nonunion, exostosis development, and/or significant loss of muscular strength. McKinney and coworkers have presented a useful classification system based on apophysis displacement [16]. The first three types include acute injuries and the fourth chronic outcomes.

Type I: Undisplaced avulsions
Type II: Avulsions displaced up to 2 cm
Type III: Avulsions displaced more than 2 cm
Type IV: Symptomatic nonunions and painful exostoses

11.5 Conservative Treatment

Most avulsion fractures of the pelvis may be effectively managed according to the nonoperative protocol set up by Metzmaker and Pappas in 1985 [4]. This protocol includes 5 stages:

Stage I. In the first 7–10 days after trauma, the pain is severe and the patient is either resting or walking with crutches and very restricted

weight bearing. Cryotherapy and NSAIDs are used to relieve the symptoms.

Stage II. In the second decade, the patient, still on crutches, is assisted in gentle active and passive exercises. The pain should be slowly subsiding.

Stage III. In the third decade after injury, the pain should be minimal, active and passive range-of-motion (ROM) exercises are encouraged, and crutches are progressively dismissed.

Stage IV. In the second month after injury, the lesion is healing with significant callus. The patient is allowed to begin a very light athletic training.

Stage V. If no complications occurred so far, the athlete may restore his standard training 2 months after injury.

11.6 Surgical Treatment

Only a few cases are eligible for surgery at the time of the first observation (Table 11.1), while it might be a viable option whenever the conservative approach fails [16]. All the painful outcomes may require surgical treatment (type IV), while severely displaced acute injuries (type III) may be considered suitable if the consequent shortening of the attached muscle or

Table 11.1 Site- and type-specific indications

	Type I	Type II	Type III	Type IV
IT	C	C*	C*	S
AIIS	C	C	S/C	S
ASIS	C	C	C	S
SCPS	C	C	C	S
IC	C	C	C	S
LT	C	C	C	S
GT	C	C	S	S

C conservative, *S* surgical
*S in case of sciatic nerve damage

the prominent profile of the detached apophysis could lead to a significant functional impairment. For instance, a post-traumatic elevated GT may result in abductor mechanism dysfunction with Trendelenburg gait and extra-articular impingement with limitation of abduction. Thus, open reduction and internal fixation of type III GT avulsions are often advocated [17]. The recent recognition of the subspine impingement after AIIS displaced avulsion fracture might suggest prompt reduction and fixation of type III AIIS injuries in youngsters participating in competitive sports requiring full hip ROM. Lastly, all the patients showing a sciatic nerve damage secondary to a displaced IT avulsion (types II or III) are candidate for timely fixation and nerve revision. As for the technique of fixation, most reports agree about using one or two half-threaded screws with or without washer, the diameter being adjusted according to the fragment size (from 4 to 6.5 mm).

Even though open reduction and screw fixation provide superior anatomical restoration in displaced injuries, and this may improve the post-injury level of performance, there is no consensus about the possibility that surgical treatment allows faster return to sport.

References

1. Sundar S, Carty H (1994) Avulsion fractures of the pelvis in children: a report of 32 fractures and their outcome. Skeletal Radiol 23:85–90
2. Rossi F, Dragoni S (2001) Acute avulsion fractures of the pelvis in adolescent competitive athletes: prevalence, location and sports distribution of 203 cases collected. Skeletal Radiol 30:127–131
3. Vandervliet EJ, Vanhoenacker FM, Snoeckx A, Gielen JL, Van Dyck P, Parizel PM (2007) Sports-related acute and chronic avulsion injuries in children and adolescents with special emphasis on tennis. Br J Sports Med 41(11):827–831
4. Metzmaker JN, Pappas AM (1985) Avulsion fractures of the pelvis. Am J Sports Med 13(5):349–358
5. Bencardino JT, Palmer WE (2002) Imaging of hip disorders in athletes. Radiol Clin N Am 40:267–287
6. Boutin RD, Russell CF, Steinbach LS (2002) Imaging of sports-related muscle injuries. Radiol Clin N Am 40:333–362
7. Pisacano RM, Miller TT (2003) Comparing sonography with MR imaging of apophyseal injuries of the pelvis in four boys. AJR Am J Roentgenol 181(1):223–230
8. Dhinsa BS, Jalgaonkar A, Mann B, Butt S, Pollock R (2011) Avulsion fracture of the anterior superior iliac spine: misdiagnosis of a bone tumour. J Orthop Traumatol 12(3):173–176
9. Miller A, Stedman GH, Beisaw NE et al (1987) Sciatica caused by an avulsion fracture of the ischial tuberosity. J Bone Joint Surg Am 69(1):143–145
10. Spinner RJ, Atkinson JL, Wenger DE, Stuart MJ (1998) Tardy sciatic nerve palsy following apophyseal avulsion fracture of the ischial tuberosity: case report. J Neurosurg 89(5):819–821
11. Dosani A, Giannoudis PV, Waseem M, Hinsche A, Smith RM (2004) Unusual presentation of sciatica in a 14-year-old girl. Injury 35(10):1071–1072
12. Larson CM, Kelly BT, Stone RM (2011) Making a case for anterior inferior iliac spine/subspine hip impingement: three representative case reports and proposed concept. Arthroscopy 27(12):1732–1737
13. Boome DM, Thompson JD (2000) Apophyseal fracture of the greater trochanter. South Med J 93:832–833
14. Mbubaegbu CE, O'Doherty D, Shenolikar A (1998) Traumatic apophyseal avulsion of the greater trochanter: case report and review of the literature. Injury 29:647–649
15. O'Rourke MR, Weinstein SL (2003) Osteonecrosis following isolated avulsion fracture of the greater trochanter in children: a report of two cases. J Bone Joint Surg Am 85(10):2000–2005
16. McKinney BI, Nelson C, Carrion W (2009) Apophyseal avulsion fractures of the hip and pelvis. Orthopedics 32(1):42
17. Wood JJ, Rajput R, Ward AJ (2005) Avulsion fracture of the greater trochanter of the femur: recommendations for closed reduction of the apophyseal injury. Injury Extra. 36:255–258

The Knee: Ligamentous Tears

12

Francesco Falciglia, Antonio Di Lazzaro
and Vincenzo Guzzanti

Knee ligament tears have increased over the past two decades and anterior cruciate ligament (ACL) injury is the most common in skeletally immature patients, because of the popularity of competitive athletic activities among adolescents. Shea et al. [1] looked at insurance claims over a five-year period for soccer players aged 5–18 years and noted that knee injuries constituted 22 % of all injuries, while ACL injuries accounted for 31 % of the total knee injury claims. Incidence of ACL injuries in skeletally immature patients is reported between 0.5 and 3 % in several studies [2]. The frequency of ACL injury increases steadily starting between the ages of 10 and 12 [3]. Kellenberger and Von Laer [4] noted, in a review of 330 patients with knee injuries, that 80 % of the patients with tibial eminence avulsions were younger than 12 years old, whereas 90 % of the patients with non-osseous ACL lesions were older than 12. As females approach skeletal maturity, and

certainly upon reaching it, they have a two- to eightfold greater risk of ACL rupture than do males. However, while still skeletally immature, boys have a higher incidence than girls.

12.1 Embryology

At the eighth week of fetal development, the knee develops between the mesenchymal rudiments of the femur and the tibia. Vascular mesenchyme becomes isolated within the joint and is the precursor of the cruciate ligaments and menisci. These tissues become immature fibroblasts, which soon develop into the cruciate ligaments. The anterior and posterior cruciate ligaments (PCL) become separate structures at the 18th week of development. Congenital anomalies of the knee appear early in fetal development [5]. Abnormalities in ligament development can lead to congenitally unstable knees. In the absence of cruciate ligaments, the intercondylar eminence of the tibia is aplastic because these structures have a role in shaping the femoral condyles and tibial plateau. Ipsilateral limb deformities are always associated with congenital anomalies of the knee [6].

F. Falciglia · A. Di Lazzaro
Department of Orthopedics, Pediatric Hospital
Bambino Gesù, S. Onofrio square 4, 00165 Rome,
Italy
e-mail: francesco.falciglia@opbg.net

A. Di Lazzaro
e-mail: antonio.dilazzararo@opbg.net

V. Guzzanti (✉)
Department of Orthopedics, Pediatric Hospital
Bambino Gesù, University of Cassino and Southern
Lazio, S. Onofrio square 4, 00165 Rome, Italy
e-mail: vguzzanti@yahoo.it

12.2 Anatomy

The distal femoral epiphysis is formed from a single nucleus of ossification that is present at birth and is the first epiphysis in the body to ossify. The nucleus of ossification of the proximal tibia appears at 2 months of age, while the secondary center of ossification appears between 10 and 14 years of age and unites with the proximal tibial epiphysis at 15 years. Proximal tibial physis fuses from the center out to the periphery and from posterior to anterior [7]. The distal femoral physis grows at a rate of 8–10 mm per year. It contributes about 40 % of the growth of the lower extremity. In contrast, the proximal tibial physis grows about 6 mm per year. It contributes about 30 % of the growth of the lower extremity. The distal femoral physis closes at 13 years of age in girls and 15 years in boys [8], while the proximal tibial physis closes at 14–15 years of age. The joint capsule that inserts from the proximal tibial epiphysis to the posterior aspect of the distal femoral epiphysis incompletely surrounds the knee. The medial collateral ligament (MCL) attaches the medial distal femoral physis, from the medial epicondyle to the medial tibia, deep to the gracilis and semitendinosus. The lateral collateral ligament (LCL) attaches the lateral distal femoral physis, from the lateral epicondyle to the proximal fibula. The adductor magnus muscle attaches on the medial portion of the femoral metaphysis. The gastrocnemius and the plantaris muscles attach on the posterior portion of the distal femoral metaphysis, just proximal to the physis.

The weaker strength of the physeal plate and the anatomic locations of the ligamentous origins and insertions may result in a physis injury rather than a pure ligament injury. The synovial fold surrounding the ACL originates on the lateral wall of the intercondylar notch at its posterior border and inserts anterior to the tibial spine. In children and adolescents, the distance between the superior margin of the ACL insertion and the femoral physis was only 3 mm and there was no significant change in this relationship with growth of the femur [9, 10]. The direction of the ACL within the knee results in its fibers being twisted approximately 90° as the knee moves from flexion to extension. The fibers can be differentiated into the anteromedial bundle and the posterolateral bundle. The anteromedial bundle shortens and the posterolateral bundle lengthens in extension, while in flexion the anteromedial bundle lengthens and the posterolateral bundle shortens. The middle genicular artery is the primary blood supply, while the inferior medial and lateral genicular arteries provide indirect blood supply.

The PCL is stronger, but shorter and less oblique in its direction, than the ACL. It is attached to the posterior intercondyloid fossa of the tibia, and to the posterior extremity of the lateral meniscus, and passes upward, forward, and medialward, to be fixed into the lateral and front part of the medial condyle of the femur. The PCL can be differentiated in an anterolateral and posteromedial bundle. The anterolateral bundle shortens in flexion and the posteromedial shortens in extension.

The MCL, the lateral ligament complex (fibular collateral ligament, popliteus tendon, and popliteofibular ligament), and the joint capsule constitute the capsule–ligamentous constraints. The MCL and LCL contribute to the primary stability of the knee during valgus and varus stress. The ACL is the primary restraint to anterior translation, while the PCL is the primary restraint to posterior translation.

12.3   Mechanism of Injury

12.3.1   ACL Injury

ACL tear often occurs during participation in athletic activities, with the two typical mechanisms being twisting and direct trauma [11, 12]. Sports that include cutting, jumping, and rapid changes in direction and velocity, such as soccer, basketball, and football, can expose players to an ACL injury. It is reported in the literature that combined valgus knee stress and decreased hip flexion in prepubescent subjects are important components in the pathomechanics of the injury [13]. Therefore, to reduce the rate of ACL injury in adolescent and children athletes, training and sport-specific skills are very important. When the foot is fixed while the leg sustains a deforming force, an ACL injury can result. The direction of tibial displacement can describe the deforming force. The ACL is stretched over the PCL when the tibia is adducted and internally rotated. The ACL is stretched over the lateral femoral condyle when the tibia undergoes a valgus stress with external rotation.

12.3.2 PCL Injury

Motor vehicle accidents are the most frequent cause of PCL tear, but athletic activities can also be responsible [14]. The typical mechanism of injury in athletics is a fall on a flexed knee while the foot is in a plantar-flexed position, which produces a posterior displacement of the tibia in relation to the femur. Another mechanism is a direct blow to the anterior portion of the tibia, while the knee is flexed. In severe trauma, a PCL rupture is often associated with other ligamentous injuries and is due to varus or valgus deforming stress combined with rotatory forces.

12.3.3 MCL and LCL Injuries

One of the most common injuries during athletic events is the MCL tear. The mechanism of injury is a rapid valgus movement from a direct blow to the lateral aspect of the knee. Patients report a history of pain and a sensation in the knee of "medial opening." Another mechanism of MCL injury is a direct valgus stress on the knee.

The isolated LCL injury is uncommon and results from a varus overstress to the knee [11].

12.4 Diagnosis

12.4.1 Clinical Examination

The diagnosis of an acute knee injury in skeletally immature patients requires a history and physical examination, integrated with imaging studies which are essential for accurate diagnosis. Clinical diagnostic accuracy is lower than in adults because of the physiological laxity in young patients.

Evaluation of laxity and range of motion in acute injuries is quite difficult because children are often frightened. The uninjured extremity is examined first, so the individual's physiological laxity can be distinguished from pathologic laxity [6, 15]. The use of an arthrometer such as the KT1000 or KT2000 was introduced to obtain objective data (Fig. 12.1).

A hemarthrosis, which appears a few hours after the trauma, can result from ACL injury, tibial spine avulsion, meniscal injury, osteochondral fracture, or patellar dislocation [16]. It is important to evaluate gait and alignment, range of motion, patellar apprehension and varus and valgus stability, and to palpate for tenderness over the joint line, ligamentous insertions and the borders of the patella and retinaculum. Radiographs should be performed before proceeding with the clinical laxity examination if a physeal plate injury is suspected. The order in which the laxity tests are performed is not important. The knee is evaluated in extension and at 30° of flexion for varus and valgus laxity. Anterior and posterior drawer should be checked with Lachman's test (Fig. 12.2a, b) and pivot shift evaluation, taking into account that children present hyperlaxity, which decreases with maturity [15]. Positive anterior drawer results, with Lachman's and flexion rotation drawer tests, indicate an ACL injury. A positive pivot

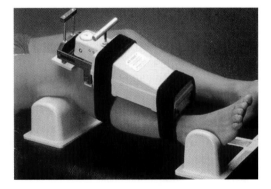

Fig. 12.1 The arthrometer KT2000 allows to compare both laxity of the injured and normal contralateral knee

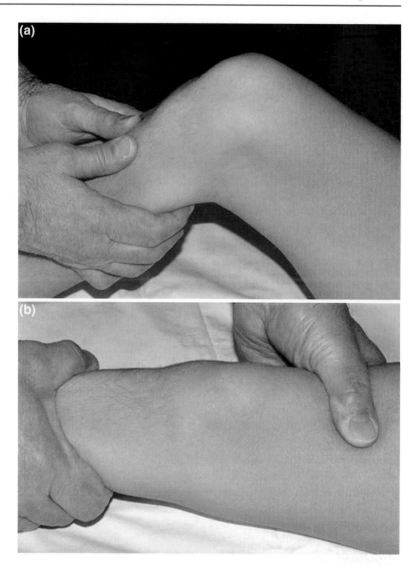

shift, jerk, or Losee's test, which in a chronic
case reproduces the patient's symptoms, suggests that an ACL injury is responsible for
symptoms of instability. However, it must be
remembered that jerk test can be positive during
the growth in patients of hyperlaxity. The
Lachman–Trillat test and with the quadriceps
active drawer test are performed to evaluate the
PCL. McMurray's test or Apley's test may also
help detect meniscal injury. It is important to
remember that all of these tests can be difficult
to perform in acute situations.

12.4.2   Imaging

Anteroposterior, lateral, oblique, tunnel, and
skyline (patellar profile) radiographs of the
knee are necessary to rule out bony injuries
such as tibial eminence avulsions (Fig. 12.17a,
b), Segond fractures, physeal injuries
(Fig. 12.3a, b), or osteochondral fractures.
Changes of the intercondylar notch and tibial
eminences may be indicative of ACL agenesis
(Fig. 12.4). Survey radiographs are comple-
mented by dynamic radiographs (Fig. 12.3b).

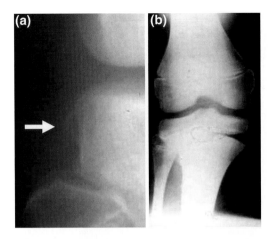

Fig. 12.3 **a** Segond fracture (*white arrow*) in an anteroposterior radiograph; **b** a valgus stress radiogram showing a physeal injury of the proximal tibial growth plate (from Guzzanti [58], with permission)

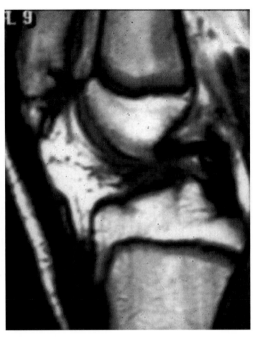

Fig. 12.5 Magnetic resonance imaging of a complete ACL tear

12.4.3 Injury of Collateral Ligaments

The medial structures are more frequently affected than the lateral or posterolateral structures, but the latter create more problems of instability. Though not frequent, lesions of the middle third of the MCL are observed in the adolescent period of growth. The clinical examination should be directed to evaluate both compartments [11]. It is always advisable to perform a radiographic examination as it can show a detachment of the ligament with an osteochondral fragment. If the fragment is only chondral and radiolucent, the X-ray is negative and the exact diagnosis is made when chondral fragment was matured as chondro-osseous fragment, unlike the Pellegrini–Stieda lesion.

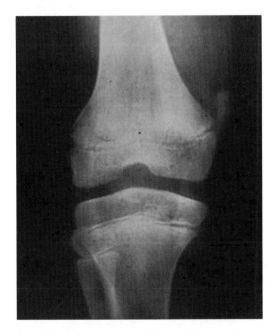

Fig. 12.4 The X-ray shows failure evidence of intercondylar eminence of the tibia due to the congenital absence of ACL

Magnetic resonance imaging (MRI) is utilized to further clarify the diagnosis (Fig. 12.5). Results are more accurate 10–15 days after the trauma [17].

In these cases, dynamic radiographs with valgus (Fig. 12.6a, b) and varus stress are necessary to evaluate the different degrees of ligamentous tears and to differentiate this type of injury from physeal injury (Fig. 12.3b). In the presence of swelling and patellar ballottement, arthrocentesis is recommended. If the latter is

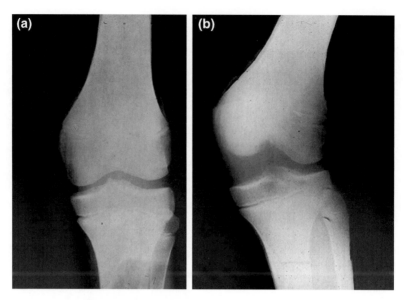

Fig. 12.6 **a** Static and **b** dynamic (valgus stress) radiographs showing a severe injury of MCL (from Guzzanti [58], with permission)

positive for hemarthrosis, we must suspect the presence of associated lesions (of the capsule, of the meniscus, of the ACL, or, if drops of fat are present in the blood, of the epiphyseal nuclei).

The treatment for isolated acute injuries of the medial or LCLs is usually conservative, consisting of immobilization in a brace at about 30° of flexion for 4–5 weeks. Only in cases with associated lesions (Fig. 12.7a, b), surgical repair is recommended [11]. The persistence of residual laxity after plaster cast treatment has been

observed in patients with complex lesions. Ligament injuries that occurred in children had repair capabilities but also exhibited similar problems as those observed in adults. The presence of an osteochondral detachment in the medial, lateral, or posterolateral compartment should induce the evaluation of the extent of tears and of the fragment stability (possibly with dynamic radiography) before deciding between conservative and surgical treatment.

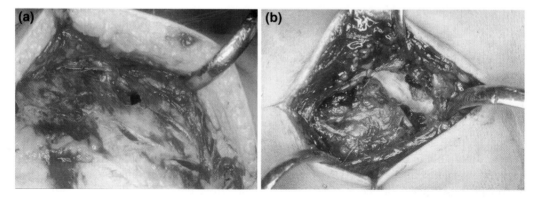

Fig. 12.7 Intra-operative features of **a** medial collateral ligament tear of the knee (patient with associated ACL and lateral meniscus tears and of **b** lateral collateral ligament tear of the knee with an injury of the posterolateral corner

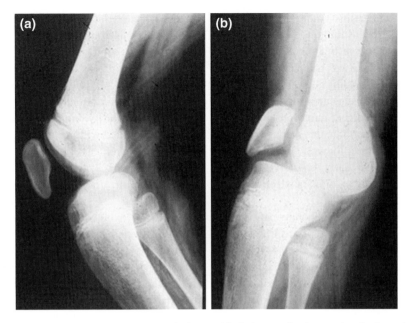

Fig. 12.8 **a** Congenital absence of ACL on lateral view and **b** during maximal extension the knee shows a severe instability

12.5 FAILURE: Anterior Cruciate Ligament

12.5.1 Congenital (Absence or Hypoplasia of the ACL)

The presence of anterior knee instability without a significant history of trauma in a child should raise suspicion of a congenital absence or hypoplasia of the ACL. Failure to find radiographic evidence of the intercondylar eminence is a useful tool for diagnosis (Fig. 12.4). The diagnosis of complete absence of the ACL is easier in the rare cases associated with other malformations. Agenesia may be combined with other anomalies of the lower limbs like proximal femoral hypoplasia and femur and/or tibia hypoplasia. The agenesia may be accompanied by severe instability in extension (Fig. 12.8a, b), requiring surgical treatment. The young age of the patients raises the same technical and biological problems that will be discussed in the following paragraph (acquired ACL injuries).

12.5.2 Acquired

12.5.2.1 ACL Injuries

Although it has been reported that the osteochondral structures have less resistance to stress than the capsule and ligaments in the growth period, isolated ACL injuries are being reported in adolescents with increasing frequency. This stems from a wider, more intense, and earlier participation of children in sporting activities and in increased diagnostic accuracy achieved with MRI and arthroscopy.

The ACL tear is classified as partial, total (proximal, distal, or middle third), and with bone avulsion. Partial tears and intercondylar eminence avulsion may lead to abnormal knee hyperlaxity secondary to ACL over distension that predisposes to secondary meniscal injuries.

Total ACL tears in skeletally immature patients create a difficult choice of treatment for patients, families, and treating physicians. The controversy regards operative timing and surgical technique, as the challenge is to perform a procedure that provides good clinical results for stability without damaging the physeal and epiphyseal growth plates. Traditionally, delayed anatomic ACL reconstructions were preferred [18] with non-operative treatment consisting of physical therapy, bracing and activity modification. The recent literature uniformly indicates that non-operative management of ACL tears in children results in a higher rate of instability that may progress to intra-articular damage, including meniscal tears [19]. Recently, there has been increased interest in early operative management to restore stability in skeletally immature knees.

Still, in the skeletally immature patient, the placement of physeal and epiphyseal drill holes and the passage of tendon grafts through them raise biological issues [20, 21]. Some reports suggest that the proximal tibial physis can be drilled without consequence, provided the lesion is central [12, 22]. Despite these reports, there are still uncertainties concerning drill hole magnitude and the safe ratio of the tunnel area of the femoral and tibial physis and of the tunnel area of the femoral and tibial epiphysis.

Data from rabbits and dogs indicate that the tolerable ratio of experimental physeal transgression must be calculated before surgery [23–25]. Moreover, Meller et al. [26] elucidated the following principles to avoid growth disturbances after a ACL reconstruction in skeletally immature sheep: (1) the tibial tuberosity should be spared to prevent genu recurvatum; (2) thermal damage to the growth plates should be avoided; (3) a small diameter drill should be used in the center of the growth plate; (4) a soft tissue graft should be used; (5) graft fixation should be achieved far from the growth plates; (6) the perforated growth plates should be filled with a soft tissue graft; and (7) the graft should be moderately pretensioned before fixation. As the studies in animals do not provide a directly transferable approach to this type of surgery in human adolescents, due care and the necessary adjustments must be considered.

In recent years, various intra-articular techniques have been adapted to the particular biological situation of young patients, following the known technique applied in adults. The goal is to provide ligament reconstruction following the biomechanical principles that suggest graft fixation in both anatomic areas of ACL insertion. This makes it impossible to avoid the involvement of the epiphysis and/or the physis of the knee. For these reasons, management of these injuries requires familiarity with methods of determining maturity, with the basic science of physeal injury and with the options available for appropriate treatment of athletic adolescents. Patients must be evaluated preoperatively for physiological maturity by assessment of Tanner stage [27], bone age [28], and remaining growth of the lower extremity [29], derived from the total growth and lower limb growth prediction based on assessment of chronologic age, bone age, parents' heights, patient's standing height, and patient's sitting height. Moreover, it is important to evaluate, preoperatively, limb length inequality (Fig. 12.9a–c), or axial deviation (Fig. 12.10) using standing lower limb X-ray.

In Tanner stage 1 patients, lower extremity growth projection is considered to be 50 % of total projected height. In Tanner stages 2 and 3 patients, lower extremity growth potential represents 40 % of total projected height. In Tanner stages 4 and 5 patients, lower extremity growth potential is 15–20 % of the total eventual height. Patients can be stratified as being at high, intermediate, or low risk of developing longitudinal and angular deformities after transphyseal ACL reconstruction.

High-risk patients are preadolescents who are in Tanner stage 1 and have a bone age of 11 years for girls and 12 years for boys and whose lower extremity growth potential exceeds 7 cm. These patients have not started their accelerated phase of adolescent growth, and radiographs show open distal femoral and proximal tibial physes [21] (Fig. 12.11a, b).

The intermediate-risk patients are in Tanner stages 2 or 3 and have a bone age of 13 years for girls and 15 years for boys and a lower extremity growth potential of 1.5–7 cm. They are at varying stages of their adolescent rapid growth phase, and radiographs show distal femoral and proximal tibial physes that are still open [30] (Fig. 12.12a, b).

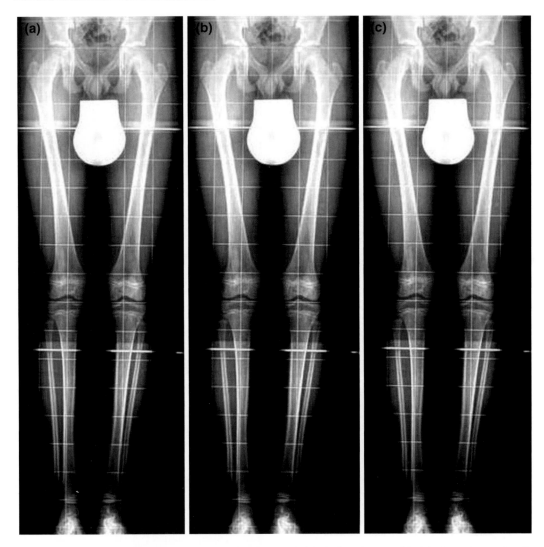

Fig. 12.9 Lower limb standing radiographs in the preoperative evaluation of patients with ACL tear: **a** example of patient with no limb length inequality or axial deviations; **b** case with right femur longer than the contralateral side; and **c** a patient showing the right femur and tibia longer than the contralateral ones

Low-risk patients are in Tanner stages 4 or 5, have a bone age of 14.5 years for girls and 16 for boys, are past their adolescent rapid growth phase, and have a lower extremity growth potential of less than 1.5 cm. Radiographic images in these patients show almost closed or closed distal femoral and proximal tibial physes [30] (Fig. 12.13a, b).

The basic science of physeal injury includes the knowledge of theoretical percentage of the total physeal area transgressed by a transphyseal femoral tunnel. This percentage must be calculated from the transverse plane with a CT scan or more commonly with MR, and from the frontal plane by anteroposterior knee radiographs, as described in experimental [23] and clinical studies [31].

Today, plans for surgical partial transphyseal reconstruction without clinical growth disturbances can be performed if the femoral physeal tunnel percentage area is <7 % in the frontal plane and <1 % in the transverse plane [31] (Fig. 12.14a, b).

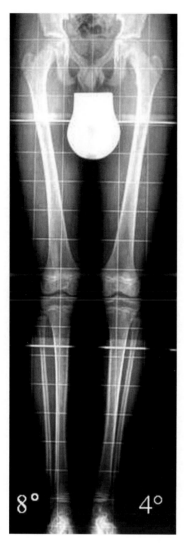

Fig. 12.10 Lower limb standing radiograph in the preoperative evaluation of patient with ACL tear showing a difference between femoral-tibial valgus angle: 8° on the a right side (*side of the tear*) and 4° on the left side (*non affected side*)

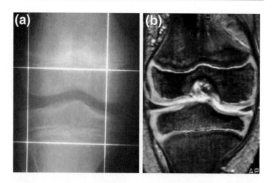

Fig. 12.11 a X-ray and **b** MR show wide open distal femoral and proximal tibial physes in a patient, male, with Tanner stage 1 and bone age of 12 years

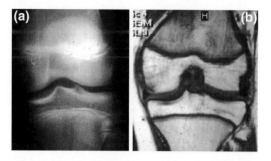

Fig. 12.12 a X-ray and **b** MR show open distal femoral and proximal tibial physes in a patient, male, with Tanner stage 2 and bone age of 13 years

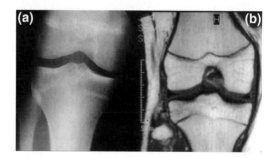

Fig. 12.13 a X-ray and **b** MR show closing distal femoral and proximal tibial physes in a patient, female, with Tanner stage 4 and bone age of 15 years

These considerations are relevant because patients in the high-risk group cannot be treated by transphyseal methods without risk of growth disturbances because, in a high percentage of them, the calculated physeal area of the drill hole is <7 % in the frontal plane or <1 % in the transverse plane. The same reason requires the avoidance of this type of operation in Tanner stages 2 or 3 patients in which the percentage of calculated damage is over the limits mentioned.

Despite these considerations, various isometric intra-articular ACL reconstruction proposed does not consider and/or document the biological limits described. That renders most experiences not reproducible. Some authors violated both the tibial and femoral physes (complete transphyseal techniques) [32–34] and

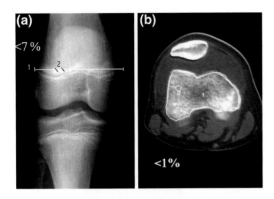

Fig. 12.14 Preoperative evaluation in a case of ACL tear: (**a**) Anteroposterior radiograph in which is possible to calculate the percentage of lesion caused by a tunnel of 6 mm in diameter *2* respect to the length of the growth plate *1*; (**b**) CT slide in which is possible to measure the percentage between the area of the growth plate *1* and the area of lesion caused by a tunnel of 6 mm of diameter *2*. To be safe the lesion of growth plate must be <7 % on A-P X-ray view (**a**) and <1 % on CT scan (**b**)

others just one physis (tibial or femoral) and one epiphysis (femoral or tibial) (partial transphyseal technique) [12, 19]. These patients could have been treated using physeal-sparing techniques [35–37]. In theory, these techniques should minimize the risk of growth disturbances or angular deformities by avoiding violation of the physes. Though a number of retrospective studies exist, with the majority achieving excellent results, there is a lack of prospective or comparative data that would advocate the superiority of one method over another. Macintosh and Darby [38] described good results using a portion of the iliotibial band looped around the lateral femoral condyle through the knee and attached distally to the proximal tibial metaphysis to reconstruct the ACL. This technique has been modified by others for use in skeletally immature patients. A recent systematic review identified six studies using modifications of this physeal-sparing extra-osseous reconstruction technique, none of which led to growth deformities at an average of 47.3 months after surgery. Patients had a mean age of 12.1 years [39].

Another all-epiphyseal technique was introduced by Guzzanti et al. [35], in which the semitendinosus and gracilis tendons were passed through a 6-mm eccentric tunnel drilled through the proximal tibial epiphysis between the physis

and articular surface with an exit at the tibial eminence. After a drill site was prepared in the distal femoral lateral epiphysis at the femoral notch, a staple was inserted into the femoral epiphysis and the hamstring tendons were looped through the staple (Fig. 12.15a). Five preadolescents (Tanner stage 1), with a minimum of 4 years of follow-up, demonstrated excellent stability and no leg length discrepancy or angular deformity (Fig. 12.15b).

Other studies have also shown that all-epiphyseal techniques can be safe and efficacious [36, 40]; however, there is one report of growth disturbance following ACL reconstruction using an epiphyseal femoral tunnel [41]. This last contradictory result requires consideration of new solutions, including alternative femoral fixations [42].

In the intermediate-risk group, the so-called partial transphyseal techniques involving one physis and one epiphysis may be performed [12, 21, 30, 43]. Growth characterization by preoperative clinical evaluation (history, physical examination, Tanner staging) and radiographic imaging methods (bone age, teleroentgenograms, radiographs, CT, and MRI) allows identification of patients in Tanner stages 2 and 3 with significant remaining lower extremity growth (≥5 cm). The calculated values of the percent area of physeal involvement produced by a transphyseal approach also aid in decisions about tunnel sites, sizes, and graft size.

Guzzanti et al. [31] claimed that violating the distal femoral physis with a drill hole and graft insertion would be acceptable if the injured area was less than 7 % in the frontal (calculated with an AP radiograph) and less than 1 % in the transverse plane of the total femoral physeal area (calculated with CT). Stable, isometric graft fixation is achieved without adverse sequelae with a 6-mm femoral physeal tunnel and 6-mm tibial epiphyseal tunnel. A femoral, rather than a tibial, physeal tunnel is chosen because experimental data from rabbits showed two of 18 cases developed tibia valga and one of 18 cases developed a shortened tibia after transphyseal tibial tunneling [23]. For this reason, an eccentric 6-mm drill hole was made through the proximal tibial epiphysis between the physis and articular

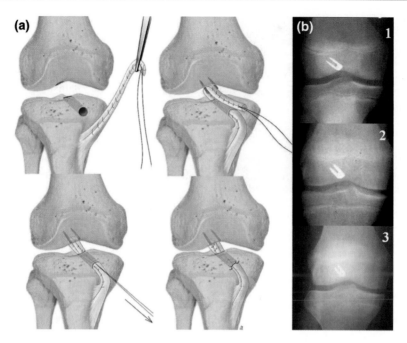

Fig. 12.15 **a** Schematic drawing of the physeal-sparing technique. The semitendinosus and gracilis tendons are passed through a 6-mm eccentric tunnel drilled through the central proximal tibial epiphysis. After a drill site prepared in the distal femoral lateral epiphysis at the femoral notch, a staple is inserted into the femoral epiphysis and the hamstring tendons are looped through a staple. The graft is sutured and fixed to tibial periosteum. (from Guzzanti [59], with permission). **b** X-rays show the position of the staple one month postoperative *1* and at three *2* and at five years *3* of follow-up. Note progressive incorporation of the staple into the lateral femoral condyle without signs of growth disturbance (from Guzzanti et al. [35], with permission)

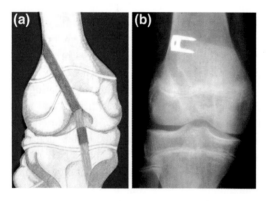

Fig. 12.16 **a** Schematic drawing of the partial transphyseal procedure. Semitendinosus and gracilis tendons, proximally detached, pass through 6 mm tunnels, one in the tibial epiphysis and the other in the femoral epiphysis and physis (from Guzzanti et al. [31], with permission). **b** X-ray at 38 months follow-up without growth disturbances

surface with the exit at the tibial eminence (Fig. 12.16a, b). Moreover, it should be kept in mind: to drill only one time the transphyseal tunnel and to perform it by hand to avoid thermal injury [33]; care should be taken to avoid potential injury to the perichondral ring [44]; the perforated growth plate should be filled with a soft tissue graft; tibial tuberosity should be spared to prevent genu recurvatum [26]; autologous semitendinous and gracilis tendons should be select as graft because of their distinct advantages in growing patients [45]. A series of surgical reports in which the femoral and tibial physes are violated (complete transphyseal methods) are reported in this intermediate-risk group [46, 47]. However, these authors do not report the percentage of lesions caused in their patients, making the techniques not repeatable.

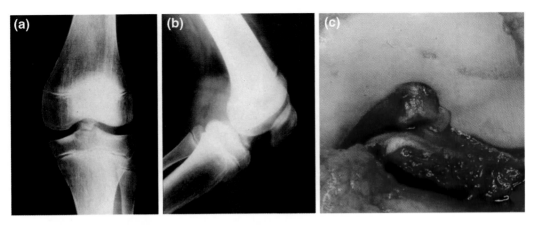

Fig. 12.17 **a** Anteroposterior and **b** lateral radiographs show an intercondylar tibial eminence avulsion (from Guzzanti [58], with permission); **c** Features of the lesion at surgery

The low-risk group of patients is treated with the same standard complete transphyseal methods used in adults because the potential for postoperative growth disturbances in this group is minimal or non-existent.

12.5.2.2 Failure of the ACL Associated with the Intercondylar Eminence Fracture

Tibial eminence avulsions are more common in children, because of the presence of an incompletely ossified tibial nucleus. The activities causing this fracture include motor vehicle accidents, sports injuries, and falls that cause hyperextension, hyperflexion, and/or rotation [48, 49]. Hyperextension and rotation are commonly related as in bicycle or motorbike injuries when the leg is extended to the floor for balance, while the body rotates around the leg during skidding or turning tight corners. In children, the ACL stretches prior to avulsion of the tibial spine and results in laxity [50].

Zaricznyj [48] stressed the importance of adequate reduction in all cases in which there is a lifting eminence, reducing the residual ACL laxity, especially for younger patients. Moreover, the author emphasized that a dislocation can determine residual atrophy and functional alteration of the ligament.

The association of eminence fracture with other ligament injuries has also been highlighted by other authors [11, 51]. Bradley et al. [51] described the association of MCL tear with injury to the middle third of the ACL in six patients under 12 years old. Clanton et al. [11] reported that five of nine children under 14 years old with collateral ligament injury had an intercondylar eminence fracture. In four of these five cases, there was also an ACL injury.

Therefore, when radiographs show an intercondylar eminence lesion, the diagnosis of associated ligamentous injury must be considered. It is therefore necessary to include stress radiography in the evaluation. MRI and/or arthroscopy is useful to confirm ligament injuries and to show meniscal or chondral lesions.

Tibial eminence avulsions can be classified into four types depending on displacement. Type I is undisplaced, Type II is partially displaced or hinged, Type III is completely displaced [52], and Type IV refers to comminuted fractures [48]. Conservative treatment with casting or a brace is recommended for Type I avulsions and reducible Type II avulsions. For displaced or irreducible fractures, open reduction and internal fixation achieve good outcomes and allow direct removal of meniscal or intermeniscal ligament entrapments (Fig. 12.17a–c).

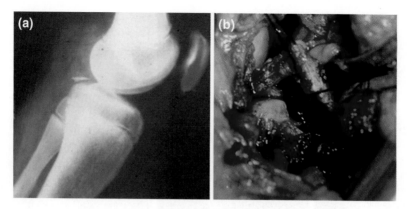

Fig. 12.18 **a** Lateral radiograph of a retrospinal surface avulsion with PCL injury and **b** operative findings

To stabilize the avulsed fragment, a physeal-sparing approach with short screw or suture fixation with a minimal (2 mm) tibial transepiphyseal or transphyseal tunnel is recommended. Suture fixation has the advantage of not requiring hardware removal, but it must be secure enough for early mobilization. Various methods of fixation, such as sutures [53], Kirschner wires or Steinman pins [54], and screws [49] can be applied using arthroscopic techniques.

12.5.3 PCL Injuries

Injuries to the PCL, whether partial, total (proximal, distal, or middle third), or with bone avulsion (Fig. 12.18a, b), are not frequent in children. However, a complete tear, if it occurs, can lead to marked laxity over time (Fig. 12.19a, b).

Radiographic examination is useful for revealing the osteochondral avulsion and any associated metaphyseal fractures of the tibia. As

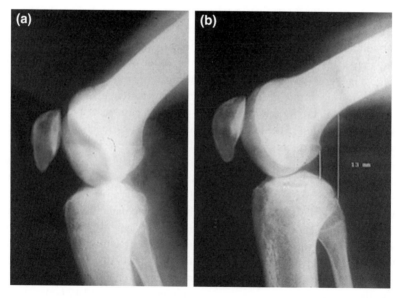

Fig. 12.19 Lateral radiograph (**a**) and dynamic X-ray posterior drawer test (**b**) showing a laxity due to a chronic PCL lesion

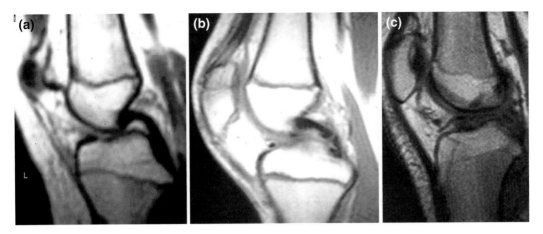

Fig. 12.20 Magnetic resonance imaging of normal PCL (**a**), partial PCL lesion (**b**), and complete PCL tear (**c**)

in children, the detached fragment may be all cartilaginous, MRI is recommended for confirmation of diagnosis (Fig. 12.20a–c). Sanders et al. [55] reported cases characterized by the detachment of the femoral insertion with the cartilaginous fragment. The possible presence of associated ligamentous and/or meniscal injuries can be confirmed by MRI or arthroscopy.

In general, PCL distal avulsion involves the posterior surface of the tibial plateau (the PCL attaches to the posterior intercondyloid fossa of the tibia).

Although few reported cases exist in the literature, surgical treatment is suggested. Crawford [56] claims to have had good results in a child patient with a PCL proximal avulsion using surgery, but an unfavorable result in another case that was treated conservatively. Mayer et al. [57] confirmed an adverse outcome in an 11-year-old patient treated conservatively.

References

1. Shea KG, Pfeiffer R, Jo HW, Curtin M, Apel PJ (2004) Anterior cruciate ligament injury in pediatric and adolescent soccer players: an analysis of insurance data. J Pediatr Orthop 24(6):623–628
2. Bales CP, Guettler JH, Moorman CT 3rd (2004) Anterior cruciate ligament injuries in children with open physes: evolving strategies of treatment. Am J Sports Med 32:1978–1985
3. Gianotti SM, Marshall SW, Hume PA, Bunt L (2009) Incidence of anterior cruciate ligament injury and other knee ligament injuries: a national population-based study. J Sci Med Sport 12:622–627
4. Kellenberger R, von Laer L (1990) Nonosseous lesions of the anterior cruciate ligaments in childhood and adolescence. Prog Pediatr Surg 25:123–131
5. Arnoczk SP, Warren RF (1988) Anatomy of the cruciate ligaments. In: Fedgin JA (ed) The cruciate ligament. Churchill Livingstone, New York, pp 179–195
6. DeLee JC, Curtis R (1983) Anterior cruciate ligament insufficiency in children. Clin Orthop Relat Res 172:112–118
7. Ogden JA, Tross RB, Murphy MJ (1980) Fractures of the tibial tuberosity in adolescents. J Bone Joint Surg 62A:205–215
8. Anderson M, Green WT, Messner MB (1963) Growth and predictions of growth in the lower extremities. J Bone Joint Surg 45A:1–14
9. Larsen MW, Garrett WE Jr, Delee JC, Moorman CT (2006) Surgical management of anterior cruciate ligament injuries in patients with open physes. J Am Acad Orthop Surg 14(13):736–744 (Review)
10. Behr CT, Potter HG, Paletta GA Jr (2001) The relationship of the femoral origin of the anterior cruciate ligament and the distal femoral physeal plate in the skeletally immature knee. An anatomic study. Am J Sports Med 29(6):781–787
11. Clanton TO, DeLee JC, Sanders B et al (1979) Knee ligament injuries in children. J Bone Joint Surg 61A:119–123
12. Lipscomb AB, Anderson AF (1986) Tears of the anterior cruciate ligament in adolescents. J Bone Joint Surg 68A:19–28
13. Noyes FR, Barber-Westin SD, Fleckenstein C et al (2005) The drop-jump screening test: difference in lower limb control by gender and effect of

neuromuscular training in female athletes. Am J Sports Med 33:197–207

14. Cross MJ, Powell JF (1984) Long-term followup of posterior cruciate ligament rupture: a study of 116 cases. Am J Sports Med 12:292–297

15. Falciglia F, Guzzanti V, Di Ciommo V, Poggiaroni A (2009) Physiological knee laxity during pubertal growth. Bull NYU Hosp Jt Dis 67(4):325–329

16. Luhmann SJ (2003) Acute traumatic knee effusions in children and adolescents. J Pediatr Orthop 23:199–202

17. Major NM, Beard LN Jr, Helms CA (2003) Accuracy of MR imaging of the knee in adolescents. AJR Am J Roentgenol 180:17–19

18. Woods GW, O'Connor DP (2004) Delayed anterior cruciate ligament reconstruction in adolescents with open physes. Am J Sports Med 32(1):201–210

19. Henry J, Chotel F, Chouteau J, Fessy MH, Berard J, Moyen B (2009) Rupture of the anterior cruciate ligament in children: early reconstruction with open physes or delayed reconstruction to skeletal maturity? Knee Surg Sports Traumatol Arthrosc 17:748–755

20. Janarv P, Nystrom A, Werner S, Hirsch G (1996) Anterior cruciate ligament injuries in skeletally immature patients. J Pediatr Orthop 16:673–677

21. Lo IK, Kirkley A, Fowler OJ, Miniaci A (1997) The outcome of operatively treated anterior cruciate disruptions in the skeletally immature child. Arthroscopy 13(5):627–634

22. Koman JD, Sanders JO (1999) Valgus deformity after reconstruction of the anterior cruciate ligament in a skeletally immature patient. A case report. J Bone Joint Surg 81(A):711–715

23. Guzzanti V, Falciglia F, Gigante A, Fabbriciani C (1994) The effect of intra-articular ACL reconstruction on the growth plate of rabbits. J Bone Joint Surg 76B:960–963

24. Stadelmaier DM, Arnoczky SP, Dodds J, Ross H (1995) The effect of drilling and soft tissue grafting across open growth plate. A histological study. Am J Sports Med 23:431–435

25. Janarv PM, Wikstrom B, Hirsch G (1998) The influence of transphyseal drilling and tendon grafting on bone growth: an experimental study in the rabbit. J Pediatr Orthop 18:149–154

26. Meller R, Kendoff D, Hankemeier S, Jagodzinski M, Grotz M, Knobloch K, Krettek C (2008) Hindlimb growth after a transphyseal reconstruction of the anterior cruciate ligament: a study in skeletally immature sheep with wide-open physes. Am J Sports Med 36:2437–2443

27. Tanner JM (1989) Foetus into man: physical growth from conception to maturity, 2nd edn. Castlemead Productions, Ware

28. Greulich WW, Pyle SI (1959) Radiographic Atlas of Skeletal development of the hand and wrist, 2nd edn. Stanford University Press, Stanford

29. Dimeglio A (1984) La Croissance en Orthope' die. EMC Paris, Appareil locomoteur.14009, A10, 3:1–8

30. Pressman AE, Letts RM, Jarvis JC (1997) Anterior cruciate ligament tears in children: an analysis of operative versus nonoperative treatment. J Pediatr Orthop 17:505–511

31. Guzzanti V, Falciglia F, Stanitski CL (2003) Pre-operative evaluation and anterior cruciate ligament reconstruction technique for skeletally immature patients in Tanner stage 2 and 3. Am J Sports Med 31(6):941–948

32. Liddle AD, Imbuldeniya AM, Hunt DM (2008) Transphyseal reconstruction of the anterior cruciate ligament in prepubescent children. J Bone Joint Surg 90B:1317–1322

33. Gebhard F, Ellermann A, Hoffmann F, Jaeger JH, Friederich NF (2006) Multicenter-study of operative treatment of intraligamentous tears of the anterior cruciate ligament in children and adolescents: comparison of four different techniques. Knee Surg Sports Traumatol Arthrosc 14(9):797–803

34. Hui C, Roe J, Ferguson D, Waller A, Salmon L, Pinczewski L (2012) Outcome of anatomic transphysealanterior cruciate ligament reconstruction in Tanner stage 1 and 2 patients with open physes. Am J Sports Med 40(5):1093–1098

35. Guzzanti V, Falciglia F, Stanitski CL (2003) Physeal-sparing intraarticular anterior cruciate ligament reconstruction in preadolescents. Am J Sport Med 31(6):949–953

36. Lawrence JT, Bowers AL, Belding J, Cody SR, Ganley TJ (2010) All-epiphyseal anterior cruciate ligament reconstruction in skeletally immature patients. Clin Orthop Relat Res 468(7):1971–1977

37. Nikolaou P, Kalliakmanis A, Bousgas D, Zourntos S (2011) Intraarticular stabilization following anterior cruciate ligament injury in children and adolescents. Knee Surg Sports Traumatol Arthrosc 19(5):801–805

38. MacIntosh D, Darby T (1976) Lateral substitution reconstruction. In: Proceedings of universities, colleges, councils and associations. J Bone Joint Surg 58B: article 142

39. Vavken P, Murray MM (2011) Treating anterior cruciate ligament tears in skeletally immature patients. Arthroscopy 27(5):704–716

40. Chicorell AM, Nasreddine AY, Kocher MS (2011) Physeal-sparing anterior cruciate ligament reconstruction with iliotibialband. Clin Sports Med 30(4):767–777

41. Lawrence JT, West RL, Garrett WE (2011) Growth disturbance following ACL reconstruction with use of an epiphyseal femoral tunnel: a case report. J Bone Joint Surg 93(A):1–6

42. Stanitski CL (1995) Anterior cruciate ligament injury in the skeletally immature patient: diagnosis and treatment. J Am Acad Orthop Surg 3(3):146–158

43. Andrews M, Noyes FR, Barber-Westin SD (1994) Anterior cruciate ligament allograft reconstruction in the skeletally immature athlete. Am J Sport Med 22:48–54

44. Kocher MS, Saxon HS, Hovis WD, Hawkins RJ (2002) Management and complications of anterior cruciate ligament injuries in skeletally immature patients: survey of the Herodicus Society and The ACL Study Group. J Pediatr Orthop 22(4):452–457

45. Anderson AF (2003) Transepiphyseal replacement of the anterior cruciate ligament in skeletally immature patients. A preliminary report. J Bone Joint Surg Am 85-A(7):1255–1263

46. Kocher M, Smith JT, Zoric B, Lee B, Micheli LJ (2007)Transphyseal anterior cruciate ligament reconstruction in skeletally immature pubescent adolescents. J Bone Joint Surg 89(12)A: 2632–2639

47. Kumar S, David A, Hunt DM (2013) Transphyseal anterior cruciate ligament reconstruction in the skeletally immature. J Bone Joint Surg 95A:1–6

48. Zaricznyj B (1977) Avulsion fracture of the tibial eminence: treatment by open reduction and pinning. J Bone Joint Surg 59A:1111–1114

49. Hunter RE, Willis JA (2004) Arthroscopic fixation of avulsion fractures of the tibial eminence: technique and outcome. Arthroscopy 20:113–121

50. Park HJ, Urabe K, Naruse K, Aikawa J, Fujita M, Itoman M (2007) Arthroscopic evaluation after surgical repair of intercondylar eminence fractures. Arch Orthop Trauma Surg 127:753–757

51. Bradley GW, Shives TC, Samuelson KM (1979) Ligament injures in the knee of children. J Bone Joint Surg 61A:588–591

52. Meyers MH, McKeever FM (1970) Fracture of the intercondylar eminence of the tibia. J Bone Joint Surg 52A:1677–1684

53. Huang TW, Hsu KY, Cheng CY, Chen LH, Wang CJ, Chan YS et al (2008) Arthroscopic suture fixation of tibial eminence avulsion fractures. Arthroscopy 24:1232–1238

54. Jung YB, Yum JK, Koo BH (1999) A new method for arthroscopic treatment of tibial eminence fractures with eyed Steinmann pins. Arthroscopy 15:672–675

55. Sanders WE, Wilkins KE, Neidre A (1980) Acute insufficiency of the posterior cruciate ligament in children. J Bone Joint Surg 62A:129–130

56. Crawford AH (1976) Fractures about the knee in children. Orthop Clin North 7(A):639–656

57. Mayer PJ, Michelli LJ (1979) Avulsion of the femoral attachment of the posterior cruciate ligament in an eleven-year-old-boy. J Bone Joint Surg 61:431–432

58. Guzzanti V (2010) Le lesioni legamentose del ginocchio. In: Sessa S, Villani C (eds) Ortopedia e traumatologia. Monduzzi editore, Parma, pp 313–317

59. Guzzanti V (2006) Technical note-24-3 ACL reconstruction: all Epiphyseal technique with semitendinosus and gracilis tendon. In: Micheli LJ, Kocher MS (eds) The pediatric and adolescent knee. Saunders, Elsevier, Philadelphia

The Knee: Meniscal Lesions

13

Piero Volpi, Matteo Cervellin, Corrado Bait,
Emanuele Prospero, A. Redaelli and Alessandro Quaglia

The knee is a complex joint structure, composed of various elements that together functionally regulate and stabilize the articulation, protecting it from external stress and regulating homeostasis. In this complex mechanism, the menisci have a very important role, both as joint stabilizers and being elements involved in load transmission and distribution between the femoral condyle and the tibial plateau.

The menisci are C-shaped at the axial plane (more or less closed depending on whether lateral or medial, respectively), with slightly concave upper surfaces and flat undersides that match their respective interfaces with the femoral condyles and tibial plateau. They act as adapters and their capacity to uniformly distribute loads and absorb shock on the joint surface is extremely important; the menisci cover about two-thirds of the tibial plateau surface. Some studies have shown that after partial meniscectomy of approximately 10 % of the meniscus surface the load on the articular heads increased 65 %. After subtotal meniscectomy, the load increase is 200 % [1]. Hence, the importance of conservative surgery when

treating meniscal fibrocartilage, particularly in young people.

The menisci are anchored to the tibia and femur by means of a group of ligaments. The medial meniscus is attached to the joint capsule; tibial insertion is via the intermeniscal ligament at the anterior horn and the insertional ligament that reaches the intercondylar plateau of the tibia. The lateral meniscus enters the joint capsule except at the level of the hiatus, resulting more mobile than the medial; the intermeniscal ligament joins the anterior horn to the tibia; the Wrisberg and Humphrey ligaments anchor the posterior horn to the medial femoral condyle and the insertional ligaments to the intercondylar side of the tibia.

The internal structure of the meniscus is microscopically heterogeneous with specific characteristics according to the forces to which it is submitted. The peripheral portion is rich in collagen fibers that are radially and longitudinally aligned, granting high resistance capacity to the centrifugal forces. The middle, avascular portion is richer in GAG and H_2O, giving resistance to compressive forces, while collagen fibers are here numerically less represented and organized.

It is therefore evident that the importance of conserving as far as possible these structures, especially in young people, to avoid overloading and instability that can lead to cartilaginous tears and early arthritic degeneration [2–5].

Regrettably, menisci are fibrocartilagenous structures with scarce self-healing properties and a scarce cellular component. This is due to the

P. Volpi (✉) · M. Cervellin · C. Bait · E. Prospero ·
A. Redaelli · A. Quaglia
Sports Traumatology and Knee Surgery, Humanitas
Clinical and Research Center, Manzoni, 20089
Rozzano, MI, Italy
e-mail: piero.volpi@humanitas.it

M. Cervellin
e-mail: matteo.cervellin@humanitas.it

V. Guzzanti (ed.), *Pediatric and Adolescent Sports Traumatology*,
DOI: 10.1007/978-88-470-5412-7_13, © Springer-Verlag Italia 2014

fundamental peripheral vascularization; the vascular contribution coming from the medial superior and inferior genicular arteries for the medial meniscus, and from the lateral genicular artery for the external meniscus, is distributed to the menisci through a capillary network limited to the most peripheral portion, namely the *red zone*. During the fetal period and until birth, meniscal vascularization presents more distributed, but during growth (starting from the end of the first years), it progressively drops until limitedly represented in the mural area (red–red zone) at the end of growth. Moreover, meniscal vascularization has topographic characteristics, resulting more concentrated at the meniscal horn level, with respect to the body. Nutritional contribution to the more central tissues (white–white and red-white) is guaranteed by the diffusion of synovial fluid, favored by the alternation of loading and unloading that allows a sort of "sponge effect." In the pre-adolescent age, however, the vascularized area is variable and can also involve those two-thirds in which the adults are avascular.

Some studies in dogs show how injuries to areas with a vascular supply can evolve toward recovery, while it is not possible to repair lesions in avascular areas [6, 7].

Indeed, the potential recovery of a meniscal tear depends on various factors: first of all on the age of the patient ; in younger patients with greater vascularization, the prognosis for meniscal repair is better [8–10]. The topography of the tear influences results of meniscal sutures; sutures of tears located at the anterior or posterior horn are reported in the literature with more favorable results [11, 12]. Moreover, the type of tear influences results of meniscal repair; longitudinal or bucket-handle tears, which present greater integrity of the circumferential fibers, have greater possibility of recovery than complex or radial lesions [13–15]. Meniscal sutures associated with ACL reconstruction in the same surgical time present better results than isolated meniscal sutures [16–19], probably in relation to greater bleeding. Lastly, it is our belief that tear timing is also important; some authors achieved better results in meniscal sutures performed within 6 weeks from the trauma [20].

So, on the one hand, vascular anatomy and its changes, which alternate from neonatal period to adolescence, would explain the difficult recovery of meniscal lesions involving the white zone and, on the other, they must guide the surgeon toward a suitable therapeutic approach for young patients, which should lead for the most part to conservative options to protect the integrity and favor the recovery of meniscal tears in the adolescent population.

Meniscal injuries in children and adolescents, which today represent 5 % of all meniscal injuries, are on the increase [21]. The reason for this increased incidence may be traced to the rise in participation in contact sports such as football, basketball, volleyball, of a growing number of pre-adolescents with more intense training requirements and rhythms, such as to justify the term "knee abuser." Furthermore, improvement in diagnostic tools enable a more precise diagnosis, despite MRI in growing subjects would seem to have less sensitivity than for fully grown adults (62 % vs. 92 %), maintaining, however, a good specificity (90 % vs. 87 %) [22–25].

These are traumatic injuries to the knee which present with a physiologically greater ligamentous laxity than that in adults, where the menisci are submitted to cutting and compressive forces, obviously more so when practicing intense physical activity. The lesions may be isolated or associated with ligament injuries, most commonly with ACL injury. The medial meniscus is the most frequently involved, because it is more rigidly connected to the joint capsule and the tibial plateau and then subjected to higher forces.

Meniscal injury in young patients is a critical event for the future of the joint. As previously mentioned, partial or subtotal meniscectomy would expose the joint cartilage to excessive force, inevitably leading to torn cartilage and early arthritic processes. This is why it is necessary to treat this type of meniscal pathology with the most conservative approach possible, always considering meniscal suturing as first surgical choice.

13.1 Anatomy of the Injuries

As for adults, meniscal injuries in children and adolescents can be defined by their appearance and orientation, as well as by localization and vascularization of the injury. Based on their shape and course, they can be classified into *vertical, horizontal,* and *complex*. Vertical injuries, in turn, are divided into radial and longitudinal, and they involve the meniscus from the tibial to the femoral side. Longitudinal injuries usually affect the outside margin of the meniscus, where the collagen fibers usually take a longitudinal course; they are more frequent in young, active patients and can lead to bucket-handle tears should the fragment become trapped between the femur and tibia, frequently luxating in the intercondylar notch. Longitudinal tears occurring in the red–red zone are often potentially repairable, especially in young subjects, whereas radial lesions have a course from the free margin toward the periphery with limited repair capabilities; they mainly affect the posterior body and horn of the lateral meniscus and the posterior horn of the medial meniscus. They are usually located in the white–white zone where the collagen fibers generally take a radial course.

Horizontal tears comprise complete or incomplete fissuring (flap); these affect mainly adults over 40 years of age. The tear divides the meniscus into two separate pieces, tibial, and femoral, one of which can turn over and form a flap.

Meniscal tears, however, are better understood and classified during arthroscopic examination that allows to choose the best treatment for the specific case. In agreement with Noyes [26], the meniscus is divided into three portions:
- anterior third.
- medial third
- posterior third
  and further divided into
- Vascularized peripheral portion (zone RED–RED)
- Partially vascularized median portion (zone RED–WHITE)

- Inner portion or freeboard avascular (zone WHITE–WHITE)

The orientation of the lesion is another critical component in choosing the appropriate treatment, we recognize the following:
- horizontal tears
- radial tears
- longitudinal tears
- complex lesions (set of multiple fracture lines).

This classification makes it possible in a simple and effective means to establish immediately which are the "reparable" injuries and which ones must be "sacrificed" with a meniscectomy.

Lastly, discoid meniscus tears should be mentioned in the morphologic classification. This anatomic variation typically affects the lateral meniscus and has a prevalence in the literature of 6–14 % approximately. When intact and asymptomatic, it is best left alone. In the presence of a lesion, symptoms are typically represented by joint pain, catching and locking. The most frequent injury is a double radial lesion: in case of tears, typically involving the more mobile, excess tissue interposed between the femur and tibia, it will be necessary to regulate the meniscus in an attempt to reproduce the normal shape of a healthy meniscus. Some authors arthroscopically remove the excess tissue and suture the outer portion [27] (Figs. 13.1, 13.2).

13.2 Diagnosis

A correct approach to diagnosing meniscal injuries in children cannot primarily disregard an accurate anamnesis, despite often, just because of age, younger children do not know how to report the incident triggering. In young patients, in fact, injuries are of a traumatic nature; "young," vascularized, elastic menisci not affected by degenerative injury. It is therefore important to pursue a traumatic event and make an early diagnosis in order to have a good chance of recovery.

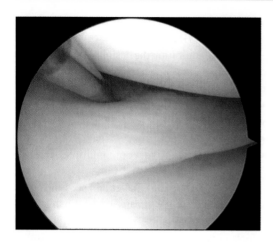 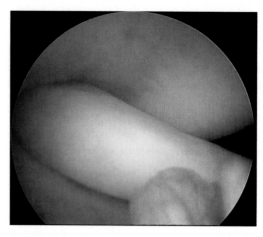

Fig. 13.1 RR longitudinal lesion at posterior horn of medial meniscus

Fig. 13.2 Bucket-handle meniscal lesion

The second step is a careful and scrupulous clinical evaluation, starting with observing deambulation to detect any lameness or extension deficit during step. Secondly, establish the morphotype of the knee. Test the range of motion of the knee, if painful in flexion and extension, if there is a limitation (mechanical or analgesic) of the extension, which may be indicative for a bucket handle lesion. Check for hemarthrosis or effusion, especially in the acute phase.

It is essential to assess knee stability, especially in the presence of a history of distortion, by testing the central pivot, the stability of medial and lateral compartments. It is important to assess any patellofemoral pain, patellar instability, eventual malalignment of the extensor mechanism. Specific meniscal tests are then performed: palpatory check for pain at the medial and lateral joint line; usually, the first test is performed in suspected meniscal tear, and it is positive in 60–80 % in the presence of a lesion. McMurray's test is carried out with the patient in a supine position making abduction/extrarotation and adduction/intrarotation movements of the foot with the knee at various degrees of flexion. A positive test produces a click, or causes pain; it is not a very sensitive test. Apley's test is performed with the patient in a prone position with knee flexed at 90°, exerting pressure on the foot and intra-extra-rotating the foot; the test is positive, if pain is provoked.

During the Steinmann test, the patient is sitting on the couch with the leg pendant and knee flexed at 90°, internal rotation and external rotation cause pain. The Finocchietto's test is positive for lesions of the posterior horn of the medial meniscus; with the knee flexed to 90° with patient supine and the foot on the bed, it exerts traction on the tibia with both hands, you will appreciate an anterior subluxation of the tibia and click due to contact between the posterior horn of the medial meniscus and medial femoral condyle. In the Ege test, the patient should perform a flexion–extension of the knee in the load, feet first in internal rotation, then in external rotation and it is positive in the case of pain. In the Thessaly' test, the patient should perform internal and external rotation of the knee in monopodalic load, with varying degrees of flexion (5° and 20°), the test is positive if pain, click or failure. Finally, in *bounce home test,* the patient requires to actively extend the knee and then performed a further extension by the examiner; in the presence of meniscal lesions, the patient will experience pain.

13.3 Radiology

Diagnostic imaging, if it is reported to sprain, is expected to begin execution of X-rays in anterior/posterior and lateral of both knees; this to show the presence of fractures of the tibial spines, osteochondral detachment, intra-articular loose bodies, bone detachment, epiphyseal fractures, falling in the differential diagnosis in case of painful or blocked knee following a sprain. In meniscal lesions, X-rays are usually negative, so the second step to perform is the MRI of the affected knee. The diagnosis of meniscal injury must be completed with MRI which is the gold standard in diagnostic radiology for this type of pathology in children and adolescents. It is important to remember that MRI should be used as adjunct to confirm and not substitute a correct and scrupulous clinical assessment.

Healthy menisci show no signal at MRI and are seen as black, with no signal in their proper context. Meniscal vascularization is more represented in children than in adults, and at MRI, it shows as a signal in the context of the peripheral portion of the meniscus, not to be confused with degenerative areas or tears. New technologies supply us with equipment able to elaborate images at a high resolution, with good sensitivity and specificity in the diagnosis of meniscal fibrocartilage disorders.

The joint is graded within the three space levels (axial, coronal, and sagittal) and with diverse weights (T1, T2, and fat suppression), enabling an extremely detailed three-dimensional evaluation of the anatomical structures. These images must always be scrupulously assessed personally by the orthopedic surgeon and, fundamental for a correct diagnosis, compared with the clinical examination observed. In this way, a complete picture can be obtained and the images correctly interpreted at MR.

Therefore, much important information can be gleaned from the magnetic resonance concerning lesion topography, which can be localized at the medial or lateral meniscus or both, and may involve the posterior or anterior horn, or the meniscal body.

Moreover, the various types of injury (horizontal, vertical, or bucket handle) and the presence of dislocated meniscal fragments in a discoid meniscus can be recognized. You will need to assess the presence of joint effusion,

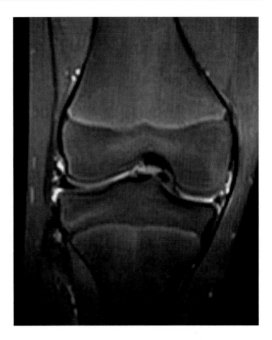

Fig. 13.3 Bucket-handle lesion of medial meniscus (MRI)

excluding lesions of the remaining articular structures (ACL, PCL, MCL, LCL, popliteus tendon), osteochondral lesions and osteochondral detachments.

A study by Kocher et al. shows that MRI in children and adolescents has a sensitivity of 67 and 79 % in the diagnosis of meniscal lesions to ML and MM, respectively, while specificity of 92 % [28]. This confirms that the RM cannot be separated from the evaluation clinic but must integrate and possibly confirm a clinical suspicion (Fig. 13.3).

13.4 Treatment

Until the early 1970s and 1980s, a meniscal tear in an adolescent, or young child, condemned the joint to secure early arthritic degeneration; in fact, meniscal tears were treated with open meniscectomy. However, already in 1940, [29] the first consequences related to meniscectomy were observed and reported. So the importance of the menisci was gradually recognized and their role as shock absorbers and stabilizers joint, stimulating in search of surgical techniques and devices that allow to keep as much as possible this important joint structures.

The modern arthroscopy has revolutionized the concept of meniscectomy toward a concept of selective meniscectomy, in which the meniscus could be assessed, palpated, and regularized at the free margin and possibly repaired. However, as mentioned above, a selective meniscectomy increased load forces on the articular cartilage, predisposing to degenerative processes of the affected area.

The choice of treatment in meniscal injuries of children and adolescents is an important moment for the future of the joint. The therapeutic decision is different in children than in adults both for the most serious long-term consequences that may occur as a result of meniscectomy, both for the higher capacities that there are in younger menisci. This choice depends on several factors, mainly the age. We repeat that the meniscus during the prenatal phase is richly vascularized, at 9 months of age the third central became avascular and at 10-year blood supply began to be gradually restricted to the third peripheral, taking on the characteristics adult. The type of injury, the extent, depth, location, quality of meniscal tissue, the timing of the injury, the functional demands of the patient, associated injuries, and a previous meniscal surgery are all critical factors in choosing surgical.

Conservative treatment (abstention) is reserved for incomplete lesions, affecting less than 50 % of the thickness of meniscal, and for small stable lesions (<3 mm) near to the meniscal wall. These lesions usually repertate during diagnostic arthroscopy, often associated with ACL reconstruction procedure, have the best chance of spontaneous recovery.

In diagnosis and treatment, an accurate arthroscopic evaluation of the lesion is, therefore, essential.

Though, today, radiological techniques provide detailed images, information about stability and depth, diriment in the therapeutic choice, can be clearly learned only inspecting the lesion with the use of the feeler.

Indications for the surgery are established, and the range of possibilities available to the surgeon are as follows:

- Suture
- Selective meniscectomy
- Subtotal meniscectomy
- Meniscal replacement

The procedures most frequently implemented are the suture and selective meniscectomy, reserving the other in cases fortunately rare.

13.4.1 Meniscal Repair

It is clearly important to save or restore, if possible, the integrity of the structures in order to long-term preserve the joint by the articular cartilage damage. The best candidate for meniscal suture is a young patient with longitudinal lesion size <15 mm, recent, localized at RR area of healthy tissue without previous surgery on the same meniscus, with an associated ACL injury [30]. On the contrary, sutures are not recommended for degenerative menisci, with older injury than 6 months, complex lesion, near WW.

In recent years, particular attention has been paid to development of the meniscal sutures, leading to improvements both in terms of surgical techniques and the surgical device. Today, the sutures are performed in arthroscopy with *outside-in, inside-out,* and *all-inside* techniques.

The *inside-out* sutures are versatile and allow suturing of all regions of the medial and lateral meniscus. Using non-absorbable wires (PDS 2-0) mounted on flexible needles, the suture is practiced with the aid of cannulas (single or double) inserted from the opposite portal to the compartment meniscus to be sutured. Through the cannula, needles are first passed in the central part of meniscal injury entering from the femoral side, then through the lesion and peripheral meniscus. Is usually required a skin incision from which to retrieve the needles and the wire; the suture is knotted to the capsule. Despite its versatility, this technique presents neurovascular risk and requires incisions to retrieve the suture.

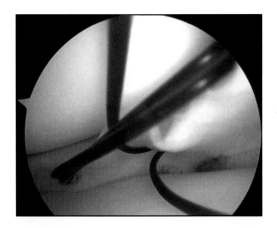

Fig. 13.4 Passage of the two threads during horizontal outside-in meniscal suture with PDS thread. On the right the shuttle thread

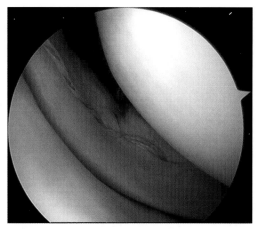

Fig. 13.5 Suture of posterior horn of medial meniscus with all-inside technique

The *outside-in* sutures are indicated mainly for lesions of the anterior or middle of the meniscus; a 18G spinal needle is introduced percutaneously under arthroscopic control, through which a monofilament suture (PDS 0) is inserted and the suture crosses the lesion in a vertical or horizontal way; a second wire loop is passed into the lesion and using it as shuttle take, the suture outside of the skin where is knotted on the joint capsule. It is a safe and inexpensive technique with reduced risks. The disadvantages are as follows: difficulty for injury to the posterior horn, the risk of iatrogenic injury to the meniscus from multiple attempts to needle placement.

The *all-inside* sutures are mainly used for the posterior portion of the meniscus; these systems have undergone a great evolution in recent years, today having a number of devices with specific characteristics. The technique involves the introduction, through arthroscopic portals, the suture constituted by a rigid part, which is positioned, through the central portion of the meniscus and the lesion, in the most peripheral meniscal side. This component is connected to a high resistance not-absorbable suture, which is tensioned with a normal knot pusher and locked with a pre-assembled node. These systems can currently provide multiple sutures without leaving the articulation with an obvious advantage in cases of large bucket-handle lesions. They are also better adaptable for suture posterior horn lesions, hardly reachable with the other techniques.

The all-inside techniques, however, have some risks: they use of non-absorbable fixation systems that can break in and mobilize joint. Furthermore, there is a risk of deepening too, over the posterior capsule, causing neurovascular lesions, particularly in small knees (Figs. 13.4, 13.5, 13.6, 13.7).

13.4.2 Meniscectomy

In cases, after a careful arthroscopic evaluation, the hypothesis of more conservative meniscal repair can be discarded, and the choice of treatment will fall on meniscectomy that in the category of patients in question should be more selective as possible.

In the case of radial tears, in WW area, we will proceed with sharp instruments (straight or angled basket depending on the portion meniscal concerned) and possibly with shaver by regulating the meniscal margin and restoring a natural and uniform shape. It is important, after finishing regularization, check to exclude other injuries or residual instability that would compromise the result and predispose to new lesions.

In cases, radial lesion deepen to the wall, you can perform a selective meniscectomy in the WW and suture the peripheral portion.

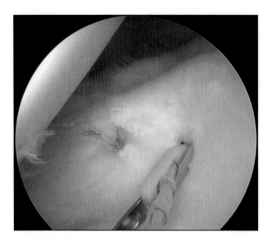

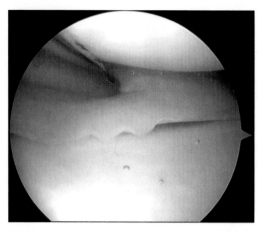

Fig. 13.6 Suture of posterior horn of medial meniscus with all-inside technique

Fig. 13.7 Knot tightening during all-inside suture

Flaps injuries are usually not repairable, and therefore, it is necessary to remove the flap at the bottom and stabilize the residual rim. These are sometimes difficult injuries to recognize because the flap may tip over and join the tibial surface of the meniscus, remaining ride. Even in this case the careful exploration with the feeler is crucial for accurate diagnosis and to not miss flap lesion that certainly would cause pain to the patient.

Longitudinal WW or longitudinal complex lesions have not potentially chance of healing; therefore, it is necessary to remove the lesion and stabilize the residual margin and evaluate the residual meniscus that is stable and does not hide other injuries.

Probably, the most serious meniscal injury is the complex bucket handle , in which the meniscus has a bucket-handle lesion aggravated by other vertical or horizontal lesions that contraindicate the suture. In these cases, it is necessary to remove the lesion often reaching a subtotal meniscectomy. In a young knee, the lesion has been removed and a subtotal meniscectomy will be considered in the future as a second surgery to restore the integrity of the joint (meniscal transplantation and meniscal scaffold).

13.5 Rehabilitation

It is important to make some considerations about the phase of functional recovery and return to sport after a knee surgery in children. First, compliance during rehabilitation may be less than in an adult, bringing sometimes the immature patient to make the imprudence's or sometimes not diligently follow the indications provided. Also, during the phase of muscular strengthening, workloads certainly cannot be managed as in an adult, to avoid overload problems on an immature skeleton. It is therefore important that these patients be closely monitored by the physiotherapist in the rehabilitation and parents that the surgeon should instruct.

The immediate post-operative includes cryotherapy, functional rest, keeping knee estende; the lens reduces swelling, pain, and avoid wrong postures.

The post-operative program is different depending on the surgical procedure performed, and for this reason, it is essential that the therapist interact with surgeon before approaching the treatment, to obtain information about the surgery performed, the weight bearing , the timing recovery ROM and about other possible information that only the surgeon who performed the procedure can provide.

After a selective meniscectomy, it grants a load-tolerant since the first day, possibly with the aid of crutches in the early hours. Rehabilitation after partial meniscectomy can generally progress as tolerated with no substantial contraindications or limitations. The goals are reduce pain and effusion, recover quickly ROM and gait pattern, maintain or recover the muscles strength, and proprioceptive neuromuscular achieve full recovery. Immediately begin isometric exercises pro quadriceps without and the gradual recovery of flexion and extension, up to full recovery of the ROM within the first week. Stationary cycling is granted 8th day, compatibly with swelling and pain. From day 15 start with swimming crawl, FKT in water for neuromuscular recovery. From the 3rd week start strengthening open and closed kinetic chain. The running will be granted to the 4th week or just recovered muscle strength.

Timing of progression during the recovery phase should be based on functional criteria [31, 32], i.e., during progression of recovery the previous steps must be overcome without complications, without joint effusion and pain.

Regarding the protocol post-operative in meniscal repair, in the literature, we found different opinions both about the load and the ROM. The standard protocols usually provide 4–6 weeks of discharge with the aid of 2 crutches to avoid excessive tension forces that the weight could cause the suture; return to a full load from the 6th week. As regards the recovery of flexion-entension is recommended a ROM of 0–60° for the first 4 weeks, followed by 0–90° for an additional 2 weeks, to progress subsequently to a complete recovery of the ROM. Following recovery of complete load and full ROM, proceed to the neuromuscular recovery, running and return to sports after 4–6 months [33].

Some authors use an accelerated recovery protocol after meniscal repair [34–36] which allows immediate weight bearing and progressive recovery of the ROM from the beginning,

claiming that earlier application of controlled stress to the repaired meniscus may enhance its functionality [37–39].

References

1. Baratz ME, Fu FH, Mengato R (1986) Meniscal tears: the effect of meniscectomy and of repair on intraarticular contact areas and stress in the human knee. A preliminary report. Am J Sports Med 14:270–275
2. Chatein F, Robinson HA, Adeleine P, Chambat P, Neyret P (2001) The natural history of the knee following arthroscopic medial meniscectomy. Knee Surg Sports Traumatol Srthrosc 9(1):15–18
3. Fairbank TJ (1948) Knee joint changes after meniscectomy. J Bone Joint Surg Am 30B(4):664–670
4. Noble J, Turner PG (1986) The function, pathology, and surgery of the meniscus. Clin Orthop Relat Res 210:62–68
5. Soballe K, Hansen AJ (1987) Late result after meniscectomy in children. Injury 18(3):182–184
6. Arnoczky SP, Warren RF (1983) The microvasculature of the meniscus and its response to injury. An experimental study in the dog. Am J Sports Med 11:131–141
7. King D (1990) 1936 The healing of semilunar cartilages. Clin Orthop Relat Res 252:4–7
8. Noyes FR, Barber-Westin SD (2002) Arthroscopic repair of meniscal tears extending into the avascular zone in patients younger than twenty years of age. Am J Sports Med 30(4):589–600
9. Bach BR Jr, Dennis M, Balin J, Hayden J (2005) Arthroscopic meniscal repair: analysis of treatment failures. J Knee Surg 18(4):278–284
10. Wilmes P, Lorbach O, Brogard P, Seil R (2008) Complication with all-inside devices used in reconstructive meniscal surgery. Orthopade 37(11):1088
11. Arnoczky SP, Warren RF (1982) Microvasculature of the human meniscus. Am J Sports Med 10(2):90–95
12. Day B, Mackenzie WG, Shim SS, Leung G (1985) The vascular and nerve supply of the human meniscus. Arthroscopy 1(1):58–62
13. Messner K, Gao J (1998) The menisci of the knee joint. Anatomical and functional characteristics, and a rationale for clinical treatment. J Anat193 (Pt 2):161–178
14. Laprell H, Stein V, Petersen W (2002) Arthroscopic all-inside meniscus repair using a new refixation device: a prospective study. Arthroscopy 18(4):387–393
15. Haas AL, Schepsis AA, Hornstein J, Edgar CM (2005) Meniscal repair using the FasT-Fix all-inside meniscal repair device. Arthroscopy 21(2):167–175

16. Cannon WD Jr, Vittori JM (1992) The incidence of healing in arthroscopic meniscal repairs in anterior cruciate ligament-reconstructed knees versus stable knees. Am J Sports Med 20(2):176–181

17. Tenuta JJ, Arciero RA (1994) Arthroscopic evaluation of meniscal repairs. Factors that effect healing. Am J Sports Med 22(6):797–802

18. Jensen NC, Riis J, Robertsen K, Holm AR (1994) Arthroscopic repair of the ruptured meniscus: one to 6.3 years follow up. Arthroscopy 10(2):211–214

19. Kimura M, Shirakura K, Hasegawa A, Kobuna Y, Niijima M (1995) Second look arthroscopy after meniscal repair. Factors affecting the healing rate. Clin Orthop Relat Res 314:185–191

20. Kirk JA, Ansell BM, Bywaters EG (1967) The hypermobility syndrome. Muscoloskeletal complaints associated with generalized joint hypermobility. Ann Rheum Dis 26(5):419–425

21. Willis RB (2006) Meniscal injuries in children and adolescents. Oper Tech Sports Med 14:197–202

22. Chang CY, Huang TF, Ma HL, Hung SC (2004) Imaging evaluation of meniscal injury of the knee joint: a comparative MRI imaging and arthropscopic study. Clin Imaging 28:372–376

23. Mc Dermott MJ, Gillingham BL, Hennrikus WL (1998) Correlation of MRI and arthroscopic diagnosis of knee pathology in children and adolescents. J Pediatr Orthop 18:675–678

24. King SJ, Carty HM, Brady O (1996) Magnetic resonance imaging of knee injuries in children. Pediatr Radiol 26:287–290

25. Zobel MS, Borrello JA, Siegel MJ, Stewart NR (1994) Pediatric Knee MR imaging: pattern of injuries in the immature skeleton. Radiology 190:397–401

26. Noyes FR, Barber-Westin SD (2009) Meniscus tears: diagnosis, repair techniques and clinical outcomes. In: Noyes knee disorders: surgery, rehabilitation and clinical outcomes. Saunders, Philadelphia, pp 733–771

27. Ahn JH, Lee SH, Yoo JC, Lee YS, Ha HC (2008) Arthroscopic partial meniscectomy with repair of the peripheral tear for symptomatic discoid lateral meniscus in children: results of minimum 2 years of follow-up. Arthroscopy 24(8):888–898

28. Kocher MS, DiCanzio J, Zurakowski D, Micheli LJ (2001) Diagnostic performance of clinical examination and selective magnetic resonance imaging in the evaluation of intrarticular knee disorders in children and adolescents. Am J Sports Med 29:292–296

29. Fairbank TJ (1948) Knee joint change after meniscectomy. J Bone J Surg 30B(4):664–670

30. Brown TD, Davis JT (2006) Meniscal injury in the skeletally immature patient. In: Micheli LJ, Kocher MS (eds) The pediatric and adolescent knee. Elsevier, Philadelphia, pp 236–259

31. Kvist J (2004) Rehabilitation following anterior cruciate ligament injury: current recommendation for sports partecipation. Sports Med 34(4):269–280

32. Cavanaugh JT, Killian SE (2012) Rehabilitation following meniscal repair. Curr Rev Musculoskelet Med 5(1):46–58

33. Kraus T, Heidari N, Sveilik M, Schneider F, Sperl M, Linhart W (2012) Outcame of repaired unstable meniscal tears in children and adolescent. Acta Orthop 83(3):261–266

34. Kozlowski EJ, Barcia AM, Tokish JM (2012) Meniscus repair: the role of accelerated rehabilitation in return to sport. Sports Med Arthrosc 20(2):121–126

35. Barber FA (1994) Accelerated rehabilitation for meniscus repairs. Arthroscopy 10:206–210

36. Barber FA, Click SD (1997) Meniscus repair rehabilitation with concurrent anterior cruciate reconstruction. Arthroscopy 13:433–437

37. Gillquist J, Oretorp N (1982) Arthroscopic partial meniscectomy: technique and long term results. Clin Orthop 167:29–33

38. The National Athletic Trainers' Association Inc (2001) Journal of Athletic Training 36(2):160–169 www.journalofathletictraining.org

39. Brindle T, Nyland J, Johnson DL (2001) The meniscus: review of basic principles with application to surgery and rehabilitation. J Athletic Training 36(2):160–169

The Knee: Osteochondritis Dissecans

14

Marie-Lyne Nault and Mininder S. Kocher

Osteochondritis dissecans is an acquired, potentially reversible idiopathic lesion of subchondral bone characterized by osseus resorption, collapse, and sequestrum formation with or without articular cartilage involvement and instability [1, 2].

The potential etiologies include the following: inflammation, genetic predisposition, spontaneous osteonecrosis, and repetitive trauma. König postulated that the inflammation theory in 1988 and hence the term_ENREF_3 [3] "osteochondritis" for the inflammation of the osteochondral joint surface, but subsequent histologic studies could not support this theory_ENREF_4 [4]. Instead, the majority of histologic studies found subchondral bone necrosis [5–10]. Concerning the genetic predisposition theory, Petrie et al. failed to demonstrated a familial inheritance with only 1, 2 % of first degree relative with radiologic OCD [11].

Currently, the most accepted etiology is repetitive trauma. Aichroth showed that among his patients with OCD, 60 % were involved in high-level competitive sports [12]. A multicenter study carried out by the European Pediatric Orthopedic Society reports that 55 % of patients with OCD were involved in regular sports activities [13]. The repetitive trauma theory is defined as repetitive microtrauma to subchondral bone that may lead to focal stress reaction and eventually stress microfracture. Persistent loading to this injured area prevents healing and leads to the subchondral bone necrosis seen in histologic studies [4, 14]. Further loading can lead to non-union and fragment separation. However, despite multiples publications on OCD, etiology is yet to be determined.

In 51–80 %, the location of the OCD in the knee is in the lateral aspect of the medial femoral condyle [13, 14]. Less frequent site involved are as follows: central medial femoral condyle (19 %), lateral femoral condyle (15–20 %), medial aspect of medial femoral condyle (7 %), patella (7 %), and trochlea (1 %) [13, 14]. The male/female ratio is 3:2, and bilateral involvement is between 12.6 and 30 % [13, 15].

14.1 Presentation

Two different presentations exist; the OCD can be an incidental radiographic finding in the course of investigation for another problem or the patient, and typically, an adolescent between 11- and 13-year old presents with an activity-related joint line knee pain. The symptoms depend on the stage at presentation. A history of swelling and mechanical symptoms, such as

M.-L. Nault · M. S. Kocher (✉)
Division of Sports Medicine, Department of Orthopedic Surgery, Boston Children's Hospital, Harvard Medical School, 300 Longwood Avenue, Boston, MA 02115, US
e-mail: Mininder.kocher@childrens.harvard.edu

M.-L. Nault
e-mail: Marie-lyne.nault@childrens.harvard.edu

popping and locking, suggested the possibility of lesion instability [16]. In their series, Cahill et al. reported 80 % of the patient having mild pain since 14 months with or without mild limp after sports activities [16]. Helfi et al. reported 32 % with no or little pain at presentation, 21.2 % moderately painful with activity, and 46.7 % markedly painful (pain at rest or mild activity) in their series of 509 affected knees [13].

On physical exam, there might be a small joint effusion and subtle limp. Palpating the joint line along the OCD lesion may reproduce the pain or elicit tenderness. The contralateral knee must be carefully examined as well. When the diagnosis is suspected, further imaging investigation must be done.

14.2　Imaging

The majority of OCD can be identified on plain radiographs, when four views are obtained: anteroposterior (AP), lateral, intercondylar notch (tunnel), and patellar skyline views (or merchant view) Fig. 14.1. The tunnel view best shows the classic posterolateral OCD of the medial femoral condyle [2].

On plain radiographs, irregular center of ossification can be incorrectly diagnosed as OCD. An irregular center of ossification is a non-pathologic irregularity of ossification seen predominantly in children under 10-year old. MRI can help to differentiate between both

diagnoses as edema in surrounding bone marrow and abnormal signal in overlying cartilage will be seen in OCD and not in irregular center of ossification [2].

When OCD diagnosis is made on plain radiograph, an MRI is generally obtain to evaluate more specifically the OCD, as its size, location, and character most importantly stability and state of the articular cartilage [17] (Fig. 14.2). Establishing the stability status is important for prognostic and treatment planning. An unstable lesion can be defined as either fractured cartilage or separation of the underlying subchondral bone [17]. Some authors believed that stable OCD have a better prognostic in terms of the resolution of symptoms [18].

Four criteria have been described on T2-weighted MR images that are associated with instability: (1) high signal line beneath the lesion, (2) focal defect in the articular cartilage, (3) fracture of the articular cartilage, (4) the presence of subchondral cyst [19]. A recent study evaluated the sensitivity and specificity of those criteria for adult OCD and juvenile OCD (OCD in immature patients) [20]. They found specificity and sensitivity of 100 % for adult OCD and a specificity of 100 % and specificity of 11 % for juvenile OCD that was when the four criteria were applied. Thus, MRI is valuable for diagnostic purpose and follow-up, but it remains inaccurate to determine instability, especially in juvenile OCD. Alternative would

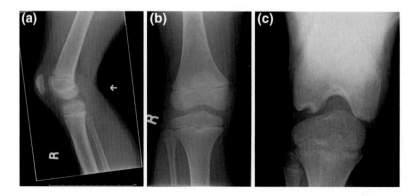

Fig. 14.1 Lateral (**a**), anteroposterior (**b**) and intercondylar notch view (**c**) of an OCD of the lateral femoral condyle. We can appreciate how the lesion is well seen on the intercondylar notch view compared with anteroposterior view

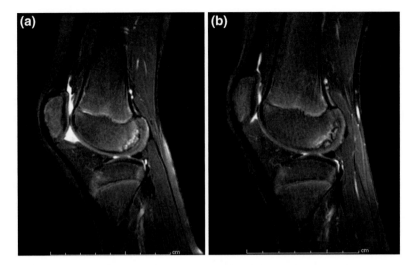

Fig. 14.2 Sagittal T2 MRI view of an 11-year-old boy. **a** At his initial visit, clinical symptoms and MRI were concordant with a stable OCD lesion, and he was treated conservatively. **b** Sagittal view one year later. The OCD lesion increased in size, and this is an example of a failed conservative treatment. This patient was then treated with drilling

be to obtain an MR arthrography to evaluate loss of cartilage continuity in cartilage mantle [21]. A break in the cartilage will result in joint fluid accumulation between the OCD and underlying bone and interfered with fragment revascularization and healing.

14.3   Classification

Different classifications exist for OCD lesion, and it can be based on radiologic imaging, MRI imaging, or arthroscopic evaluation.

Berndt and Hardy described a radiologic classification initially for talar dome OCD but subsequently used for knee OCD [22]: stage 1, involvement of a small area of compression of the subchondral bone; stage 2, partially detached osteochondral fragment; stage 3, completely detached fragment that remains in the underlying crater; stage 4, complete detachement/loose body.

DiPaola et al. [23] described an MRI-based classification: stage 1, no break in articular cartilage or thickening of articular cartilage; stage 2, articular cartilage breached, low signal rim behind fragment indicating fibrous attachment;

stage 3, articular cartilage breached with high signal T2 changes behind fragment suggesting fluid behind the lesion; stage 4, loose body with defect of articular surface.

Guhl et al. [24] described the arthroscopic classification of OCD: stage 1, irregularity and softening of cartilage, no fissure, no definable fragment; stage 2, articular cartilage breached, not displaceable; stage 3, definable fragment, displaceable, but still attached partially by some cartilage (flap lesion); stage 4, loose body and defect of the articular surface.

O'Connor et al. [25] evaluated the accuracy of the MRI classification compared with the arthroscopic classification. When following the DiPaola classification criteria [23], 28 out of 33 cases (85 %) were accurately correlated with the arthroscopic findings. This is of great importance to establish the stable or unstable status of the OCD lesion and plan the appropriate treatment.

14.4   Management

A recent report by the American academy of orthopedic surgeons (AAOS) based on evidence-

based literature on OCD management in immature and mature patients failed to established
strong guidelines. Concerning treatment, all
questions lead to inconclusive evidence except
for skeletally immature and mature patient with
symptomatic and salvageable unstable OCD
should be offered a surgical treatment, which
was a consensus from the work group in the
absence of evidence [18]. The next section on
management will present the different option
available, and the author preferred one.

14.5   Conservative Management

A trial of non-operative treatment is generally
accepted for OCD in skeletally immature patient
even though there are no prospective studies that
support this recommendation.

Conservative management protocols vary
among authors, but the underlying principle is
the same: limit the repetitive impact loading on
the OCD. That can be done by activity restriction alone, simple hinge brace, unloader brace,
casting or splinting. Brace and activity restriction allow knee range of motion and some
authors believe that motion is good for cartilage
nutrition and healing [1, 14, 26]. Duration of
non-operative treatment varies from 3 to 18
months in the different protocols [1], after failure of 6 months of non-operative treatment,
surgical option should be considered [2].

Our preference is to allow knee motion but
protect weight bearing until the child is able to
ambulate without pain. This first step often takes
4–6 weeks. We then progress to weight bearing
as tolerated in an unloader brace and start
physical therapy for knee motion and strengthening. A second MRI is obtained after 3–4
months of conservative treatment, and if OCD
lesion healing signs are seen, subsequent healing
assessment is done clinically or radiographically. If symptoms worsen or warrant further
evaluation, the MRI may be repeated. A supervised return to full activities in the unloader
brace is permitted if the child is pain free after
3 months of treatment.

14.6   Surgical Management

Indication for the surgical treatment of OCD
recognized by the AAOS is a symptomatic salvageable unstable or displace OCD lesion. Their
extensive literature review could not concluded
for or against surgical treatment of stable
symptomatic OCD lesion that failed conservative treatment or for any specific cartilage repair
technique in unsalvageable OCD lesion [18].
Those recommendations cannot support a specific treatment based on evidence-based literature, but still patients need treatment and our
indications for operative treatment are as follows: (1) all patients with detached or unstable
lesions, (2) symptomatic patients approaching
physeal closure (within 6–12 months), and (3)
stable lesions that have not healed after 6–9
months of non-operative management [1, 14].

For stable OCD lesion that failed conservative management, most authors agree with an
arthroscopic drilling of the lesion Figs. 14.3 and
14.4. The concept underlying drilling is that
perforating the dense osseous rim help revascularization and healing of the OCD lesion. Drilling can be performed either transarticular or
intraepiphyseal. Advantage of intraepiphyseal is
non-violation of articular cartilage, but it is
technically more challenging and required fluoroscopy [27] (Fig. 14.5).

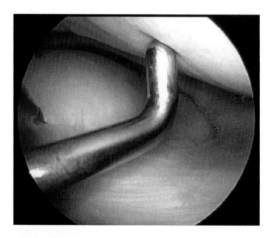

Fig. 14.3 Arthroscopic view of a stable OCD, soft
cartilage surface is appreciated with the probe

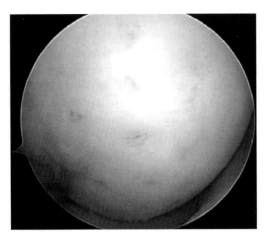

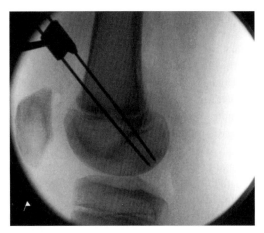

Fig. 14.4 Arthroscopic image after a transarticular drilling of a stable OCD

Fig. 14.5 Sagittal fluoroscopic view of an intraepiphyseal drilling

For unstable OCD lesion in patients with continuous or worsening symptoms, a surgical fixation treatment should be offered to the patient and family [18]. These lesions are unlikely to heal without treatment, and those patients are at higher risk of developing server early osteoarthrosis, for which limited affective treatment exist in a younger population (Fig. 14.6).

OCD lesion can first be assessed arthroscopically. If possible, the osteochondral defect is elevated and drilling and curettage of the OCD bed is performed leaving intact the cartilage surface. If the lesion is unstable but not moveable, then transarticular drilling is performed

after fixation. Option for bone graft is present, especially to restore a congruent articular surface level. Different techniques of fixation exist, including metallic headless compression screws or bioabsorbable implants like screw and pins. Another fixation technique is the use of biologic fixation with osteochondral plugs. In most cases, we now utilize bioabsorbable implants such as 1.5 or 2.4 mm bioabsorbable poly-(L-lactide) copolymer tack (Smartnail, ConMed Linvatec, Utica, NY) or a 2.7 mm bioabsorbable poly(L-lactide) screw (Bio-compression screw, Arthrex, Naples, FL). We reserve Herbert screw fixation for very large lesions in which significant compression is felt to be necessary to stimulate

Fig. 14.6 a Sagittal view of proton density MRI 3 months after an arthroscopic drilling and fixation with bioabsorbable implants. The OCD lesion is healing. **b** Coronal view of a fat sat MRI of the same patient, two bioabsorbable implants can be visualize on this view

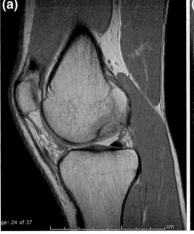

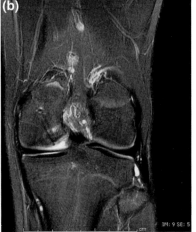

healing. Fixation can be achieved arthroscopically or with a mini-arthrotomy. Large posterior
lesions, patellar lesions, and trochlear lesions
can be difficult to access via purely arthroscopic
technique, and if visualization is inadequate, a
mini-arthrotomy should be performed on the
side corresponding to the location of the lesion.

Large, fragmented unsalvageable OCD
lesions, and long established loose bodies with
minimal or no subchondral bone must be treated
with excision and debridement. The AAOS systematic literature review could not recommend
for or against a specific cartilage technique repair
in symptomatic skeletally immature patient with
unsalvageable OCD lesion [18]. Abrasion
arthroplasty or microfracture might be performed
on the remaining exposed subchondral bone
(Fig. 14.7). For lesions with greater than 3 cm of
exposed subchondral bone, we considered a cartilage repair technique, either a chondrocyte
biopsy at the time of microfracture for potential
future autologous chondrocyte implantation or an
osteochondral autograft transplantation (OAT).

14.7   Clinical Results

14.7.1 Conservative Treatment

For conservative treatment, the rates of healing
have varied from 50 to 94 % [2]. Hefti et al.

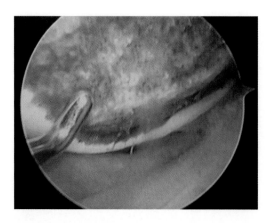

Fig. 14.7 Unsalvageable lesion after removal of cartilage and debridement. Ready for microfracture

found no significant difference between cast
treatment and others conservatives [1] methods
[13]. Wall et al. [28] reported a casting protocol
used on a series of 42 children that involved 6
weeks of cylinder cast immobilization with
weight bearing followed by unloader brace and
activity restriction. At 6 months after the
beginning of this treatment, 66 % of patient had
no pain.

In skeletally immature patients, lesion size
seems to be a prognostic factor of conservative
treatment success [28, 29]. Patients with smaller
stable OCD lesion has tendency to progress
toward healing.

14.7.2 Stable OCD

Rates of healing following arthroscopic drilling
range between 82 and 98 % [30, 32]. A recent
meta-analysis reviews the outcome of transarticular versus intraepiphyseal drilling [33]. It is
comparable in terms of radiographic healing,
and in both techniques, no complications were
reported. Kocher et al. reported a series of 30
medial femoral condyle stable OCD in skeletally
immature patients who failed conservative
treatment for 6 months and had an arthroscopic
transarticular drilling, younger age was found to
be a predictor of improved functional outcome
(Lysholm score) and radiographic healing was
achieve in all patient in an average of four, 4
months [32].

14.7.3 Salvageable Unstable OCD

Kocher et al. reported a series of 24 skeletally
immature unstable OCD treated with internal
fixation [34]. Lesion location, type of fixation
and prior surgery could not be identified as
prognostic factors for the healing rate. Furthermore, lesion stage determined with Ewing and
Voto stages [35] did not statistically significantly influence the healing rate and functional
outcome score (Lysholm score, International
knee Documentation Committee Score and
Tegner Activity Scores). Magnussen et al.

presented a series of 12 OCD stages 4 that were internally fixed and had a subsequent hardware removal at 12 weeks [36]. At 12 weeks, 11 out of 12 lesions were healed. At a mean follow-up of 9, 2 years, no patient had needed a second surgery for loose body removal and they had normal activity of daily living (Knee injury and Osteoarthritis Outcome Score). Gomoll et al. reported a series of 12 unstable Cahill and Berg [37] 2C OCD lesion that underwent fixation with compression screw [38]. At a mean follow-up of 6 years, all lesions healed and patients demonstrated excellent satisfaction with low morbidity (Lysholm Score, Knee Injury and Osteoarthritis Outcome Score, International Knee Documentation Committee Score).

14.7.4 Unsalvageable Unstable OCD

Concerning the treatment of unsalvageable OCD lesion, there is one level II study comparing microfracture to OAT in children under 18-year old with unsalvageable OCD of femoral condyle [39]. Forty-seven patients were randomized to either microfracture or OAT treatment; at an average of 4, 2 years of follow-up, the OAT procedure showed superiority to microfracture in terms of statistically significant fewer failures (9 out of 22 in microfracture group and none out of 25 in OAT group) and a statistically greater International Cartilage Repair Society Scores at 24 and 48 months for OAT group. Authors also reported that lesion size (cutoff 3 cm^2) had a statistically significant impact on ICRS Score in the microfracture group, but not significant in the OAT group.

Micheli et al. reported a series of 37 pediatrics cases of distal femur cartilage defect treated with autologous chondrocyte implantation [40]. Fourteen out of 37 were diagnosed with ODC, and 23 had undergone a prior cartilage repair procedure. Mean defect size was 5.4 cm^2. Mean follow-up period was 4.3 years, and the implantation is failed in one patient. Significant clinical improvement was measured with the Cincinnati Knee Rating System from baseline to last follow-up. They concluded that autologous chondrocytes implantation is an effective option for large cartilage defect in children and adolescents.

References

1. Kocher MS, Tucker R, Ganley TJ, Flynn JM (2006) Management of osteochondritis dissecans of the knee: current concepts review. Am J Sports Med 34(7):1181–1191
2. Edmonds EW, Polousky J (2013) A review of knowledge in osteochondritis dissecans: 123 years of minimal evolution from Konig to the ROCK study group. Clin Orthop Relat Res 471(4):1118–1126
3. König F (1888) About free body in the joints. Zeiteschr Chir 27:90–109
4. Shea KG, Jacobs JC Jr, Carey JL, Anderson AF, Oxford JT (2013) Osteochondritis dissecans knee histology studies have variable findings and theories of etiology. Clin Orthop Relat Res 471(4):1127–1136
5. Campbell CJ, Ranawat CS (1966) Osteochondritis dissecans: the question of etiology. J Trauma 6(2):201–221
6. Green WT, Banks HH (1953) Osteochondritis dissecans in children. J Bone Joint Surgery American volume (1):26–47
7. Linden B, Telhag H (1977) Osteochondritis dissecans. A histologic and autoradiographic study in man. Acta Orthop Scand 48(6):682–686
8. Milgram JW (1978) Radiological and pathological manifestations of osteochondritis dissecans of the distal femur. A study of 50 cases. Radiology 126(2):305–311
9. Uozumi H, Sugita T, Aizawa T, Takahashi A, Ohnuma M, Itoi E (2009) Histologic findings and possible causes of osteochondritis dissecans of the knee. Am J Sports Med 37(10):2003–2008
10. Yonetani Y, Matsuo T, Nakamura N et al (2010) Fixation of detached osteochondritis dissecans lesions with bioabsorbable pins: clinical and histologic evaluation. Arthroscopy: J Arthroscopic Relat Surgery 26(6):782–789 Official Publication of the Arthroscopy Association of North America and the International Arthroscopy Association
11. Petrie PW (1977) Aetiology of osteochondritis dissecans. Failure to establish a familial background. J Bone Joint Surgery 59(3):366–367 British volume
12. Aichroth P (1971) Osteochondritis dissecans of the knee. A clinical survey. J Bone Joint Surgery 53(3):440–447 British volume
13. Hefti F, Beguiristain J, Krauspe R et al (1999) Osteochondritis dissecans: a multicenter study of the European pediatric orthopedic society. J Pediatr Orthop B 8(4):231–245
14. Flynn JM, Kocher MS, Ganley TJ (2004) Osteochondritis dissecans of the knee. J Pediatr Orthop 24(4):434–443

15. Mubarak SJ, Carroll NC (1979) Familial osteochondritis dissecans of the knee. Clin Orthop Relat Res 140:131–136

16. Cahill BR (1995) Osteochondritis dissecans of the knee: treatment of juvenile and adult forms. J Am Acad Orthopaedic Surgeons 3(4):237–247

17. Wall E, Von Stein D (2003) Juvenile osteochondritis dissecans. Orthopedic Clinics North America 34(3):341–353

18. Chambers HG, Shea KG, Anderson AF et al (2012) American academy of orthopaedic surgeons clinical practice guideline on: the diagnosis and treatment of osteochondritis dissecans. J Bone Joint Surgery 18, 94(14):1322–1324 American volume

19. De Smet AA, Ilahi OA, Graf BK (1996) Reassessment of the MR criteria for stability of osteochondritis dissecans in the knee and ankle. Skeletal Radiol 25(2):159–163

20. Kijowski R, Blankenbaker DG, Shinki K, Fine JP, Graf BK, De Smet AA (2008) Juvenile versus adult osteochondritis dissecans of the knee: appropriate MR imaging criteria for instability. Radiology 248(2):571–578

21. Kramer J, Stiglbauer R, Engel A, Prayer L, Imhof H (1992) MR contrast arthrography (MRA) in osteochondrosis dissecans. J Comput Assist Tomogr 16(2):254–260

22. Berndt AL, Harty M (1959) Transchondral fractures (osteochondritis dissecans) of the talus. J Bone Joint Surgery 41-A:988–1020 American volume

23. Dipaola JD, Nelson DW, Colville MR (1991) Characterizing osteochondral lesions by magnetic resonance imaging. Arthroscopy: J Arthroscopic Relat Surgery 7(1):101–104 Official Publication of the Arthroscopy Association of North America and the International Arthroscopy Association

24. Guhl JF (1982) Arthroscopic treatment of osteochondritis dissecans. Clin Orthop Relat Res 167:65–74

25. O'Connor MA, Palaniappan M, Khan N, Bruce CE (2002) Osteochondritis dissecans of the knee in children. A comparison of MRI and arthroscopic findings. J Bone Joint Surgery 84(2):258–262 British volume

26. Hughston JC, Hergenroeder PT, Courtenay BG (1984) Osteochondritis dissecans of the femoral condyles. J Bone Joint Surgery 66(9):1340–1348 American volume

27. Edmonds EW, Albright J, Bastrom T, Chambers HG (2010) Outcomes of extra-articular, intra-epiphyseal drilling for osteochondritis dissecans of the knee. J Pediatr Orthop 30(8):870–878

28. Wall EJ, Vourazeris J, Myer GD et al (2008) The healing potential of stable juvenile osteochondritis dissecans knee lesions. J Bone Joint Surgery 90(12):2655–2664 American volume

29. Cahill BR, Phillips MR, Navarro R (1989) The results of conservative management of juvenile osteochondritis dissecans using joint scintigraphy. A prospective study. Am J Sports Med 17(5):601–605; discussion 605–606

30. Bradley J, Dandy DJ (1989) Results of drilling osteochondritis dissecans before skeletal maturity. J Bone Joint Surgery 71(4):642–644 British volume

31. Bruns J, Rayf M, Steinhagen J (2008) Longitudinal long-term results of surgical treatment in patients with osteochondritis dissecans of the femoral condyles. Knee Surgery Sports Traumatology Arthroscopy Official J ESSKA 16(5):436–441

32. Kocher MS, Micheli LJ, Yaniv M, Zurakowski D, Ames A, Adrignolo AA (2001) Functional and radiographic outcome of juvenile osteochondritis dissecans of the knee treated with transarticular arthroscopic drilling. Am J Sports Med 29(5):562–566

33. Gunton MJ, Carey JL, Shaw CR, Murnaghan ML (2013) Drilling juvenile osteochondritis dissecans: retro- or transarticular? Clin Orthop Relat Res 471(4):1144–1151

34. Kocher MS, Czarnecki JJ, Andersen JS, Micheli LJ (2007) Internal fixation of juvenile osteochondritis dissecans lesions of the knee. Am J Sports Med 35(5):712–718

35. Ewing JW, Voto SJ (1988) Arthroscopic surgical management of osteochondritis dissecans of the knee. Arthroscopy: J Arthroscopic Relat Surgery4(1):37–40 Official Publication of the Arthroscopy Association of North America and the International Arthroscopy Association

36. Magnussen RA, Carey JL, Spindler KP (2009) Does operative fixation of an osteochondritis dissecans loose body result in healing and long-term maintenance of knee function? Am J Sports Med 37(4):754–759

37. Cahill BR, Berg BC (1983) 99 m-Technetium phosphate compound joint scintigraphy in the management of juvenile osteochondritis dissecans of the femoral condyles. Am J Sports Med 11(5):329–335

38. Gomoll AH, Flik KR, Hayden JK, Cole BJ, Bush-Joseph CA, Bach BR Jr (2007) Internal fixation of unstable Cahill Type-2C osteochondritis dissecans lesions of the knee in adolescent patients. Orthopedics 30(6):487–490

39. Gudas R, Simonaityte R, Cekanauskas E, Tamosiunas R (2009) A prospective, randomized clinical study of osteochondral autologous transplantation versus microfracture for the treatment of osteochondritis dissecans in the knee joint in children. J Pediatric Orthopedics 29(7):741–748

40. Micheli LJ, Moseley JB, Anderson AF et al (2006) Articular cartilage defects of the distal femur in children and adolescents: treatment with autologous chondrocyte implantation. J Pediatric Orthopedics 26(4):455–460

The Knee: Patellofemoral Disorders

15

Marco Giordano, Angelo Gabriele Aulisa
and Vincenzo Guzzanti

Patellofemoral disorders are very common among adolescents and include a number of diseases that are not always easy to identify. *Patellar malalignment* is a clinical sign frequently observed and represents a generic and multifactorial static anatomical disorder. The direct response to this static malalignment is *patellofemoral maltracking,* which consists of abnormal sliding of the patella within the trochlear groove during flexion and extension of the knee. This may be reflected on radiological surveys [1]. As a consequence, the patellofemoral relationship is dysfunctional.

Different classifications have been proposed for dysfunctional patellofemoral malalignment. Some are based on the severity of the problem, and others on the mechanism of action or on the onset. The most well-known classification refers to how the patella sets in the femoral groove and has three main categories: patellar tilt, patellar subluxation, and patellar tilt with subluxation [2]. All of these pathological relationships must be confirmed by dynamic studies on transversal plane.

15.1 Patellofemoral Development

The embryonic outline of the lower limb appears at about 28 days of gestation.

A 37-day period then begins the endochondral ossification of the femur, tibia, and fibula together, with early differentiation of the patella and patellar tendon [3]. The secondary centers of ossification of the patella do not appear until 3–5 years of age, depending on sex [4]. The final form of the trochlea is already present in the fetus [5]. Wiberg has classified the patellar facet size into three subtypes [6].

The patella has several functions. First, it allows increasing of the lever arm of the extensor apparatus, improving the action of the quadriceps muscle using the patella as a fulcrum for a better mechanical advantage [7]. The patella also brings together the divergent forces of the four beams of the quadriceps muscle, transmitting the force to the patellar tendon and the tibial tuberosity without friction [8, 9]. Finally, this great sesamoid bone physically protects the cartilage of the femoral condyles from any traumatic frontal impacts and adds to the cosmetic contour of the knee.

15.2 Anatomy

The extensor mechanism of the knee is formed from the quadriceps, its tendon, the patella and the patellar tendon. The normal alignment of this

M. Giordano · A. G. Aulisa · V. Guzzanti (✉)
Orthopedic Department, Pediatric Hospital Bambino
Gesù, S. Onofrio square 4, Rome, 00165 Italy
e-mail: vguzzanti@yahoo.it

M. Giordano
e-mail: marco.giordano@opbg.net

A. G. Aulisa
e-mail: angelogabriele.aulisa@fastwebnet.it

V. Guzzanti (ed.), *Pediatric and Adolescent Sports Traumatology,*
DOI: 10.1007/978-88-470-5412-7_15, © Springer-Verlag Italia 2014

mechanism is in slight valgus, with the apex at the center of the knee. The patella articulates with the femoral groove beginning at approximately 20° of knee flexion, and the contact area between the patella and the femoral groove increases with greater degrees of flexion. The medial and lateral patellofemoral ligaments act as guy wires for statically stabilizing the patella in the sulcus. Medial soft tissue restraints account for resistance to lateral patellar translation in lesser degrees of flexion. At ≥30° of flexion, bony constraint affords patellofemoral stability. In the first degrees of flexion, the patella is superior to the osseous constraints of the femoral sulcus. In particular, the medial patellofemoral ligament (MPFL) acts as the primary soft tissue restraint to lateral dislocation. This ligament extends from the anterior aspect of the femoral epicondyle to the superomedial margin of the patella, lying superficial to the joint capsule and deep to the vastus medialis obliquus (VMO) [10, 11]. The fibers of the MPFL fan out and insert with the vastus medialis tendon. The medial patellotibial ligament (MPTL) acts as a secondary medial stabilizer. MPTL fibers run from the medial side of the tibia, below the joint line and medial to the patellar tendon inserting into the lower pole of the patella [12].

15.3 Patellar Tracking

In normal conditions, the patella slides freely and in a linear fashion in the trochlear groove. In these conditions, the patella follows a toroidal path from extension through flexion. Thus, a great dynamic and multidirectional stability is required. The patellar tracking is influenced by the rotation of the tibia relative to the femur, by the patellofemoral joint morphology and the direction of the tensile force of the quadriceps.

The external rotation of the tibia by 30° of flexion to extension is responsible for the lateral displacement of the tibial tuberosity [9]. This determines an angle subtended between the line of pull of the quadriceps and the direction of the patellar tendon called Q angle. Increased

femoral neck anteversion and proximal tibial external torsion makes lateral dislocation of the patella more likely because these conditions generate an increase in the Q angle.

15.4 Patellar Stability

The patella is controlled by the dynamic and static elements of the extensor mechanism and also significantly influenced by torsional and angular alignment of the proximal and distal lower extremity segments. The "dynamic elements" are the four quadriceps muscle proximally, the pes anserinus tendon medially which internally rotates the tibia and the biceps tendon laterally which externally rotates the tibia. The "Q" angle can dynamically change by hamstring activity causing that rotation. The static stabilizing elements of the extensor mechanism are the patellofemoral joint contains and congruency reflected by depth of the sulcus and fit of the patella, in the medial and lateral retinaculum, the medial and lateral patellofemorals ligaments, the medial and lateral patellotibial ligaments and the patellar ligament whose length establishes the height of the patella in relation to the femoral condyles and also transmits the forces of the quadriceps contraction to the tibia. The MPFL is the primary static stabilizer of the patella and prevents it from subluxating or dislocating laterally. Its importance in controlling lateral patellar dislocation has been well documented in several biomechanical studies [13, 14]. Cadaveric studies have shown that 50–60 % of the restraint to lateral translation is provided by the MPFL [15]. The MPTL contributes to 13 % of medial stability [12] and plays an important role as a secondary medial patellar stabilizer [16], helping the patellar tendon to limit upward displacement of the patella during strong quadriceps contraction [17].

The bone conformation of the knee contributes to static patellofemoral stability with the lateral condyle of the femur more prominent than the medial condyle. This limits lateral displacement of the patella. The femoral sulcus is flattened at its proximal part, becoming deeper in the distal portion. Therefore, it is more likely that dislocation of the patella will occur in extension or early flexion.

Dynamic forces include the quadriceps muscle and specifically the medial structures (VMO) that control the movement of the patella during the full range of motion, preventing lateral dislocation especially in early flexion. All conditions that weaken the stabilizing action of the vastus medialis may predispose to lateral dislocation of the patella. Other muscle groups (hamstrings, gastrocnemius-soleus, ankle and foot flexors and extensors) indirectly participate to the stability of the extensor mechanism of the knee [18].

15.5 Clinical Assessment

Malalignment of the lower limbs should be looked for during clinical examination. When lower limb malalignment is present, it generally is associated with patellofemoral malalignment. Skeletal changes of the static balancing of the lower limbs, even on the frontal and sagittal planes, need to be carefully recognized to assess their impact on the patellofemoral relationship. The first assessment should be performed on a standing patient to check for abnormalities of the axis of the lower limbs, like valgus or varus knee or torsional defects. The affected limb should always be compared with the contralateral

extremity. The physiologic varus or valgus deformity that occurs during skeletal growth is generally bilateral and symmetrical. Normal knee alignment changes as a child grows. Measuring the femoral–tibial angle in standing and supine positions assesses the presence of a varus or valgus deformity. A varus angle between 10 and 15° is normal in neonates. The femoral–tibial alignment becomes neutral between 14 and 20 months of age, to a maximum valgus of 10–15° by 3–3½ years of age. The normal femoral–tibial alignment of 5–7° is achieved between 6 and 8 years of age. Genu varus (bowlegs) is assessed for by placing in contact the two medial malleoli and measuring the distance between the femoral condyles. Genu valgum (knock knee) can be assessed for in the supine position by measuring the distance between the medial malleoli, with fully extended knees and the patellae facing upward and the medial femoral condyles in contact. The examiner must define the alignment in the sagittal plane to focalize a genu recurvatum or procurvatum. On the axial plane, torsional defects of the lower limbs may be present. The term "torsion" refers to a rotational change between the epiphysis of a bone. These torsional defects can be isolated or, more frequently, combined. The most common types of torsional defects in children are increased femoral anteversion combined with proximal or distal tibial external torsion (Fig. 15.1). In the coronal plane, femoral

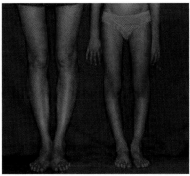 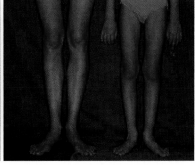

Fig. 15.1 Lower limbs malalignment in mother (35 years old) and child (6 years old). Increased anteversion of the femoral neck associated with tibial external rotation. In standing position in full extension of the knee with the feet aligned the legs appear bowed and a squinting patella is present. When the patella is maintained on coronal plane, external tibial torsion becomes clear

anteversion is defined by the angle of the femoral neck in relation to the femoral shaft. Children with isolated increased femoral anteversion have an intoeing gait that becomes evident when running. In the prone position, there is an excessive internal rotation of the hip and decreased external rotation. In the standing position with full extension of the knees and the feet aligned, the legs appear bowed and "squinting patellae" are present. Typically, the child plays sitting on his knees with the lower legs positioned laterally relative to the thighs ("frog-like position"). In most cases, the tendency to intoe becomes less evident as the femoral anteversion decreases or, in other cases, as the external tibial torsion increases.

Isolated tibial torsion, internal or external, is observed during skeletal growth. Tibial rotation can be cause of intoeing or outtoeing in children up to 3–4 years of age. Internal tibial torsion is a cause of intoed walking in childhood. In this case, patients sit down on their feet. At clinical examination, the lateral malleolus lies anterior to the medial malleolus and, in the standing position with front-facing patellae, internal rotation of the legs and feet is evident. The amount of lateral tibial torsion increases from about 5° at birth to an average of 15°/20° at maturity. Therefore, spontaneous improvement is often due to physiological skeletal growth.

Isolated external rotation of the tibia is less frequent. The child walks with the feet turning out. In the standing position with the feet aligned, the kneecaps present a convergent squint. The frequent association of marked anteversion of the femur with increased external tibial rotation can be characterized by intoeing of the knee with right assessment of the foot. The child will sit down in a frog-like position showing the disharmonic circling of the legs during running.

The presence of lower limbs malalignment associated with an abnormal patellofemoral relationship associated constitutes a diagnostic and therapeutic problem that is not always easily solved in adolescents. A complete and careful diagnostic pathway should precede any form of treatment.

15.5.1 Physical Examination of the Knee

The examiner can visually observe a squinting patellae or a bayonet deformity of the patellar tendon. With the patient sitting with his legs held out of bed, it is possible to evaluate the appearance of the patellae. In particular, cases of high patellae can be seen by examining the knees frontally. If also associated with a patellar tilt, it is possible to appreciate a squinting patella that appears like the "eyes of a grasshopper." Examination in the upright position allows evaluating the clinical Q angle between a line drawn from the anterior superior iliac spine and the center of the patella, and from this to the tibial apophysis. In a lateral view, a deformity of the sagittal profile of the knee that seems like a "camel" is frequently associated with high patella. The examination should be extended at the presence of a prominence of the anterior tibial apophysis as observed in case of Osgood–Schlatter disease. In the supine position, great attention must be given to examination of the knee (Fig. 15.2). The measure of the Q angle is repeated, and patellar tracking is checked during full flexion and extension. On palpation, patellofemoral ligament insufficiency must be ruled out and points of pain accurately monitored. Finally, it is necessary to search for all signs that may indicate a patellofemoral problem with the Fairbanks apprehension test [19], the patellar tilt

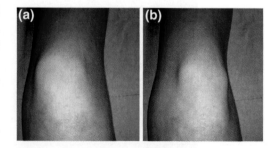

Fig. 15.2 Knee of a 12-year-old female suffering from recurrent patellar dislocation. In conditions of muscle relaxation, the patella appears normal (**a**), while the isometric contraction of the quadriceps muscle (**b**) pulls the patella laterally and patellar subluxation becomes evident

test and the Glide test [20]. During the examination, the possible presence of a valgus hindfoot or equinus deformity of the foot, which could cause alterations on patellar tracking, must also be sought. An associated pronation of the foot should be assessed for when the patient is walking. A prolonged half-squat test can evoke anterior knee pain (AKP). The comparative analysis of both lower limbs is essential and can attest to the presence of hypotrophy of the quadriceps.

15.5.2 Symptoms and Signs

Anterior knee pain is one of the symptoms that appear either isolated or combined with other symptoms. It is important to underline that a knee pain of a pediatric patient is hip pain, until proven otherwise. A more typical assessment concerns symptom characterization. When pain is isolated, it is typically undefined, poorly localized and may be exacerbated by prolonged sitting position with knee flexed, climbing the stairs, squatting or changing direction. Patients indicate the entire front of the knee as the focus of discomfort. This complaint is frequent in females. In the absence of true chondromalacia, it is unlikely to find true joint swelling, although the patient may report a sensation of a bloated knee.

Sometimes the patients may complain of a feeling of the knee "catching" or pseudolocking, which is usually transient. In these cases, it is very important to differentiate this from other causes of joint block (meniscal lesions and osteochondritis dissecans). Patients should be questioned about feelings of instability. In fact, pain is often one of the clinical signs in cases of patellar instability, especially if associated with a secondary chondromalacia.

15.6   Instrumental Assessment

Using clinical findings alone, diagnosis may be elusive in some instances. The identification and classification of symtomatic patellofemoral

malalignment requires visualization of the patellofemoral joint in early flexion, because the patella has a tendency to line up in the trochlear groove at flexion over 25–30°, even in the cases of patellofemoral malalignment. Moreover, considering that maltracking is a dynamic condition, radiographic assessment should focus on the dynamic phase. For this reason, routine anteroposterior, lateral and axial views are not specifically useful.

Therefore, if patellofemoral maltracking is clinically suspected, the adolescent knee is submitted to static and the dynamic computed tomography (CT). The static CT provides complete information about the patellofemoral relationship [2], the morphology of the femoral condyles and trochlear groove, the distance in the frontal plane between the apex of the tibial tuberosity and the bottom of the trochlear groove (TTTG) and also allows evaluation of the height of the patella. During dynamic isometric quadriceps contraction, the behavior of different types of patellofemoral malalignment (improvement and unmodified or worsening) [21] is clarified, and this confirms the observations of the past [22], when it was stressed the importance of the dynamics to various forms of instability (subluxation and dislocation).

If the knee pain is associated with the CT evidence of patellar tilt alone, it may be attributed to an excess of stability and then compatible with lateral patellar compression syndrome. In other circumstances, the knee pain is associated with CT evidence of patellar subluxation or subluxation and tilt, being only one of the symptoms of different degrees of patellar instability. The recent introduction of dynamic MRI will soon replace the use of static and dynamic CT [23].

15.7   Lateral Patellar Compression Syndrome

The syndrome is generally characterized by AKP. The patella tends to move laterally while remaining stable during the full range of motion. The lateralization forces determine the loss of the balance of the extensor mechanism of the knee resulting in a pathological shift of the patella to the lateral femoral condyle [18]. Listen carefully to the patient and correctly interpret the characteristics of the pain is always the best way to address the diagnosis.

Clinical examination is critical in the diagnosis. The tightness of the lateral retinaculum should be sought to confirm the suspicion. With the patient in a supine position, the inability to elevate the patella medially over the tangent plane of the femoral condyles (passive patellar tilt test) gives evidence of a retraction of the lateral retinaculum. With the knee flexed at 20–30° degrees, it should be possible to push the patella medially more than one-fourth of the patellar width (Glide test) [20]. The lateral retinaculum is tight if the patella moves medially less than this distance. Clinically, there are no signs of instability. Radiographic examination with axial views at different degrees of flexion has various limits like the difficulty of evaluation with quadriceps contraction, the absence of a defined reference plane for measurement, the overlapping of images and no detection of minimal rotational malpositioning [21]. CT scan and, recently, MRI are much more useful, because they allow the documentation of patellar tilt that does not improve or worsen during the dynamic test with quadriceps contraction. Conservative treatment is the first choice [24]. Rest, immobilization with brace and, occasionally, the use of anti-inflammatory drugs can sometimes be helpful. However, rehabilitation is the basis of therapy. The exercises aim to loosen the retracted lateral structures and to strengthen the medial dynamic stabilizers (vastus medialis oblique and adductors) and to restore the balance of the extensor apparatus. Surgical treatment should be considered if conservative therapy fails. When this occurs, lateral retinacular release is indicated. Sectioning of the lateral retinaculum must be accurate and complete, taking care not to leave any residual fibers in tension. At the end of the intervention, it is necessary to verify the ability to push the patella medially over two quadrants with the knee flexed at 30°. Postoperative rehabilitation starts

as soon as possible in order to avoid scar tissue formation, but return to sports activities should be avoided for at least 3–4 months after surgery.

15.8 Patellar Instability

Patellar instability is a frequent condition in children and adolescents. The instability is a dynamic clinical state that in 20 % of patients is secondary to a direct blow, whereas in a high percentage of cases is possible to individualize the presence of predisposing factors which alter the normal patellafemoral function. Both subluxation and patellar dislocation (acute or recurrent) are different degrees of patellofemoral instability syndrome.

15.8.1 Acute Patellar Dislocation

Acute patellar dislocation is the most common acute knee injury in active children and adolescents, and it may lead to functional disability and failure to return to full sports participation. The majority of injuries occur in the early adolescent age group. The incidence of primary patellar dislocation is 5.8 per 100,000, increasing in adolescents to 29 per 100,000 [25]. About 60 % of acute dislocations in younger patients occur during physical activity. The most common activities in which these injuries occur are ball sports (football, basketball, and baseball), accidental falls and gymnastics.

Traumatic patellar dislocation causes a high incidence of injuries to the MPFL. MPFL injury patterns in skeletally immature patients are different from those skeletally mature patients. The most frequent anatomical site of complete MPFL lesions in children and adolescents is the patellar attachment. The patellar insertion remains cartilaginous until 16–18 years of age, in contrast to the distal femoral attachment, making it more vulnerable and favoring avulsion fractures associated with MPFL tear rather than MPFL tear only [26]. Traumatic patellar dislocation may result in an osteochondral fracture in about 5 % of cases [27]. These are from either the lateral femoral condyle or from the patella itself, usually caused by shear forces induced by contraction of quadriceps muscle at the lateral femoral condyle during the relocation of the dislocated patella.

A complete medical history and careful clinical examination, supplemented with imaging, are essential to define the type and severity of dislocation and the presence of predisposing factors in order to plan the most appropriate treatment.

15.8.2 Mechanism of Injury

Indeed, the purely traumatic patellar dislocation is not frequent. Usually, the etiology includes predisposing factors. Up to 80 % of patients sustaining patellar dislocation have anatomic variables that predispose to lateral instability [28]. High patella, trochlear dysplasia, hyperlaxity, an increased quadriceps angle due to various torsional deformities of both the femur and the tibia, female gender, and a positive family history have all been associated with patellofemoral dislocation [25, 27, 29–31]. Acute patellar dislocation may occur from either a direct or indirect mechanism of trauma. Direct injuries result from a medial blow to the patella, which forces it laterally. Indirect trauma is more common and involves a valgus force with the foot fixed to the ground and either internal rotation of the femur or external rotation of the tibia. In this position, common in sports, the Q angle is increased and contraction of quadriceps pulls the patella laterally, exceeding the tensile strength of the MPFL. The direction of dislocation is typically lateral. Medial dislocations are uncommon and usually iatrogenic [32].

15.8.3 Clinical Presentation

At the time of initial evaluation, patients frequently report a "giving way" or "going out of joint" sensation during twisting movements of the knee. Usually, the patella has spontaneously relocated before the patient presents to the physician. On the rare occasion when the patella remains dislocated at initial evaluation (fewer than 20 % of cases), the knee is in the flexed position, and the patient has significant pain and swelling with extreme apprehension. The femoral condyles are readily palpable medially, and the patella is visualized laterally as a mass. In this case, extension of the knee will reduce the patella. The injured knee is initially examined in extension. In the acute setting, patients will often be tender in all areas of the knee, so palpation is not always useful. Later, palpation allows to identify the specifically injured areas. The physician should assess the retinacular structures, ligaments and joint lines for swelling or tenderness. After a first episode of dislocation, hemarthrosis will rapidly develop. Tenderness, often accompanied by significant medial ecchymosis, is usually encountered over the medial origin of the MPFL at the adductor tubercle or along the medial facet of the patella. If arthrocentesis reveals fat droplets in the joint fluid, an associated osteochondral fracture should be suspected. Attempts to displace the patella laterally will be prevented by the patient's apprehension.

The contralateral knee should be examined for the presence of predisposing factors. An examination of knee stability is also essential to exclude ACL injuries. The differential diagnoses include acute sprain of the medial collateral ligament, avulsion of tibial eminence, isolated osteochondral fractures, and rupture of the quadriceps or patellar tendons.

15.8.4 Imaging

With a suspected diagnosis of acute patellar dislocation, radiographic assessment should include anteroposterior, lateral and tangential views of both knees, according to the Merchant technique, in which the knee is supported at 35–45° of flexion to allow evaluation of the patellofemoral joint [33]. These radiographs may show displacement or residual lateral placement of the patella because of the disruption of the medial stabilizers (Fig. 15.3), but in most cases, the patella is reduced.

Anteroposterior views allow evaluation for the presence of possible osteochondral fragments from the medial patellar margin or the lateral femoral condyle. The lateral view allows for assessment of a high patella, based on the Insall–Salvati ratio. Oblique and notch views may be necessary to identify any loose bodies or osteochondral defects, although a significant number of these injuries are missed on plain radiographs. Stanitski el al correlated arthroscopic and radiographic findings in 48 adolescents with acute patellar dislocation. Only 23 % of these had an osteochondral lesion detected by radiographs, whereas arthroscopy found chondral or osteochondral injury in 71 % [33].

MRI is routinely indicated after acute patellar dislocation. Advancements have greatly improved the imaging capability of MRI for detecting soft tissue injury to the MPFL with a sensitivity of 85 % and an accuracy of 70 % [15, 34]. MRI is also useful for detecting chondral and osteochondral lesions and can help both diagnosis and evaluation of the extent of injury (Fig. 15.4). The classic MRI findings in acute patellofemoral

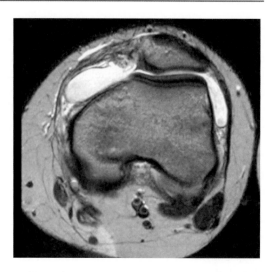

Fig. 15.4 The MPFL tear with an osteochondral fragment avulsed from patellar insertion at MRI study (from [38], with permission)

dislocations include focal impaction injuries of the lateral femoral condyle, osteochondral injuries to the medial facet and medial retinacular injuries. "Kissing lesion" bone bruises on the lateral femoral condyle and the medial patella result from lateral dislocation of the patella and its relocation. MRI may also demonstrate inflammation around the VMO and may show MPFL tears or avulsions [34]. CT scans can be useful in the acute setting for assessing the presence of osteochondral detachment.

15.8.5 Treatment

Most patients present with the patella reduced and rarely require reduction by the physician. Arthrocentesis of the joint can be performed to reduce pain. Management of the first episode of patellar dislocation is still up for debate but the conservative approach continues to be the most common, except in the presence of osteochondral lesions. Normalization of the strength and function of the quadriceps remains the gold standard of conservative treatment. After a brief period of immobilization in extension with protected weight bearing (5–10 days), the patient should initiate quadriceps isometrics,

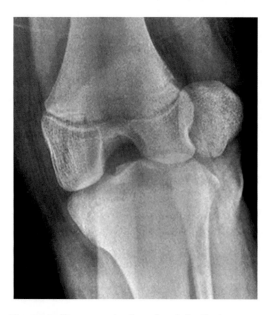

Fig. 15.3 X-ray examination of a skeletally immature patient (13-year-old girl) showing acute lateral dislocation of the patella

straight leg raises and single plane motion exercises. It is important to recover the entire quadriceps muscle in the strengthening program despite the traditional teaching, which focused primarily on the vastus medialis. As symptoms allow, the patient can progress to running and then ultimately advance to sport-specific activities.

Patellar taping and bracing have been performed as adjunctive non-operative rehabilitative techniques to medialize the patella, but recent studies have shown that they provide only symptomatic relief without actually medializing the patella [35]. However, despite the fact that a recurrent history of patellar dislocation in children and adolescents after conservative treatment has been reported to be benign, a significant number of patients will experience chronic instability, redislocation, or chronic patellofemoral pain. After non-operative treatment, redislocation rates range from 15 to 71 % [15, 25, 36]. The cause of this high frequency of redislocation is found not only in a persistent insufficiency of the MPFL secondary to its tear, but also in the presence of predisposing factors [28]. For this reason, direct reconstruction of the MPFL did not give better results than conservative treatment [25, 37]. The role of the MPFL as a guide for a static stabilizer of the patella in the sulcus was better defined [38]. In fact, biomechanical research has demonstrated that the MPFL accounts for 50–60 % of the medial soft tissue restraining force against lateral patellar subluxation or dislocation [12, 14, 39, 40]. Because of its specific function, the focus on reconstruction of the MPFL has increased in recent years. Different techniques are proposed for MPFL reconstruction, with greater attention on minimally invasive surgical approaches and respect for esthetics [16, 25, 37, 38, 40]. In addition, even MPTL insufficiency, which antagonizes the lateral displacement of the patella in measure of 13 % of patients, can facilitate redislocation [12].

Indeed, the MPTL plays an important role as a secondary medial patellar stabilizer [16], helping the patellar tendon to limit upward displacement of the patella during strong quadriceps contraction [17]. So in the presence of predisposing factors for instability such as high patella, severe Q angle (>15°), increased tibial tubercle-trochlear groove distance (TT-TG > 1.2 cm), trochlear dysplasia and hyperlaxity, the reconstruction of both the MPFL and MPTL, by combined use of ST and G, allows to achieve greater stability [41]. This approach avoiding physeal plate is utilized for recurrent dislocation of the patella and described later [38].

While surgical treatment for acute patellar dislocation remains controversial, in cases of osteochondral lesions, surgical reconstruction of the MPFL and MPTL with cartilaginous defect repair is accepted and considered the gold standard. Osteochondral fragments can be managed with either an arthroscopic approach or through a small arthrotomy. The osteochondral lesion detaches from the lateral femoral condyle or the patellar articular surface. The central and medial patellar facets are the most frequent site of injury. An arthroscopic examination allows the surgeon to accurately determine the size of the fragment, the extent of subchondral bone on the fragment, the anatomic location of the fragment and the need for fixation. The loose fragment is often far from its origin and is most easily retrieved and positioned near its bed with the arthroscope than during an arthrotomy.

Surgical management of an osteochondral fragment is critical to long-term prognosis of knee joint function. There is other treatment of choice for osteochondral lesions. Whenever possible, fragments >1.0–1.5 cm in diameter should be replaced and stabilized with headless compression screws or absorbable pins, which provide stable fixation and compression of the fragment and permit early joint motion. Microfractures, drilling, osteochondral grafting, or autologous chondrocyte implantation may be considered for various cases. More often, the bone is thin and does not allow a firm fixation. In these cases, arthroscopic removal is preferable. Postoperative management includes knee brace immobilization for 4 weeks with protected weight bearing, followed by early physical therapy for range of motion and strengthening exercises.

15.8.6 Recurrent Patellar Dislocation

In younger patients, the rate of recurrent dislocation is higher than in patients over 20 years of age [36]. These patients have frequently had a first episode of acute dislocation of the patella, and patient history is often sufficient to guide the diagnosis. Several abnormalities are responsible for this severe degree of instability in a high percentage of cases: flattened or hypoplastic lateral femoral condyle, hypoplastic or high patella, trochlear groove dysplasia (short and shallow), axial (genu valgum) and sagittal (genu recurvatum) deviations or torsional deformities of the legs (excessive femoral anteversion or external tibial torsion), lateral offset of the tibial tuberosity, generalized ligamentous laxity and contracture dysfunction of the vastus lateralis [25, 27, 29–31]. These combined anatomic and constitutional factors predispose to patella maltracking with recurrent lateral dislocation, especially in early flexion.

15.8.7 Physical Examination

From a clinical point of view, recurrent patellar dislocation may manifest as repeated episodes of patellar dislocation or, become evident after a history of AKP associated with instability symptoms. A complete medical history and careful clinical examination are essential to define the type of dislocation and should be supplemented with imaging. Clinical examination should include everything stated above for the evaluation of patellofemoral joint disorders.

15.8.8 Imaging

The use of conventional axial views at 20–30° of flexion (Laurin views), posteroanterior weight-bearing views of both knees at 45° flexion, lateral views and Merchant views are all often used in cases of recurrent patellar dislocation. However, it is preferable to use static or static and dynamic CT study [21] and MRI, which are now considered reliable methods of identifying risk factors for chronic patellar instability [23] especially in pediatric and adolescent patients. These images show different degrees of subluxated patellae or tilted *and* subluxated patellae.

15.8.9 Treatment

Conservative treatment based on a physical therapy program should be pursued to decrease the frequency of episodes of patellar instability. However, if the quality of life is undermined and expectations related to sports are disappointed, surgical treatment must be considered. In this case, the patella must be studied with imaging: often a subluxated or tilted *or only* subluxated aspect on static CT worsens during dynamic study. The choice of surgical procedure is closely related to the skeletal age of the patient, the severity of instability, the patient's sports performance and especially to any factors predisposing to instability.

In growing patients, physeal-sparing procedures are recommended. The aim of treatment for patellar instability should be to prevent repeated episodes of dislocation, give the patient the feeling of stability during activities, regain good joint function, reduce the patient's risk of injury and, preserve the esthetic appearance of the knee and reduce hospitalizations. Several techniques have been proposed for the surgical treatment of recurrent patellar dislocation in adolescents.

The distal bony realignment of the tibial tubercle is not recommended in skeletally immature patients because it can induce premature physeal closure and subsequent genu recurvatum. However, some authors have utilized distal periosteal patellar tendon realignment, either partial, as described by Goldwaith in 1904, or total, as suggested by Dal Monte in 1979 and Ippolito in 2011 [42].

In 1922, Galeazzi described an effective technique for physeal-sparing MPTL reconstruction with the semitendinosus tendon. The purpose of this technique is to direct the pull of the quadriceps in line with the intercondylar notch of the femur. This aim is also reached in reconstructing the MPTL, which contributes to establish the height of the patella in relation to the femoral condyle and also transmits the force of the quadriceps contraction to the tibia [43]. This technique was adopted and modified by Fiume in 1954, who added lateral retinacular release and medial retinacular reefing. In 1972, Baker adopted this technique but made an oblique mediolateral tunnel across the patella.

The technique requires a preoperative arthroscopic evaluation to assess for the presence of meniscal or cartilage defects. The operation is performed with the patient in a supine position, using a pneumatic tourniquet applied to the proximal thigh. A medial longitudinal parapatellar incision is made to expose the extensor apparatus. A lateral release is performed, taking care to avoid tearing the synovial membrane. After the semitendinosus tendon is identified, it is divided at the muscle–tendon junction. The tendon must be at least 12–13 cm long. An oblique 4-mm hole is drilled through the patella from the inferomedial to the superolateral side, and the tendon is passed through it from the medial to the lateral. After firmly drawing the patella medially and downward to reposition it in the trochlea, the tendon is sutured with considerable tension (Fig. 15.5). Successively the lax medial retinaculum is reefed. The knee is immobilized in a 20° flexion brace for 3 weeks. Postoperative CT scans are routinely performed to check for overcorrection, which can lead to development of a medial patellar subluxation [42]. Isometric muscle exercises of the quadriceps are started in a brace the day after the operation. Once the immobilization device is removed, continuous passive motion of the knee and volitional exercises, combined with neuromuscular electrical stimulation are started, along with exercises to strengthen the quadriceps and hamstring muscles. One month after surgery, the patient can begin knee flexion of more than 90° and progressive weight-lifting until normal function is reached. Sports activities should be avoided for 4–6 months.

In the author's experience, with 4 years of follow-up, Galeazzi's semitendinosus tenodesis modified by Baker, with adequate lateral release

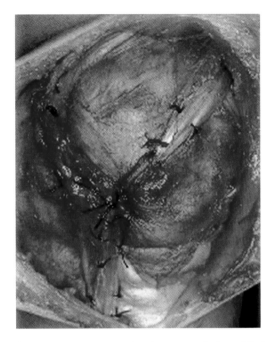

Fig. 15.5 Galeazzi's semitendinosus tenodesis modified by Baker. The semitendinosus tendon was passed through the patella in an oblique tunnel and was sutured to itself. After finding the right tension and obtaining a repositioning of the patella medially and downward, the operation is completed by lateral release and medial retinacular reefing

and medial retinacular reefing, produces good clinical mid-term results in skeletally immature patients [44]. Other studies have reported unsatisfactory results at long-term follow-up [43].

Three important factors that may influence of Galeazzi's technique results have been reported: appropriate tension before suturing the tendon to the patella, adequate lateral release and a normal joint surface of the patella at the time of surgery [30]. The data obtained with static CT at follow-up showed that the patella reached a satisfactory congruence with the trochlea in all knees that were subluxated and tilted prior to surgery [44]. However, dynamic CT showed that this technique is unable to counter the tendency of upward displacement of the patella, or to prevent subluxation and tilting of the patella in patients with high patella preoperatively [44]. The maintenance of this malalignment in dynamic conditions could lead to a risk of chondromalacia and perhaps explains the poor results reported by other authors at long term follow-up [45]. These results require the development of new technical solutions. In recent years, it has been published that the MPFL accounts for 50–60 % of the medial soft tissue restraining force against lateral patellar subluxation or dislocation [15], and this has increased interest in surgical reconstruction of the MPFL alone [39, 46]. Even if the indications for the reconstruction of the MPFL are not yet fully clarified [47], it may reach good results alone in the absence of predisposing factors for instability. However, the presence of an excessive Q angle or a high patella may complicate the outcome of this technique, as suggested by Mountney [48]. This report stated that patellofemoral joint stability problems are rarely straightforward and may be influenced by other factors such as articular geometry, alignment of the lower limb, rotational deformities, patellar height and ligamentous laxity [48]. Because of these considerations, the presence of a high patella, a high Q angle or other risk factors should put to increase stability and obtain better results at follow-up [25, 39, 40, 49] reconstructing both MPFL and MPTL.

The choice to reconstruct both the MPFL and MPTL ligaments is based on the reported importance of the MPFL as a primary medial patellar stabilizer [13, 14, 50] and of the MPTL as an accessory stabilizer [16] and patellar height regulator during strong quadriceps contraction [17]. The use of combined MPFL/MPTL reconstruction using the ST tendon and G autograft augmentation contributes to maintain patellar stability in opposition to the stress occurring during the growth period. This neo-ligament consisting of two tendons gives greater resistance against to ligamentous laxity and to the high patella and/or abnormal TTTG that often characterize recurrent patellar dislocation in skeletally immature patients. The surgical technique (Fig. 15.6a and b) requires a preoperative arthroscopic evaluation to assess for the presence of meniscal or cartilage defects and

involves four mini-incisions. First, a transverse skin incision is made medial to the anterior tibial apophysis to identify the insertion of the pes anserinus tendons. After dissection, the harvested semitendinosus and gracilis tendons are sutured, preserving the distal insertion site. A second mini-incision is made just medial to the inferior patellar apex. An additional 2-cm incision is made at the superomedial border of the patella. A longitudinal 2-mm Kirschner nail is driven into the medial third of the patella. A distal-to-proximal intraosseous longitudinal, 4-mm diameter tunnel is created. Once the tunnel is expanded to a diameter of 4.5 mm, the ST and G tendons are passed over the tibial growth plate and through the soft tissue and are brought distal to proximal into the patellar tunnel. A fourth skin incision is made to expose the femoral adductor tubercle. The proximal portions of the ST and G tendons are tunneled into the medial parapatellar subfascial soft tissue. The ST and G tendons are tensioned at 30°–45° of flexion [44] and fixed at the middle of the edge of the adductor tubercle of the medial femoral condyle by a titanium suture anchor (Arthrex Corkscrew suture anchor with needles: 5 × 12.1 mm with two size-0 fiber wires). The ST and G autografts are secured to the periosteum of the proximal pole of the patella with a bioabsorbable suture. Patellar stability is checked in full knee extension, allowing congruent smooth tracking of the patella. The knee is then positioned in a 20° flexion brace for 3 weeks. Postoperative CT scan is performed to check for overcorrection. Isometric quadriceps muscle exercises are started in the brace the day after surgery. Once immobilization is removed, controlled passive motion of the knee and neuromuscular electrical stimulation are started, along with quadriceps and hamstring muscle strengthening exercises. One month after surgery, knee flexion of more than 90° and progressive weight bearing are allowed. Sports activities are restricted for 4–6 months. The technique, which does not require a lateral release and/or medial retinaculum reefing, is in continuity with Galeazzi's procedure but also represents a theoretical and practical improvement to it.

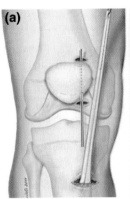 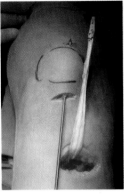 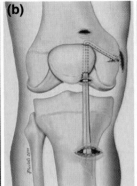 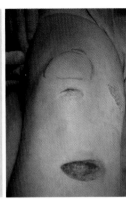

Fig. 15.6 Combined MPFL/MPTL reconstruction by ST tendon and G autograft augmentation by mini-incisions: **a** the harvested semitendinosus and gracilis tendons prepared preserving the distal insertion site with longitudinal 2-mm Kirschner nail driven into the medial third of the patella (from [38], with permission); **b** the proximal portions of the ST and G tendons are passed into the 4 mm longitudinal patellar tunnel avoiding tibial proximal growth plate, tunneled into the medial parapatellar subfascial soft tissue, tensioned at 30° to 45° of flexion and fixed in the medial condylar femoral insertion area of MPFL by a titanium suture anchor (from [38], with permission)

However, if the predisposing factors for patellar instability could exceed the strength carried by the ST and G tendons during growth, at the end of skeletal growth, distal non-physeal-sparing alignment techniques could be adopted to perform a definitive surgical correction.

15.9 Anterior Knee Pain

Anterior knee pain is a non-specific symptom commonly seen in the pediatric and adolescent populations and should be considered a "working diagnosis" until a specific diagnosis is made [1]. Several causes may create AKP and the correct clinical approach is "always looking for the cause." If a child reports knee pain, hip patholologies typical for the age should be ruled out first [synovitis, slipped capital femoral epiphysis, Legg-Calvè-Perthes disease, necrosis of the femoral epiphysis, tumors, juvenile idiopathic arthritis (JIA)]. Articular disorders that may occur with AKP are divided into four subgroups: (1) *intra-articular disorders* (a) synovial causes (trauma, JIA, plica syndrome); patellar causes (patellar lateral pressure syndrome, chondromalacia, chondral lesions, osteochondritis dissecans, shape dysplasia); (b) intercondylar notch causes

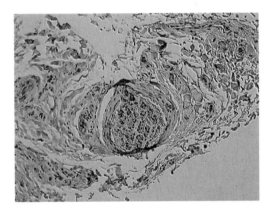

Fig. 15.7 Histological appearance of retinacular nerve excised for biopsy during a lateral release procedure. Nerve demyelination and fibrosis are highlighted, similar to those typical of Morton's interdigital neuroma (personal observation)

(fat pad, ganglia, hematoma, ruptured ACL); (c) femoral causes (osteochondritis dissecans); (2) *extra-articular disorders* (capsule, collateral ligaments, subcutaneous tissues, retinacular stress) [51], Fig. 15.7, tendons and/or apophysis (Osgood–Schlatter, Sinding-Larsen-Johansson, patellar tendinitis, iliotibial band tendinitis), quadriceps atrophy; (3) *articular disorders* (reflex sympathetic dystrophy, chondroma, osteoid osteoma); (4) *para-articular disorders* (benign and malignant tumors).

The surgical treatment of a patient with AKP must be performed after the whole diagnostic algorithm. Anterior knee pain can be attributed to lateral patellar compression only if patellofemoral malalignment (usually a tilt) is documented. If a specific cause cannot be found for the adolescent's anterior knee pain, it is defined as idiopathic.

References

1. Stanitski CL (1995) Management of patellar instability. J Pediatr Orthop 15(3):279–280
2. Schutzer SF, Ramsby GR, Fulkerson JP (1986) Computed tomographic classification of patellofemoral pain patients. Orhop Clin North Am 17:235–248
3. Sledge CB (1966) Some morphologic and experimental aspects of limb development. Clin Orthop Relat Res 44:241–64
4. Tria AJ Jr, Klein KS (1992) An illustrated guide to the knee, in anatomy. Churchill Livingstone, New York, p 4
5. Wamsley R (1939) The development of the patella. J Anat 74:360–369
6. Wiberg G (1941) Roentgenographic and anatomic studies on the femoro-patellar joint. Acta Orthop Scand 12:319–410
7. Kaufer H (1971) Mechanical function of the patella. J Bone Joint Surg Am 53(8):1551–1560
8. Fulkerson JP, Hungerford DS (1990) Biomechanics of the patellofemoral joint, in disorders of the patellofemoral joint. The Williams and Wilkins Co., Baltimore, pp 25–41
9. Hungerford DS, Barry M (1979) Biomechanics of the patellofemoral joint. Clin Orthop Relat Res 144:9–15
10. Feller JA, Feagin JA Jr, Garrett WE Jr (1993) The medial patellofemoral ligament revisited: an anatomical study. Knee Surg Sports Traumatol Arthrosc 1:184
11. Warren LF, Marshall JL (1979) The supporting structures and layers on the medial side of the knee: an anatomical analysis. J Bone Joint Surg Am 61:56
12. Panagiotopoulos E, Strzelczyk P, Herrmann M, Scuderi G (2006) Cadaveric study on static medial patellar stabilizers: the dynamizing role of the vastus medialis obliquus on medial patellofemoral ligament. Knee Surg Sports Traumatol Arthrosc 14:7–12
13. Conlan T, Garth WP, Lemons JE (1993) Evaluation of the medial soft-tissue restraints of the extensor mechanism of the knee. J Bone Joint Surg Am 75(5):682–693
14. Desio SM, Burks RT, Bachus KN (1998) Soft tissue restraints to lateral patellar translation in the human knee. Am J Sport Med 26:59–65
15. Arendt EA (2009) MPFL recontruction for PT instability. The soft (tissue) approach. Orthop Traumatol Surg Res 95S:S97–S100
16. Hautamaa PV, Fithian DC, Kaufman KR, Daniel DM, Pohlmeyer AM (1998) Medial soft tissue restraints in lateral patellar instability and repair. Clin Orthop Relat Res 349:174–182
17. Arendt EA (2007) Anatomy and biomechanics of the patellar ligaments. Tecniche chirurgiche in ortopedia e traumatologia 5:13–18
18. Stanitski CL (2003) Patellar instability in the skeletally immature patient. In: Delee JC, Drez D, Miller MD (eds) DeLee and Drez's orthopaedic sports medicine, vol 2. WB Saunders, Philadelphia, pp 1749–1760
19. Fairbank HA (1937) Internal derangement of the knee in children and adolescents: (section of Orthopædics). Proc R Soc Med 30(4):427–432
20. Kolowich PA, Paulos LE, Rosenberg TD, Farnsworth S (1990) Lateral release of the patella: indications and contraindications. Am J Sports Med 18(4):359–365
21. Guzzanti V, Gigante A, Di Lazzaro A, Fabbriciani C (1994) Patellofemoral malalignment in adolescents computerized tomographic assessment with or without quadriceps contraction. Am J Sports Med 22:55–60
22. Lavermicocca A (1922) Un fenomeno del ginocchio nella lussazione abituale della rotula. XIII Congr Soc It Ort
23. Lomasney LM, Demos TC, Neveu M, Fedors NH, Tonino P, Cheung LW (2013) Functional data for the diagnosis of patellofemoral laxity obtained by MRI during quadriceps isometric contraction. Orthopedics 36(1):e13–8
24. Cook JL, Micheli LJ (2006) Pediatric lateral retinacular release with medial plication under arthroscopic control. In: Micheli L, Kocher MS (ed) The pediatric and adolescent knee. Saunders Elsevier, Philadelphia, pp 163–166
25. Palmu S, Kallio PE, Donnel ST, Helenius I, Nietosvaara Y (2008) Acute patellar dislocation in children and adolescents: a randomized clinical trial. J Bone Joint Surg 90A:463–470
26. Felus J, Kowalczyk B (2012) Age-related differences in medial patellofemoral ligament injury patterns in traumatic patellar dislocation: cases series of 50 surgically treated children and adolescent. Am J Sports Med 40(10):2357–2364
27. Rorabeck CH, Bobechko WP (1976) Acute dislocation of the patella with osteochondral fracture: a review of eithteen cases. J Bone Joint Surg Br 58:237–240
28. Buchner M, Baudendistel B, Sabo D, Schmitt H (2005) Acute traumatic primary patellar dislocation: long-term results comparing conservative and surgical treatment. Clin J Sport Med 15(2):62–66
29. Hawkins RJ, Bell RH, Anisette G (1986) Acute patellar dislocations: the natural history. Am J Sports Med 14:117–120

30. Oliva F, Ronga M, Longo UG, Testa V, Capasso G, Maffulli N (2009) The 3-in-1 procedure for recurrent dislocation of the patella in skeletally immature children and adolescents. Am J Sports Med 37:1814–1820

31. Joo SY, Park KB, Kim BRK, Park HW, Kim BR, Park HW (2007) The "four-in-one" procedures for habitual dislocation of the patella in children. J Bone Joint Surg Br 89(12):1645–1649

32. Hughston JC, Deese M (1988) Medial subluxation of the patella as a complication of lateral retinacular release. Am J Sports Med 16:383–388

33. Stanitski CL, Paletta GA Jr (1998) Articular cartilage injury with acute patellar dislocation in adolescents: arthroscopic and radiographic correlation. Am J Sports Med 26:52–55

34. Sanders T, Loredo R, Grayson D (2001) Computed tomography and magnetic resonance imaging evaluation of patellofemoral instability. Operative Tech Sports Med 9(3):152–163

35. Gigante A, Pasquinelli FM, Paladini P et al (2001) The effects of patellar taping on patellofemoral incongruence: a computed tomography study. Am J Sports Med 29:88–92

36. Larsen E, Lauridsen F (1982) Conservative treatment of patellar dislocations: influence of evident factors on the tendency to redislocation and the therapeutic result. Clin Orthop Relat Res 171:131–136

37. Nietosvaara Y, Paukku R, Palmu S, Donnel ST (2009) Acute patellar dislocation in children and adolescent. Surgical technique. J Bone Joint Surg 91A(Suppl 2):139–145

38. Giordano M, Falciglia F, Aulisa AG, Guzzanti V (2012) Patellar dislocation in skeletally immature patients: semitendinosous and gracilis augmentation for combined medial patellofemoral and medial patellotibial ligament reconstruction. Knee Surg Sports Traumatol Arthrosc 20(8):1594–1598

39. Brown GD, Ahmad CS (2008) Combined medial patellofemoral ligament and patellotibial ligament reconstruction in skeletally immature patients. J Knee Surg 21:328–332

40. Drez D Jr, Bradley Edwards T, Williams CS (2001) Results of medial patellofemoral ligament reconstruction in the treatment of patellar dislocation. Arthroscopy 17:298–306

41. Giordano M, Falciglia F, Aulisa AG, Poggiaroni A, Guzzanti V (2011) Acute patellar dislocation in adolescent. J Sport Traumat 28(2–3):63–65

42. Savarese E, Bisicchia S, Carotenuto F, Ippolito E (2011) A technique for treating patello-femoral instability in immature patients: the tibial tubercle periosteum transfer. Musculoskelet Surg 95(2):89–94

43. Letts RM, Davidson D, Beaule P (1999) Semitendinosus tenodesis for repair of recurrent dislocation of the patella in children. J Pediatr Orthop 19:742–747

44. Aulisa AG, Falciglia F, Giordano M, Savignoni P, Guzzanti V (2012) Galeazzi's modified technique for recurrent patella dislocation in skeletally immature patients. J Orthop Sci 17(2):148–155

45. Grannatt K, Heyworth BE, Ogunwole O, Micheli LJ, Kocher MS (2012) Galeazzi semitendinosus tenodesis for patellofemoral instability in skeletally immature patients. J Pediatr Orthop 32(6):621–625

46. Buckens CF, Salis DB (2010) Reconstruction of the medial patellofemoral ligament for treatment of patellofemoral instability. A systematic review. Am J Sports Med 38:181–188

47. Nomura E, Inoue M, Kobayashi S (2007) Long term follow-up and knee osteoarthritis change after medial patellofemoral ligament reconstruction for recurrent patellar dislocation. Am J Sports Med 1851–1859

48. Mountney J, Senavongse W, Amis AA, Thomas NP (2005) Tensile strength of the medial patellofemoral ligament before and after repair or reconstruction. J Bone Joint Surg 27B:36–40

49. Balsamo LH, Gerbino PG (2006) Semitendinosus tenodesis to the patella for recurrent lateral subluxation of the patella. In: Micheli LJ, Kocher M (eds) The pediatric and adolescent knee. Saunders Ed., pp 169–173

50. Amis AA, Firer P, Mountney J, Senavongse W, Thomas NP (2003) Anatomy and biomechanics of the medial patellofemoral ligament. Knee Sept 10(3):215–220

51. Stanitski Cl (1994) Anterior knee pain. In: Stanitski CL, DeLee JC, Drez D Jr (ed) Pediatric and adolescent sports medicine. Saunders, Philadelphia, p 336

Ankle and Foot: Osteochondritis Dissecans of the Talus

16

Sandro Giannini, Roberto E. Buda, Marco Cavallo, Francesco Castagnini, Gherardo Pagliazzi and Francesca Vannini

16.1 Definition

Osteochondritis dissecans (OD) of the talus is a disease affecting the subchondral bone and secondarily the articular cartilage, which may cause the formation of a loose body [1, 2].

16.2 Epidemiology

OD occurs in the convex-shape parts of the joint surface, as knee, elbow, and ankle: ankle is the third most frequently affected site (4 %) after knee and elbow. It represents the first cause of loose bodies of the ankle joint in pediatric population. The estimated prevalence of OD in the talus is around 0.002:100,000 in the overall

S. Giannini (✉) · R. E. Buda · M. Cavallo ·
F. Castagnini · G. Pagliazzi · F. Vannini
First Clinic of Orthopedics and Traumatology,
Rizzoli Orthopedic Institute, University of Bologna,
Via Pupilli 1, 40136 Bologna, Italy
e-mail: sandro.giannini@ior.it

R. E. Buda
e-mail: roberto.buda@ior.it

M. Cavallo
e-mail: marco.cavallo@ior.it

F. Castagnini
e-mail: francescocastagnini@hotmail.it

G. Pagliazzi
e-mail: gpagliazzi@libero.it

F. Vannini
e-mail: france_vannini@yahoo.it

population, nevertheless the data are controversial due to frequent asymptomatic cases and wrong diagnoses [2]. Children under 10 years of age are usually spared, while OD usually occurs in patients from 10 to 40 years old, with a peak in the second decade of life, especially at the skeletal maturity. When this disease occurs before physeal closure, it is called juvenile OD; if the skeletal maturity is reached, it is called adult OD. It is generally accepted that the younger is the patient, the better is the course, and the outcome, even if this is confuted by a recent study [3, 4]. OD in the ankle is generally smaller than in the knee, and it is more difficult to diagnose and to heal.

In the general and in the pediatric population, males are more affected than females (2:1), although this trend is about to change because young females practicing sports activities are on the increase. Medial lesions, particularly in the middle and posterior third, are more frequent than lateral ones (60–20 %) [5]. Bilateral lesions are rare.

16.3 Etiology, Pathology, and Natural History

The etiology of OD is still debated. Traumatic, vascular, genetic, endogenous, and infective causes have been implicated [6–9]. Although the etiology is still unclear, the epidemiology shows that the association between OD and traumas is remarkable, mostly with regard to lateral lesions. Nevertheless, medial lesions,

V. Guzzanti (ed.), *Pediatric and Adolescent Sports Traumatology*,
DOI: 10.1007/978-88-470-5412-7_16, © Springer-Verlag Italia 2014

which are the most frequent and larger in size, are not connected to trauma, probably claiming a sort of predisposition. Hence, trauma and predisposition are generally linked together: according to Bauer's hypothesis [10], the higher is the mechanical pressure, the lower is the predisposition required. Sprains which involve forced supination or pronation are the most important traumatic cause (they are traced in 90 % of cases), especially when added to overweight or ligamentous laxity. In particular, strenuous and repetitive high-impact physical activity, cause of continuous micro-traumas, strongly relates to OD, while an acute osteochondral lesion on the site of OD is a rare finding.

Nowadays, the genetic etiology is supported by some case reports [7, 11]. It is likely that OD does not run in families, even if a recent study states that a missense mutation in aggrecan may lead to an autosomal-dominant transmission.

Vascular etiology, dealing with embolism, is widely accepted, in combination with single or repetitive traumas. Correlation with an infective etiology is weak. Steroid therapies and systemic lupus erythematous (SLE) are signaled as other remote causes of OD.

Many authors consider OD as an aseptic bone necrosis [6–8, 11]. Although some old studies did not find any sign of necrosis or ischemia, recent histo-pathological findings in the knee seem to support this theory. After the damage, a process of healing from the surrounding bone usually follows and, sometimes, could succeed in restoring the tissue. Nevertheless, some factors, like mechanical ones, may lead to an incomplete healing: thus, the bone is not integrated due to interposition of a sclerotic tissue providing a barrier to blood supply. Consequently, subchondral stem cells are definitively blocked from regenerating and healing the lesion site. Nevertheless, the continuous surface of hyaline cartilage and the sclerotic tissue anchor the fragment, preventing the detachment and the formation of a loose body. Cartilage can be only secondarily involved in OD, softening and loosing GAGs and chondrocytes. Eventually, the severe damages do not permit to hold the

fragment any longer, resulting in a loose body in the articular environment.

Even if juvenile OD is usually a benign disease, in contrast to adult OD prognosis, the lesion may even evolve to a clinical evident ankle deformity and instability. Progression to osteoarthritis is usually remote, apart when the tissues are largely necrotic [12]. A study on the natural history of OD, performed using clinical and MRI evaluations, shows that the progress of the disease is similar to the hypothesis supported by the histological findings. If the fragment is not displaced, in the presence of viable cartilage, the percentage of healing is very high and the surgery is not required. On the contrary, vascularization is severely restrained in case of displaced fragments, suggesting surgery as the only way to heal the lesion.

The stability of the joint and the small size of the lesions seem to be the other important positive prognostic features [13–16].

16.4 Clinical Evaluation

The OD is frequently reported by young patients following a major trauma or a normal physical activity [5, 17].

The OD can be asymptomatic. The symptoms are sometimes slight, leading patients to the physician's attention after many months. The most common patient's complaint is a mild chronic pain, present in more than 90 % of the cases: walking on uneven grounds may increase symptomatology. Sometimes, morning stiffness is recorded. Occasional ankle swelling and weakness accompany pain. Patients may also complain for locking , catching, clicking, suggesting the presence of a loose body. They may remark inability to load on the joint.

Palpation often evokes tenderness on posterior-medial or anterior-lateral areas of the talus, without ligament involving. The range of motion may be limited, although a normal finding is equally or even more probable. The patient may limp or at least show an antalgic gate.

Anterior drawer and talar tilt test should be performed as sprains usually underlie OD.

16.5 Imaging

Routine X-ray may show the lesion, but OD can easily be undiagnosed. Oblique and plantar-flection projections are useful to improve the detecting rate of posterior lesions. OD may appear as a pseudocystic area in which opacity and subsiding may be present. Sometimes, it is more similar to an abrasion or a dent over a rim of sclerosis. Still radiographic assessment shows limited sensitivity (68.5 %).

MRI is the gold standard for OD diagnosis [2, 14–16, 18]. It can stage the damage in detail, detecting the extension and the exact location of the lesion, the state of cartilage, and the presence of loose bodies. Frequent findings are decreased signal intensity on T1-weighted images and increased intensity on T2-weighted images: they suggest synovial fluid under the fragment, or, according to other authors, a high vascularized granulation tissue. Although literature confirms that MRI data are strictly related to arthroscopic ones (sensitivity: 92 %, specificity: 55 %), still false positive may be detected in juvenile OD, especially in assessing the instability of the fragments. In a recent study [2], MRI finds that 21 out of 23 lesions were unstable: the arthroscopic assessment was coincident in only 10 cases. The pattern of the misdiagnosed fragment was a hyper-intensity signal at fragment-bone interface, revealing a lower MRI detection rate at Berndt-Hardy third stage. Some authors [16] consider this signal a trace of edema which, if not stemmed, could lead to an unstable lesion. Probably, MRI detecting power may be inferior than expected, mostly at the onset of the disease, at the Berndt-Hardy third stage, and in younger patients. Another study states that, in children population, MRI in the knee significantly correlates with arthroscopic findings: the hyper-intensity signal should not be considered to evaluate stability, or a breach in articular surface (detected by T1-weighted imaging) should be added to raise the reliability [16].

Moreover, MRI may be helpful in diagnosing other possible coexisting conditions, in particular calcaneus stress fractures or diffuse cartilage thinning and synovitis.

Recently, MRI arthrography, using gadolinium to improve the definition of overlying cartilage and the separation of the fragment, was proposed as a tool to highlight the presence of granulation tissue. This may be helpful in doubtful cases [3].

CT scan may give information on the lesion and in particular on the bony state, contributing to a precise clarification of the lesion, still it is not free of invasivity, especially in young patients [19].

Scintigraphy with technetium is supposed to be valuable for diagnosing OD, but it is not helpful for choosing the right treatment as it is not good for determining fragment instability. Some argue that adolescents should be excluded because of lower reliability.

The advent of MRI has put scintigraphy as a second choice diagnostic means [19].

16.6 Classification

The first classification, based on X-ray findings, was originally proposed by Berndt-Hardy for osteochondral lesions of the talus and then adapted to OD [12]. In the first stage, a small area of compression of subchondral bone can be detected. When an osteochondral fragment is partially detached, it is classified as second stage; if completely isolated, but not displaced, it is categorized as third stage. The fourth stage requires a loose body.

Berndt and Hardy remains to date the only classification specifically adapted for OD of the ankle; all the other classifications available on the ankle regard osteochondral lesions. Berndt and Hardy is the reference classification even for osteochondral lesions: later, occurred the modifications based on the arthroscopic findings [20] and the addition of a stage describing a subchondral cyst [21]. The last classifications rely on MRI findings [22, 23]. An interesting classification considering the acute and chronic lesions and their related treatments was made by Giannini [24, 25]. The acute lesions are divided in two stages, with the fragment size <1 or >1 cm^2. The chronic lesions are divided in 4 groups: the zero stage encompasses the injuries with preserved joint surfaces. In the first stage, the lesion is inferior to 1.5 cm^2. The second stage is divided in two subgroups according to the depth (5 mm) of the lesions, which are >1.5 cm^2. In the third stage, only massive injuries are admitted.

Otherwise, different classifications have been proposed for OD in the knee: among them, Guhl suggested an arthroscopic classification [26], Di Paola presented an MRI classification [30], and ICRS in particular is widely used [24]. Substantially, differences among classifications are very limited. A more recent MRI classification divides lesions into "stable" and "unstable" [15]. In the first stage, only stable lesions are encountered: bone signal is changed and some cartilage swelling is appreciable. The second and the third stages encompass stable fragmentation. From an in situ bone fragment, along with a linear high T2-weighted signal or a possible bone cyst (second stage), the cartilage starts degenerating, presenting some focal signal intensity changes (third stage). The fourth A and B stages are reserved for unstable fragment: linear high T2-weighted signal is extended as far as the cartilage, which, in the end, may be lost.

16.7   Treatment

The goal of treatment is the preservation of articular cartilage and the healing of the damage as soon as possible, as the progression to growth plate closure turns a juvenile OD into an adult OD, with a poorer prognosis. Conservative treatment is the favorite option in case of a stable and small-sized fragment, despite the long time needed to heal completely [28].

There is general agreement in literature recommending that a stable, small lesion in a patient far from skeletal maturity should be treated conservatively [5, 10, 12, 17]. Even the site of the lesion should be taken into account, as some surgical choices may need osteotomy, at

risk of harming the outcome, causing dysmetria or deviation when growth plates are not closed. Surgery is recommended when conservative outcome is not satisfactory, the fragment is displaced or large, and the lesion cannot be expected to heal without perforation of the base (due to sclerosis or depth of the base).

Higuera [12] treated 68 % of his patients conservatively (most of them were classified in the Berndt-Hardy stage three): cast and no weight bearing were recommended for at least six weeks, followed by three months of active movements with no load bearing. In only one case, the unsatisfactory outcome after conservative treatment required surgery. The surgical procedures performed were bone marrow stimulation and/or fixation, followed by a short period of immobilization and subsequently active movements with no weight bearing allowed. 94 % of the patients, including those surgically treated, achieved excellent or good clinical results, meaning no pain or only during exercise, and a full, or minimally restricted, range of movement. 68.5 % of radiological results were classified as excellent or good.

Letts and Perumal [5, 17] suggested similar treatments, showing encouraging results.

Drilling [29] presents several advantages in case of non-healing stable lesions. Using a Kirschner wire, the talus is drilled in order to create channels into subchondral bone through which bone marrow cells can penetrate the articular space and heal the lesion by stimulating neovascularization and bony union of the fragment. Drilling may be performed anterograde or retrograde. The anterograde approach runs the pin through the medial malleolus into the lesion. This approach may damage cartilage overlying the lesion. The retrograde approach instead spares cartilage and physes, penetrating the talar dome from the head of the talus, avoiding ankle surfaces. This method is more technically demanding and may cause displacement of the fragment and soft tissue injury. No evidences are reported about superiority of one of these techniques over the other. In both cases, healing is reported in 90 % of the cases after treatment.

Lesions which cannot be expected to heal with drilling (excessive sclerosis or previous failed procedure) are susceptible to fragment excision, microfractures, mosaicplasty, osteochondral autograft transplantation, autologous chondrocyte implantation (ACI), or bone marrow-derived cells transplantation [13].

Arthroscopic approach is preferred if possible. In juvenile OD, due to the small dimensions of the joint and the open growth plates, which have to be preserved by limiting traction and stress on the joint, dedicated instrumentation is required.

Fragment excision is questioned: considering multiple works about knee and ankle, this technique can provide only satisfactory short-term results, as a remarkable risk of sequelae may be present at long-term follow-up. As fragment viability has been assessed, a fixation of the fragment may be a sensible way to restore joint surfaces, sparing ankle osteoarthritis risks [30].

Microfractures show encouraging short-term results [31]. No evidences sustain long-term reliability, although no studies focusing specifically on ankle OD are available to our knowledge. At mid-term follow-up, clinical and MRI deterioration of outcomes are evident, mostly if compared to osteochondral autologous transplantation [32]. The healing of the lesion through fibrocartilage makes this treatment a choice for small-sized lesions only. 41 % of failure after microfractures is reported in the OD of the knee [32].

Mosaicplasty or OATS can be performed arthroscopically in the knee but requires typically an open approach to the ankle. The hyaline cartilage is restored, but with fibrocartilage filling the gaps between the plugs, resulting in poor quality and poor long-term outcome. In addition, only small-sized lesions (1–5 cm^2) can be repaired due to limited donor area, and donor-site morbidity is a possible complication. Besides, a stable shoulder is fundamental to reach a stable fixation of the plugs. Dedicated instrumentations help this procedure, which is quite technically demanding, especially in the ankle. The designed donor site is usually a non-weight-bearing area of the ankle or, more frequently, of the knee [32, 33]. Similar clinical results and the same rate of donor-site disease are reported using these techniques. Reports regard mainly OD in the knee or osteochondral lesions in the ankle.

ACI on collagen membrane [34] have been experimented as a reconstructive technique after a prior surgery for knee OD. The juvenile OD recovered very well after the surgery, with encouraging clinical results not depending on the dimensions of the lesions. The arthroscopic findings at 1-year follow-up demonstrated a fibrocartilage repair in a half of the cases, and a mixture of cartilages with hyaline and fibrous kinds in the other half. ACI in the ankle instead has been proposed only in osteochondral lesions, with encouraging results [35].

The "one step" mononucleated bone marrow cells transplantation [24, 25] has been recently proposed for OD in the knee and osteochondral lesions of both knee and ankle. This technique uses the multi-potential ability of nucleated cells, present in the bone marrow, in association with PRF to regenerate both the cartilage and the bone component of the OD lesion.

Cells are collected from spongy bone of the posterior iliac crest and concentrated directly in the operating room in order to isolate the nucleated cells like stem cells, bone marrow resident cells, monocytes, and lymphocytes. While the process of concentration takes place, an ankle arthroscopy is performed, removing possible detached fragments and clearing the lesion until healthy tissues are reached. Then, 2 ml of the concentrated cells are loaded on a scaffold (like the hyaluronate or collagen membrane) previously modeled on the measures obtained during arthroscopy. Through a specific delivery device, the biomaterial is positioned on the lesion. Then, PRF is sprayed on the lesion in order to fasten the implant and promote the growth and the differentiation of the cells. A non-weight-bearing period follows surgery. Four weeks after surgery, muscular reinforcement, swimming, and walking exercises precede the full bearing, starting ten weeks after surgery. After 6 months, light running is permitted, and 10 months after the surgery, high-impact sports

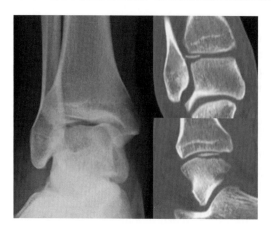

Fig. 16.1 Preoperative X-ray and CT scan of a 15-year-old male affected by acute lesion with a detached fragment, bigger than 1 cm. Clinically, the ankle was painful and swelled

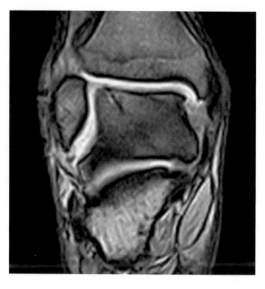

Fig. 16.2 An arthroscopic fixation of the fragment with reabsorbable pins was performed. MRI after six months and X-ray after 12 months show an excellent result. Pain and swelling are no longer present and the patient is satisfied

are allowed. Good clinical and radiological outcomes have been achieved also in juvenile OD of the talus, but the results are still unpublished.

Our preferred surgical guidelines are focused on Giannini's classification, specifically proposed for osteochondral lesions of the talus [25]. Excluding those OD cases requiring conservative treatment, in acute OD cases, when the fragment is more than 1 cm, fixation should be performed, using reabsorbable pins, possibly with arthroscopic technique (Figs. 16.1, 16.2).

Microfractures are advised in those lesions incapable to heal but smaller than 1.5 cm^2 (comparable to chronic type I): still, such small OD is to be considered rare in our experience. Regenerative techniques should be taken into account in those lesions, more than 1.5 cm^2 incapable to heal, according to the treatment proposed for chronic grade II and IIA. In the recent past, our experience has been addressed to chondrocyte implantation. To date, the "one step" technique is preferred. It has to be noticed that OD is frequently to be considered as IIA lesions, due to the large involvement of the subchondral bone usually present. In this case, our choice is to fill the lesion with cancellous bone or DBM before the scaffold implantation (Figs. 16.3, 16.4, 16.5).

When the lesions are extremely large and with an incomplete talar anatomy disruption, a partial fresh allograft is possibly the most reasonable solution. Lyon et al. described the use of this technique in the treatment of juvenile OD in the knee (not all patients were skeletally immature) [37]. The clinical and radiological results were promising. No data exist for this technique in the OD of the ankle, but a paper describing this technique in ankle osteochondral lesions reported satisfactory results [36].

16.8 Conclusion

Juvenile OD of the talus is a rare disease, affecting subchondral bone and, secondarily, articular cartilage in a skeletal immature population, usually sited in the medial part of the talus. An aseptic bone necrosis is the most accredited pathogenesis whose natural healing is probably blocked by micro-traumas, causing an osteochondral injury. Clinically, asymptomatic cases are possible, but a mild chronic pain is usually present, often accompanied by swelling,

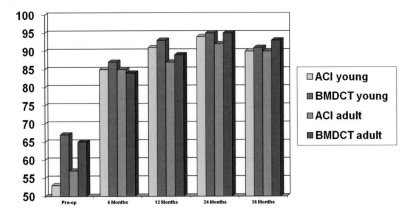

Fig. 16.3 Clinical comparison between autologous chondrocyte implantation (*ACI*) and bone marrow-derived cell transplantation (*BMDCT*), using AOFAS score. No differences between young and adult population have been recorded after three years of follow-up

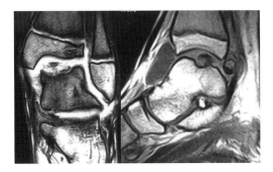

Fig. 16.4 A 12-year-old female affected by OD. Clinically, she had pain and could not bear sports activity and walking on uneven grounds. MRI showed a IIA lesion according to Giannini's classification. She underwent arthroscopy and bone marrow-derived cells transplantation

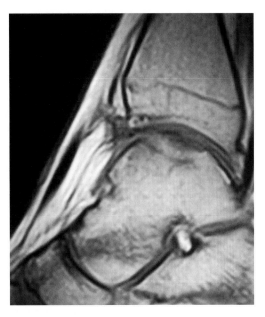

Fig. 16.5 Control MRI of the same patient one year after the treatment. The implant stimulated the regeneration. The bone lesion is filled with newly formed bone, while cartilage is on the way to the healing. Clinically, the pain is rarely present and the patient is back to high-impact sport activity

stiffness, or locking. A specific classification is not available following the radiographic Berndt and Hardy's. The most suitable treatment is conservative in the first stages of the disease and it is generally the first step to attempt especially in younger patients. A loose body is instead an indication to surgical fixation, while drilling or regenerative procedures are based on the subchondral bone sclerosis and surgeons experience and preferences. Drilling is suitable to permit a healing of the lesion with minimal surgical trauma, microfractures are to be considered only for small-sized injuries. Mosaicplasty and osteochondral autograft may cause donor-site morbidity and are scarcely reported in OD; furthermore, the indication is controversial due to the need of a stable shoulder for plugs implantation. Regenerative techniques and fresh allografts are granting good results in osteochondral lesions and few reports of OD among larger case series are available, but further studies are required to describe the results obtained in this specific disease alone.

References

1. Bruns JBP (1998) Osteochondrosis dissecans. Arthroskopie 11:166–176
2. Heywood CS, Benke MT, Brindle K, Fine KM (2011) Correlation of magnetic resonance imaging to arthroscopic findings of stability in juvenile osteochondritis dissecans. Arthroscopy 27(2):194–199
3. O'Connor MA, Palaniappan M, Khan N, Bruce CE (2002) Osteochondritis dissecans of the knee in children. A comparison of MRI and arthroscopic findings. J Bone Joint Surg Br 84(2):258–262
4. Zwingmann J, Südkamp NP, Schmal H, Niemeyer P (2012) Surgical treatment of osteochondritis dissecans of the talus: a systematic review. Arch Orthop Trauma Surg 132(9):1241–1250
5. Perumal V, Wall E, Babekir N (2007) Juvenile osteochondritis dissecans of the talus. J Pediatr Orthop 27(7):821–825
6. Steinhagen J, Niggemeyer O, Bruns J (2001) Etiology and pathogenesis of osteochondrosis dissecans tali. Orthopade 30(1):20–27
7. Petrie PW (1977) Aetiology of osteochondritis dissecans. Failure to establish a familial background. J Bone Joint Surg Br 59:366–367
8. Suckel A, Hoyer M, Raab C, Wünschel M (2012) Osteochondrosis dissecans and osteochondral lesions of the talus: clinical and biochemical aspects. Sportverletz Sportschaden 26(2):91–99
9. Uozumi H, Sugita T, Aizawa T, Takahashi A, Ohnuma M, Itoi E (2009) Histologic findings and possible causes of osteochondritis dissecans of the knee. Am J Sports Med 37(10):2003–2008
10. Bauer M, Jonsson K, Lindén B (1987) Osteochondritis dissecans of the ankle. A 20-year follow-up study. J Bone Joint Surg Br 69(1):93–96
11. Hammett RB, Saxby TS (2010) Osteochondral lesion of the talus in homozygous twins: the question of heredity. Foot Ankle Surg 16(3):e55–e56
12. Higuera J, Laguna R, Peral M, Aranda E, Soleto J (1998) Osteochondritis dissecans of the talus during childhood and adolescence. J Pediatr Orthop 18(3):328–332
13. Wall E, Von Stein D (2003) Juvenile osteochondritis dissecans. Orthop Clin North Am 34(3):341–353
14. Wall EJ, Vourazeris J, Myer GD, Emery KH, Divine JG, Nick TG, Hewett TE (2008) The healing potential of stable juvenile osteochondritis dissecans knee lesions. J Bone Joint Surg Am 90(12):2655–2664
15. Hughes JA, Cook JV, Churchill MA, Warren ME (2003) Juvenile osteochondritis dissecans: a 5-year review of the natural history using clinical and MRI evaluation. Pediatr Radiol 33(6):410–417
16. Samora WP, Chevillet J, Adler B, Young GS, Klingele KE (2012) Juvenile osteochondritis dissecans of the knee: predictors of lesion stability. J Pediatr Orthop 32(1):1–4
17. Letts M, Davidson D, Ahmer A (2003) Osteochondritis dissecans of the talus in children. J Pediatr Orthop 23(5):617–625
18. Pill SG, Ganley TJ, Milam RA, Lou JE, Meyer JS, Flynn JM (2003) Role of magnetic resonance imaging and clinical criteria in predicting successful nonoperative treatment of osteochondritis dissecans in children. J Pediatr Orthop 23(1):102–108
19. Moktassi A, Popkin CA, White LM, Murnaghan ML (2012) Imaging of osteochondritis dissecans. Orthop Clin North Am 43(2):201–211
20. Pritsch M, Horoshovski H, Farine I (1986) Arthroscopic treatment of the osteochondral lesions of the talus. J Bone Joint Surg 68A:862–865
21. Loomer R, Fisher C, Lloyd-Smith R, Sisler J, Cooney T (1993) Osteochondral lesions of the talus. Am J Sports Med 21:13–19
22. Taranow WS, Bisignani GA, Towers JD, Conti SF (1999) Retrograde drilling of osteochondral lesions of the medial talar dome. Foot Ankle Int 20(8):474–480
23. Hepple S, Winson IG, Glew D (1999) Osteochondral lesions of the talus: a revised Classification. Foot Ankle 20:789–793
24. Vannini F, Battaglia M, Buda R, Cavallo M, Giannini S (2012) "One step" treatment of juvenile osteochondritis dissecans in the knee: clinical results and T2 mapping characterization. Orthop Clin North Am 43(2):237–244
25. Giannini S, Buda R, Cavallo M, Ruffilli A, Cenacchi A, Cavallo C, Vannini F (2010) Cartilage repair evolution in post-traumatic osteochondral lesions of the talus: from open field autologous chondrocyte to bone-marrow-derived cells transplantation. Injury 41(11):1196–1203
26. Guhl JF (1982) Arthroscopic treatment of osteochondritis dissecans. Clin Orthop 167:65–74
27. Dipaola J, Nelson DW, Colville MR (1991) Characterising osteochondral lesions by magnetic resonance imaging. Arthroscopy 7:101–104
28. Lam KY, Siow HM (2012) Conservative treatment for juvenile osteochondritis dissecans of the talus. J Orthop Surg (Hong Kong) 20(2):176–180
29. Gunton MJ, Carey JL, Shaw CR, Murnaghan ML (2012) Drilling Juvenile Osteochondritis Dissecans: Retro- or Transarticular? Clin Orthop Relat Res. doi: 10.1007/s11999-011-2237-8
30. Pascual-Garrido C, Tanoira I, Muscolo DL (2010) Viability of loose body fragments in osteochondritis dissecans of the knee. A series of cases. Int Orthop 34:827–831

31. Salzmann GM, Sah BR, Schmal H, Niemeyer P, Sudkamp NP (2012) Microfracture for treatment of knee cartilage defects in children and adolescents. Pediatr Rep 4(2):e21

32. Gudas R, Simonaityte R, Cekanauskas E, Tamosiunas R (2009) A prospective, randomized clinical study of osteochondral autologous transplantation versus microfracture for the treatment of osteochondritis dissecans in the knee joint in children. J Pediatr Orthop 29:741–748

33. Sasaki K, Matsumoto T, Matsushita T, Kubo S, Ishida K, Tei K, Akisue T, Kurosaka M, Kuroda R (2012) Osteochondral autograft transplantation for juvenile osteochondritis dissecans of the knee: a series of twelve cases. Int Orthop 36(11):2243–2248

34. Krishnan SP, Skinner JA, Carrington RW, Flanagan AM, Briggs TW, Bentley G (2006) Collagen-covered autologous chondrocyte implantation for osteochondritis dissecans of the knee: two- to seven-year results. J Bone Joint Surg Br 88(2):203–205

35. Giannini S, Buda R, Vannini F, Di Caprio F, Grigolo B (2008) Arthroscopic autologous chondrocyte implantation in osteochondral lesions of the talus: surgical technique and results. Am J Sports Med 36(5):873–880

36. Hahn DB, Aanstoos ME, Wilkins RM (2010) Osteochondral lesions of the talus treated with fresh talar allografts. Foot Ankle Int 31(4):277–282

37. Lyon R, Nissen C, Liu XC, Curtin B (2012) Can fresh osteochondral allografts restore function in juveniles with osteochondritis dissecans of the knee? Clin Orthop Relat Res. doi: 10.1007/s11999-012-2523-0

Ankle and Foot: Acute Ligamentous Tears of the Ankle

17

Francesco Falciglia, Marco Giordano and Vincenzo Guzzanti

Ankle sprains are the most common type of acute sports trauma [1]. Epidemiologic studies revealed that ankle injury accounted for 14 % of all visitors to an emergency department [2] and for 11.4 % of children and adolescent population practicing sport activity [3]. In the past decade, improved biomechanics techniques have provided a better understanding of the mechanism of injury with consequent research into sports injury prevention and management [4].

The peak incidence of ankle sprain (7.2 per 1,000 person-years) occurs in patients between 15 and 19 years of age. Over half (53.5 %) of all ankle sprains occurred in individuals between 10 and 24 years old. The peak male incidence occurred between 15 and 19 years of age with an estimated incidence rate of 8.9 per 1,000 person-years, whereas females had a peak incidence between 10 and 14 years of age with an estimated incidence rate of 5.4 per 1,000 person-years [5].

Nearly half of all ankle sprains (49.3 %) occur during athletic activity, with basketball (41.1 %), football (9.3 %), soccer (7.9 %) being associated with the highest percentage of ankle sprains [5].

After an acute ankle inversion injury, a partial rupture of the anterior talo-fibular ligament (ATFL) or an isolated capsular lesion is present in 1 % of patients [6]. A rupture of both the ATFL and the calcaneofibular ligament (CFL) occurs in 15–25 % of cases. Isolated rupture of the CFL happens in approximately 1 % of patients. Injury to the posterior talo-fibular ligament is extremely rare [7]. Isolated ligament injuries of the deltoid ligament are also infrequent. Disruption of the ankle syndesmosis occurs in 1–5 % of patients after severe inversion trauma of the ankle. It is important to underline that the cartilage rim that covers the anterior distal tibia, the anterior part of the medial malleolus and the medial talar facet can be damaged by inversion trauma.

17.1 Anatomy

The ankle is a congruent joint composed of the tibia and fibula, both of which articulate with the talus. The talus is wide anteriorly and narrow posteriorly. This provides stability when the joint is in a neutral position, as the wider part of the talus is locked securely in the joint. Stability of the ankle is provided by both the bony configuration and by ligaments. Soft tissue stability is provided mainly by the deltoid ligament on the medial side and by the ATFL, the CFL, the posterior talo-fibular ligament, and the tibio-

F. Falciglia (✉) · M. Giordano · V. Guzzanti
Orthopedic Department, Pediatric Hospital Bambino Gesù, University of Cassino and Southern Lazio, S. Onofrio Square 4, 00165 Rome, Italy
e-mail: francesco.falciglia@opbg.net

M. Giordano
e-mail: marco.giordano@opbg.net

V. Guzzanti
e-mail: vguzzanti@yahoo.it

V. Guzzanti (ed.), *Pediatric and Adolescent Sports Traumatology*,
DOI: 10.1007/978-88-470-5412-7_17, © Springer-Verlag Italia 2014

fibular syndesmosis superiorly on the lateral side [7, 8]. Dynamic stability is achieved by the peroneus brevis muscle laterally (everts the foot) and the tibialis posterior muscle medially (inverts the foot).

During ankle motion, rotation and translation around and along the movement axes occur. The ATFL is in a plane parallel to the axis of movement (flexion–extension) if the ankle is in a neutral position. This ligament, considered to be an intra-articular reinforcement of the joint capsule, is the main stabilizer on the antero-lateral aspect and is the most vulnerable to injuries [9]. Most ankle ligament injuries occur during internal rotation in the equinus position with the foot in plantar flexion, when the narrowest part of the talus is placed in the ankle mortise, so rendering the ankle the most lax. This is likely an important cause for the high prevalence of injuries of the ATFL [9–11].

The CFL originates from the anterior tip of the fibula and runs obliquely distally and posteriorly to attach to the lateral surface of the calcaneus. In some cases, the CFL attaches predominantly to the ATFL [7, 8]. In contrast to the ATFL, it is all extra-articular and separated from the fibrous capsule. The CFL is associated intimately with the postero-medial part of the peroneal tendon sheath and connects the talocrural and subtalar joints. The posterior talofibular ligament is a short, thick ligament that is tight when the ankle is in extension and lax during flexion. Injuries of this ligament are infrequent. The distal tibiofibular syndesmosis is essential for stability of the ankle mortise, and therefore for weight bearing and walking.

The main stabilizer on the medial side is the deep portion of the deltoid ligament. This ligament is fan-shaped, thick, strong, and infrequently injured. Anatomic variations in size, shape, orientation, and capsular relationship of the lateral ankle ligaments are common. Up to 75 % of subjects show some anatomic variations, most commonly of the CFL. The ATFL is divided into two separate bundles in one-third of patients. These anatomic variations should be considered when performing surgical reconstruction of ligaments [12].

17.2 Mechanism of Ankle Sprain Injury

Understanding the mechanism of injury is very important for prevention. Andersen et al. [13] reported that there were two major mechanisms of ankle inversion sprain: (1) impact by an opposing player on the medial aspect of the leg just before or at foot strike, resulting in a laterally directed force, causing the player to land with the ankle in a vulnerable inverted position; (2) forced plantar flexion when the injured player hits the opponent's foot when attempting to shoot or clear the ball. Both of these mechanisms ultimately led to rupture of the ATFL, as this ligament often sustains higher strain and strain rate values than the other ligaments in the antero-lateral ankle.

In a static cadaver study, Markolf et al. [14] reported that 41–45-Nm external rotatory torque would cause ankle failure, as defined by a major decline in torque as the foot continues to rotate, indicating a bony fracture or ligamentous rupture. However, only one quantitative investigation into ankle biomechanics during a real ankle sprain injury scenario was reported [15]. An accidental inversion sprain was analyzed, where the ankle sprain occurred in a laboratory with high-speed video capture. The ankle joint reached an inversion of 48° and an internal rotation of 10°.

A combination of forced external rotation, extension, and axial loading of the ankle causes a rupture of the ATFL [9, 10]. This can also be accompanied by a partial rupture of the deltoid ligament.

The mechanism of injury of the deltoid ligament is an excessive eversion. Injury of the ankle syndesmosis is often seen in soccer players after external rotation of the foot, in dancers after forced extension of the foot, and in alpine skiers after combined external rotation, axial compression, and forced extension [16, 17].

17.3 Classification of Acute Inversion Injuries

Many classifications have been proposed for acute sprains of the ankle and all were aimed at the research of the extent of the injury to then apply the most suitable treatment.

Ankle ligament injuries have been classified as grade I (mild), grade II (moderate), and grade III (severe) [18]. In grade I injuries, including stretching of the ligament, the loss of function is minimal and the anterior drawer and talar tilt tests are negative. In grade II injuries, there is a partial rupture of the ligaments, some loss of motion, and moderate dysfunction. Dynamic maneuvers are uncertain and there is moderate laxity. In grade III injuries, including complete rupture of the ligaments and joint capsule, there is major loss of function and reduction in motion, and dynamic maneuvers are uncertain in the acute presentation due to pain. Radiographs are often needed to rule out a fracture.

Some authors questioned the application of this classification system, as a partial rupture of the ATFL or isolated capsular lesion (grade I) is present in less than 1 % of cases after a supination injury [17] and studies show that there is no difference between the prognosis of single (grade II) or multiple (grade III) ligament ruptures [19]. However, it is important to distinguish an incomplete lesion of the ATFL without capsular damage from a complete ligament rupture, which is always associated with a capsular lesion of varying size.

Other systems for grading an acute ankle sprain have been proposed [20]. The two most basic systems are the anatomic system, which classifies the injury into three degrees based on the damaged ligaments, and the American Medical Association Standard Nomenclature System which considers the severity of the injury to the ligaments [21].

Davis and Trevino [22] presented a staging system that consisted of four grades, with some subgrading according to the pathology, the damage to the ligamentous structure and the instability, as presented clinically.

Mann et al. [20] proposed a system for practical clinical outpatient use. It is based on three parameters: pain, swelling, and inability to walk. Each parameter is rated 0–3 points (0 = none, 1 = mild, 2 = moderate, 3 = severe) and a total score is calculated: Grade I: 1–3 points, Grade II: 4–6 points, and Grade III: 7–9 points.

The various classifications proposed for acute presentation are not easy to apply. Clanton [21] suggested a system based on the treatment requested. This classification divides the injured ankle into categories of stable or unstable. The stable group is suggested to receive symptomatic treatment for pain relief. The unstable group is then divided into non-athletes (or older patients) and young active athletes. Non-athletes and older patients are suggested to receive functional treatment while the young active are suggested to receive primary surgical approach. Other authors divided skeletally immature patients into those with negative stress radiograph findings, those with positive tibio-talar stress radiograph findings, and those with subtalar instability. Those with positive tibio-talar instability are suggested to consider surgical repair of the lateral ligament complex [23, 24].

17.4 Diagnosis of Acute Inversion Injuries

The target of the diagnosis of an ankle inversion sprain is to differentiate the mild and moderate forms from severe cases to favor an adequate treatment [19]. While the therapy of a mild and moderate sprain is well defined and the conservative approach is treatment of choice, the therapy addressed to severe cases is subject to controversial. The first step is to differentiate the mild, moderate, and severe sprains. The acute mild injury is characterized by history: a minor trauma, mild swelling, the absence of hematoma, mild limping, and negative laxity tests (easy to evocate). The moderate or severe cases are clinically characterized by immediate similar signs history: acute pain with sensation of "craquement," marked limited function, patient limp and walks with aid of cannes, remarkable swelling (possibly the sign of "coquille d'oeuf" of Roberte-Jaspar [25]), pain on the antero-lateral aspect, and clinic ligamentous instability (difficult to evocate). Because of the reported poor reliability of physical examination for diagnosis of complete ligament ruptures with wide capsular involvement after inversion trauma of the ankle, stress radiography, arthrography, MRI, and ultrasonography (US) were utilized [24, 26–28]. Some of the instru-mental methods are expensive, however, and their reliability is also debated. Physical exam-ination is unreliable in the acute situation in moderate and severe cases because the anterior drawer test cannot be performed due to pain. The reliability of physical examination can be enhanced when repeated a few days after the trauma as determined in a series of 160 patients, all of whom underwent arthrography [29]. A few days after the trauma, the swelling and pain have subsided and it becomes obvious if the cause of swelling was edema or hematoma. The pain on palpation has become more localized, and the anterior drawer test can now be performed. Negative pain on palpation over the ATFL rules out acute lateral ligament rupture. However, positive pain on palpation over the ATFL cannot distinguish a complete rupture associated with wide capsular tear. Pain on palpation, in com-bination with bruising, has a 90 % chance of indicating an acute lateral ligament rupture. A positive anterior drawer test has a sensitivity of 73 % and a specificity of 97 %. A positive anterior drawer test, in combination with pain on palpation over the ATFL and bruising, has a sensitivity of 100 % and a specificity of 77 % [29]. A special mention must be to the obser-vation of the presence of a complete tear of ATFL associated with an avulsion of the chon-dral or osteochondral fragment from the fibular malleolar apex or from the talus.

Few investigators have reported the incidence of avulsion fractures among mature patients with severe inversion injury. Broström [9, 30] repor-ted it as 13 and 14 % in two different studies. The incidence of avulsion fracture was higher in a recent study [31] than in the Broström studies.

This may be because avulsion fracture of the lateral malleolus is often misdiagnosed as ankle sprain or ligament rupture because the fragments are undetected on early plain radiographs [9, 32, 33].

Vahvanen et al. [33] found avulsion fragments in 19 of 40 sprained ankles in skeletally immature patients, 11 of which were not visible radio-graphically. Chaumien [34] reported 30 % of the avulsed fragment from the lateral malleolus in a series of 19 children and adolescents affected by acute severe inversion sprain. Busconi and Pappas [32] reported that in some skeletally immature patients, conventional radiographs often fail to show avulsion fragments. Broström [9] found intra-operatively that 11 of 90 ATFL injuries (13–14 % of cases) had avulsed frag-ments. Three of these were not radiographically visible. Schütze and Maas [35] investigated 130 pediatric patients with ligamentous rupture with or without osteochondral fragments who were treated surgically. In 37 % of these patients, they found an osteochondral fragment intra-opera-tively. One-third of these could not be seen radiographically. All of these investigators have assumed that most avulsed fragments are carti-laginous in skeletally immature patients and thus are not visible on traditional radiographs until they have ossified and enlarged.

Avulsion fracture from the lateral malleolus or from the talus may be misdiagnosed because the fragment is superimposed on the lateral malleolus in mature patients on early plain radiography. In skeletally immature patients, it may be totally cartilaginous and undetectable on radiographs [32, 35]. Physical examination alone does not provide a diagnostic modality for chondral or osteochondral avulsion fragments not detected by radiographs.

Therefore, there is some difficulty to recog-nize and to differentiate complete ATFL lesions from those coupled with wide capsular lesions, with avulsion fragments, that are unstable [28] and then defined as severe cases. Ultrasound examination (static and dynamic; during anterior drawer test, and talar tilt test) has to be consid-ered for severe ankle sprain in skeletally immature patients to find the avulsion fragments

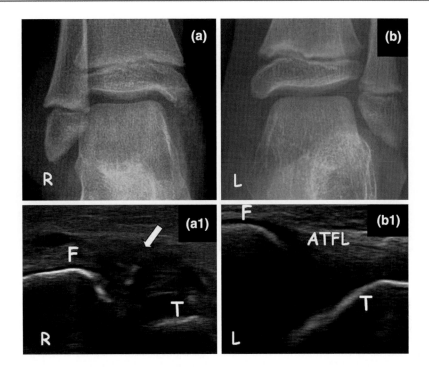

Fig. 17.1 X-Ray and static ultrasound evaluation of right ankle compared with the contralateral side. 11-year-old male. Fibula (*F*), talus (*T*), right (*R*), left (*L*), anterior talo-fibular ligament (*ATFL*). **a** X-ray of the *right* sprained ankle: radiolucency of the lateral soft tissue indicating swelling without evident signs of osteochondral avulsion. **b** X-ray of *left* non-affected ankle: normal radiographic imaging. **a1** Ultrasound of the *right* sprained ankle shows the presence of chondral avulsion from the fibula (*white arrow*) and the hematoma with an heterogenous mass where the capsular and the ATFL were injured. **b1** Ultrasound of the *left* non-affected ankle shows the normal ATFL appearance as an homogenous area between the fibula and talus

and evaluate the severity of capsular and ligament lesions [28, 32, 33, 36]. It must be underline that during the first 24–48 h after trauma, it is difficult to perform the dynamic maneuvers needed because of the pain and swelling. For these reasons, it is important to perform ultrasonographic examination at few days (3–5) after the acute trauma, to better evaluate the joint stability. In this way, it is possible to better define a stable lesion (moderate forms) from an unstable one [28, 32, 33, 36] (severe cases). The ultrasonographic sign of an introflexion of the damaged ATFL, of the capsule and, if present, of the avulsed fragment into the joint space is distinctive of an acute severe inversion sprain. The anatomic structures teared, and hematoma dip into the ankle joint through the wide capsular injury as the negative intra-articular pressure created by manual stress produces a vacuum effect (Figs. 17.1, 17.2).

Static and dynamic ultrasonography has a high sensitivity for diagnosing acute severe sprains associated with unstable ankle [28, 36, 37].

17.5 Treatment of Acute Inversion Injuries

Treatment of acute inversion sprains depends on the degree of the injury. Repeated studies and recent systematic reviews have shown that acute mild to moderate ankle sprains that include incomplete tear of the ligament or complete ligament tear with limited capsular injury and without avulsion fragments can be treated safely

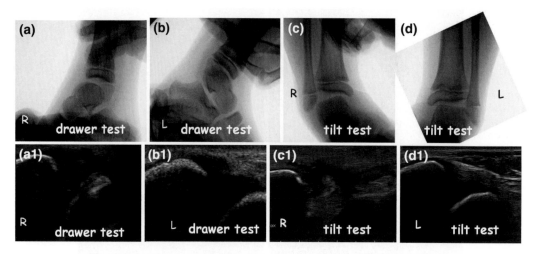

Fig. 17.2 The same patient of Fig. 17.1. X-ray and dynamic ultrasound evaluation of right sprained ankle compared with contralateral side executed under general anesthesia. **a** X-ray anterior drawer test of the *right* sprained ankle (>5 mm of anterior dislocation). **b** X-ray anterior drawer test of the *left* non-affected ankle (stable ankle). **a1** Dynamic US anterior drawer test of the *right* sprained ankle: the injured ATFL, capsule, and cartilaginous avulsed fragment deep into the joint. **b1** dynamic US evaluation of the *left* non-affected ankle does not show any abnormal images of ATFL and capsule. **c** X-ray talar tilt test of the *right* sprained ankle showing a value >10° of inclination. **d** X-ray talar tilt test of the *left* non-affected ankle does not show any abnormal degree of inclination value. **c1** Dynamic US talar tilt test of the *right* sprained ankle: the injured ATFL, capsule, and cartilaginous avulsed fragment deep into the joint. **d1** Dynamic US talar tilt test of the *left* non-affected ankle does not show any abnormal images of ATFL and capsule

with conservative treatment. Functional treatment with a short period of rest, cooling (ice), compression, and elevation to reduce edema (the RICE principle) during the first 1–3 days should always be recommended. Early weight bearing without crutches is encouraged. Active range of motion training should be started after the acute-phase treatment is completed,

The ankle rehabilitation program includes the returning to a normal range of motion associated with peroneal musculotendinous unit strengthening exercises to provide dynamic stability to the ankle combined with calf muscles and Achilles tendon exercises of flexibility to facilitate a neutral and more stable position of the ankle. Proprioceptive rehabilitation should be the final key. Deficit in proprioceptive rehabilitation has been shown to correlate with an increased incidence of ankle sprain [38], while proprioceptive exercises may decrease the risk of injury by almost 50 % [39]. Balance can be improved with exercises on wobble boards or small trampolines. The injured ligaments should be protected from new injuries during the healing phase by using external support to control the range of motion and to reduce the symptoms of functional instability. It is to remember that a gradual return to activity is dependent on progressive functional ability. One must walk before one may run, run before cut (change direction), and cut before being considered capable of playing. When all exercises are able to be carried out at full speed, return to play is allowed [40].

The results of functional treatment of these types of ankle sprains are satisfactory in most cases, and most athletes are able to return to sporting activities within a few weeks [27].

There is still controversy as to whether acute severe sprains, that is, complete tear of one or more ligaments with extensive capsular injury [21] ligament ruptures, should be treated non-surgically by active functional treatment and early mobilization, or with primary surgical

Fig. 17.3 The same patient of Figs. 17.1 and 17.2. **a** Operative findings: the cartilaginous avulsion fragment kept by Kocher clamp. **b**, **c**, and **d** Reinsertion by suture of the avulsed fragment on the fibular bone with reinforcement of capsular suture

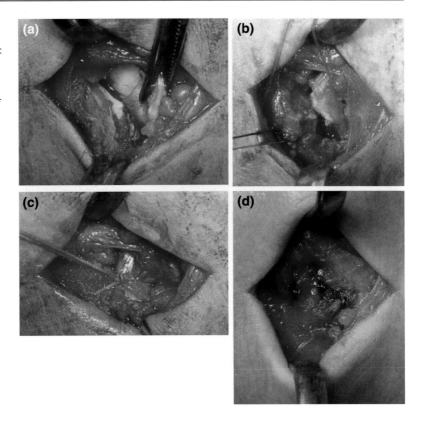

repair followed by immobilization using a plaster cast or brace. Only a few prospective, randomized, controlled studies are found in the literature [41, 42]. A relatively recent meta-analysis concluded that surgical treatment leads to superior results in the short- and medium-term in athletes, in terms of the ankle giving way and residual pain. A large, randomized, prospective trial of surgical and functional treatment of lateral ankle ligament ruptures with 6–11 years of follow-up revealed that surgical treatment leads to less residual pain and giving way than functional treatment [43].

Complete ATFL lesions are generally associated with a wide capsular tear and produce potential chronic instability unstable lesions of the ankle joint in children [33] that can be associated with various features of chronic lateral impingement [21, 44]. Chronic instability in children is sustained by ankle laxity due to insufficiency of repaired fibrous tissue, loss of proprioception, and weakness of general tendons

and is favored by constitutional ligamentous laxity, cavus foot, calcaneus varus, and varus tilt of the tarsal plafond. Moreover, repeated ankle sprains during growth risk to condition the perfect joint tarsal function as the talus morphology can be modified (Fig. 17.3a–e). Ultrasound investigation, in cases of acute inversion ankle sprain in skeletally immature patients, can help the physician to better assess the severity of the ligamentous lesion and can demonstrate a stable versus an unstable lesion. As written previously when introflexion of the ATFL and capsule into the joint is demonstrated by dynamic ultrasound, with anterior drawer and talar tilt tests, in particular especially during internal rotation, the lesion is to be considered unstable [45, 46].

In skeletally immature patients, it is important to perform a new dynamic evaluation after 3–5 days to better identify the presence of an avulsed unstable fragment that cannot be observed on radiographs. This evaluation can help determine an adequate form of treatment as

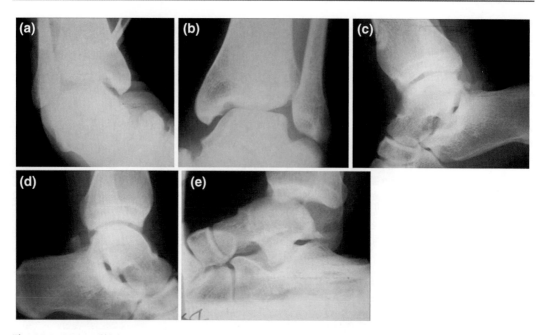

Fig. 17.4 Male of 18 yrs with chronic instability (Figs. 17.4a, e) secondary to ligament and capsule ruptures without avulsion fragment: first acute severe inversion sprain at 11 years of age and repeated sprains (twelve episodes) during 7 years. X-ray shows the abnormal talus morphology (Fig. 17.4c) if compared with non-affected side (Fig. 17.4b, d)

various authors have reported that unsatisfactory long-term results are due to the presence of avulsed fragments [32, 34]. For this reason, these lesions require surgical treatment [27, 33, 36].

As concern acute severe inversion sprains without avulsed fragments, surgical treatment can be adopted in skeletally immature patients when higher functional demands are required, or their activities necessitate perfect ankle function. Primary repair of the ligament with reconstruction of the normal anatomy even if debated offers the best resistance to the extra stresses imposed by sports activities [32, 33, 43] (Fig. 17.4) and can be considered one way to ensure a stable ankle in children with ligament rupture [33, 45, 46]. Despite the clinical and statistically significant superiority of surgical over functional treatment reported in case of acute severe ankle sprains [41], there are a number of reasons for questioning the routine use of surgery as the treatment of choice in non-athlete patients even if it is difficult to define the future choices of active children. First, delayed operative reconstruction of the injured ligaments

has been reported to generate similar results compared with acute repair, even many years after the initial injury [12]. The decision to operate on every patient with an ankle ligament injury will increase the number of patients referred for surgery and impose an unacceptable strain on the available capacity of operating theaters. Operative treatment is also associated with much higher costs. In addition, surgery enhances the risk of complications such as infection, failure of wound healing, dystrophy, and nerve damage, even if these complications can be avoided by closely following the anatomic pathways and scrupulously applying all the rules of asepsis. However, the literature lacks of randomized trials, not retrospective, and recent comparing the results of the conservative and surgical treatment applied to acute severe sprains without avulsed fragment in non-athletic skeletally immature patients. The data obtained could improve the information from the studies existing [44, 46] and dated [28, 47]. Moreover, it is hopeful that the methods of the results detection are homogeneous. Kaikkonen et al.

[41] proposed a performance test protocol with a scoring scale, to evaluate functional recovery after ankle injury. The practical consisted of three questions on subjective assessment, two clinical measurements on the ankle, two muscle strength tests, one ankle functional stability test, and one balancing test. The total score correlated very well with the isokinetic strength test of the ankle, the subjective opinion about recovery and the subjective function assessment. Thus, this protocol is practical for clinical evaluation of ankle sprain injury. Bie et al. [36] derived an ankle functional scoring system that evaluated the pain, instability, weight bearing, swelling, and gait pattern, adding together for a score up to 100.

References

1. Fong DTP, Hong Y, Chan LK, Yung PSH, Chan KM (2007) A systematic review on ankle injury and ankle sprain in sports. Sports Med 37(1):73–94
2. Fong DTP, Man CY, Yung PSH, Cheung SY, Chan KM (2008) Sport-related ankle injuries attending an accident and emergency department. Injury 39(10):1222–1227
3. Zaricznyj B, Shattuck LJ, Mast TA, Robertson RV, D'Elia G (1980) Sports-related injuries in school-aged children. Am J Sports Med 8(5):318–324
4. Chan KM, Fong DTP, Hong Y, Yung PSH, Lui PPY (2008) Orthopaedic sport biomechanics: a new paradigm. Clin Biomech 23(1 Supp):21–30
5. Waterman BR, Owens BD, Davey S, Zacchilli MA, Belmont PJ Jr (2010) The epidemiology of ankle sprains in the United States. J Bone Joint Surg 92A:2279–2284
6. Prins JG (1978) Diagnosis and treatment of injury to the lateral ligament of the ankle. A comparative clinical study. Acta Chir Scand Suppl 486:3–149
7. Golano' P, Vega J, de Leeuw PAJ, Malagelada F, Manzanares MC, Gotzens V, van Dijk CN (2010) Anatomy of the ankle ligaments: a pictorial essay. Knee Surg Sports Traumatol Arthrosc 18:557–569
8. Wiersman PH, Grifioen FMM (1992) Variations of three lateral ligaments of the ankle. A descriptive anatomical study. Foot 2:218–222
9. Brostrom L (1964) Sprained ankles. I. Anatomic lesions in recent sprains. Acta Chir Scand 128:483–495
10. Rasmussen O, Kromann-Andersen C (1983) Experimental ankle injuries. Analysis of the traumatology of the ankle ligaments. Acta Orthop Scand 54:356–362
11. Fallat L, Grimm DJ, Saracco JA (1998) Sprained ankle syndrome: prevalence and analysis of 639 acute injuries. J Foot Ankle Surg 37:280–285
12. Kannus P, Renstrfm P (1991) Treatment for acute tears of the lateral ligaments of the ankle. Operation, cast, or early controlled mobilization. J Bone Joint Surg 73A:305–312
13. Andersen TE, Floerenes TW, Arnason A, Bahr R (2004) Video analysis of the mechanisms for ankle injuries in football. Am J Sports Med 32(1 Supp):69–79
14. Markolf KL, Schmalzried TP, Ferkel RD (1989) Torsional strength of the ankle in vitro. The supination-external-rotation injury. Clin Orthop Rel Res 246:266–272
15. Fong DTP, Hong Y, Shima Y, Krosshaug T, Yung PSH, Chan KM (2009) Biomechanics of supination ankle sprain: a case report of an accidental injury event in laboratory. Am J Sports Med 37(4):822–827
16. Boytim MJ, Fischer DA, Neumann L (1991) Syndesmotic ankle sprains. Am J Sports Med 19:294–298
17. Taylor DC, Englehardt DL, Bassett FH III (1992) Syndesmosis sprains of the ankle. The influence of heterotopic ossification. Am J Sports Med 20:146–150
18. Konradsen L, Hflmer P, Sfndergaard L (1991) Early mobilizing treatment for grade III ankle ligament injuries. Foot Ankle 12:69–73
19. Van Dijk CN, Lim LS, Bossuyt PM et al (1996) Physical examination is sufficient for the diagnosis of sprained ankles. J Bone Joint Surg 78B:958–962
20. Mann G, Nysha M, Constantini N, Matan Y, Renstrom P, Lynch SA (2002) Mechanics of injury, clinical presentation, and staging. In: Nyska M, Mann G (eds) The uns table ankle human kinetics, pp 54–60
21. Clanton TO (1999) Athletic injuries to the soft tissues of the foot and ankle. In: Coughlin MJ, Mann RA (eds) Surgery of the foot and ankle. Mosby, St Louis, pp 1090–1209
22. Davis PF, Trevino S (1995) Ankle injuries. In: Baxter D (ed) The foot and ankle in sport. Mosby, St Louis, pp 147–169
23. Pijnenburg ACM, Bogaard K, Krips R, Marti RK, Bossuyt PM, van Dijk CN (2003) Operative and functional treatment of rupture of the lateral ligament of the ankle. A randomised, prospective trial. J Bone Joint Surg Br 85(4):525–530
24. van den Bekerom MPJ, Kerkhoffs GMMJ, McCollum GA, Calder JDF, van Dijk CN (2012) Management of acute lateral ankle ligament injury in the athlete. Knee Surg Sports Traumatol Arthrosc 21:1–6
25. Roberte-Jaspar A (1956) Severe sprains of the ankle. Acta Orthop Belg 22(2):132–136
26. Friedrich JM, Schnarkowski P, Rqbenacker S et al (1993) Ultrasonography of capsular morphology in normal and traumatic ankle joints. J Clin Ultrasound 21:179–187

27. Kerkhoffs GM, van den Bekerom M, Elders LAM et al (2012) Diagnosis, treatment and prevention of ankle sprains: an evidence-based clinical guideline. Br J Sports Med 46:854–860

28. Campbell DG, Menz A, Isaacs J (1994) Dynamic ankle ultrasonography: a new imaging technique for acute ankle ligament injuries. Am J Sports Med 22(6):855–858

29. van Dijk CN, Mol BW, Lim LS et al (1996) Diagnosis of ligament rupture of the ankle joint. Physical examination, arthrography, stress radiography, and sonography compared in 160 patients after inversion trauma. Acta Orthop Scand 67:566–570

30. Broström L (1965) Sprained ankles. III. Clinical observations in recent ligament ruptures. Acta Chir Scand 130:560–569

31. Naoki H, Hidekazu T, Nobumasa S, Fumio K (2007) Avulsion fracture of the lateral ankle ligament complex in severe inversion injury. Incidence and clinical outcome. Am J Sports Med 35:1144–1152

32. Busconi BD, Pappas AM (1996) Chronic, painful ankle instability in skeletally immature athletes. Ununited osteochondral fractures of the distal fibula. Am J Sports Med 24:647–651

33. Vahvanen V, Westerlund M, Nikku R (1984) Lateral ligament injury of the ankle in children. Follow-up results of primary surgical treatment. Acta Orthop Scand 55:21–25

34. Chaumien JP, Rigault P, Touzet P, Padovani JP (1986) Severe sprains of the ankle in children and adolescents. Rev Chir Orthop Rep Appar Mot 72(2):56–62

35. Schütze F, Maas U (1989) Osteochondral involvement in fibulotalar ligament ruptures. Z Kinderchir 44:91–93

36. de Bie RA, de Vet HC, Wildenberg FA, Lenssen FA, Knipschild PG (1997) The prognosis of ankle sprains. Int J Sports Med 18(4):285–289

37. Simanovsky N, Hiller N, Leibner E, Simanovsky N (2005) Sonographic detection of radiographically occult fractures in paediatric ankle injuries. Pediatr Radiol 35:1062–1065

38. Mcgiune TA, Greene JJ, Best T, Leverson G (2000) Balance as a predictor of ankle injuries in high school basketball players. Clin J Sport Med 10:239–244

39. Bahr R, Lian O, Barh IA (1997) A twofold reduction in the incidence of acute ankle sprains in volleyball after the injury prevention program: a prospective cohort study. Scand J Med Sci Sport 7(3):172–177

40. Stanitski CL (1988) Management of sports injuries in children and adolescents. Orthop Clin North Am 19(4):689–698

41. Munk B, Holm-Christensen K, Lind T (1995) Long-term outcome after ruptured lateral ankle ligaments. A prospective study of three different treatments in 79 patients with 11-year followup. Acta Orthop Scand 66:452–454

42. Povacz P, Unger SF, Miller WK et al (1998) A randomized, prospective study of operative and nonoperative treatment of injuries of the fibular collateral ligaments of the ankle. J Bone Joint Surg 80A:345–351

43. Kaikkonen A, Kannus P, Jarvinen M (1994) A performance test protocol and scoring scale for the evaluation of ankle injuries. Am J Sports Med 22(4):462–469

44. Meislin RJ, Rose DJ, Parisien JS, Springer S (1993) Arthroscopic treatment of synovial impingement of the ankle. Am J Sports Med 21(2):186–189

45. Guzzanti V (2001) Ankle ligament injuries in children. Fourth international pediatric orthopedic symposium. Orlando, USA, pp 586–587

46. Guzzanti V, Falciglia F (2012) Lesioni capsulo-legamentose acute della tibio-tarsica nell'adolescente. G.I.O.T. 37(Supp 1):S224–S229

47. Guzzanti V, Di Lazzaro A, Falciglia F (1997) Le distorsioni della tibio-peroneo-astragalica in età evolutiva. G.I.O.T. suppl. vol. XXIII fasc.3 ott.1997:483–486

48. Tol JL, Verheyen CP, van Dijk CN (2001) Arthroscopic treatment of anterior impingement in the ankle. J Bone Joint Surg 83B:9–13

Ankle and Foot: Chronic Instability

18

Sandro Giannini, Gherardo Pagliazzi, Alberto Ruffilli,
Deianira Luciani, Camilla Pungetti and Massimiliano Mosca

18.1 Introduction

Ankle sprain is a common sports-related injury that predominantly occurs in skeletally mature patients with a lower incidence in children and adolescents. However, as young athletes became more active in organized and specialized activity today, an increasing number of both acute and chronic injuries have been reported in this age group. It has been estimated that about 16–25 % of all injuries in the sport practice consists in ankle sprain [1, 2]. The majority of ankle sprains are caused by an inversion force on a plantar-flexed foot, and the anatomic structure most frequently involved is the lateral ligament complex. The lateral ankle ligament complex is compound of the anterior talo-fibular ligament

(ATFL), the calcaneo-fibular ligament (CFL), and the posterior talo-fibular ligament (PTFL). The ATFL is the weakest and the shortest of the ligaments and is the primary restraint to anterior ankle subluxation and to inversion stress in plantarflexion [3]. The CFL represents an important restraint to forces when the ankle joint is in neutral and dorsiflexed positions, while the PTFL is the strongest ligament of the lateral complex and usually is not injured with inversion sprains [4]. In dealing with younger athletes, serious acute ankle sprains typically result in physeal fractures, because ligaments are stronger than bone in the skeletally immature child [5]. Although physeal fracture is the most common consequence of an inversion injury in the young age, if the degree of the inversion stress is below the threshold required to cause a physeal fracture, attenuation or rupture of the ligaments and joint capsule may occur. Not infrequently, ligamentous lesions are underestimated or undiagnosed. The lack of appropriate treatment in acute instability may lead to a chronic instability cause of persistent pain and impairment in the young athlete. Subtalar joint instability may be also associated [6].

18.2 Diagnosis

Patients with chronic ankle instability typically show two different clinical pictures: symptoms after an acute ankle sprain, which patient refers to be a recurrent evenience; or a persistent sense

S. Giannini (✉) · G. Pagliazzi · A. Ruffilli ·
D. Luciani · C. Pungetti · M. Mosca
First Clinic of Orthopedics and Traumatology,
Rizzoli Orthopedic Institute, University of Bologna,
Via Pupilli 1, 40136 Bologna, Italy
e-mail: sandro.giannini@ior.it

G. Pagliazzi
e-mail: gpagliazzi@libero.it

A. Ruffilli
e-mail: aruffilli@tiscali.it

D. Luciani
e-mail: deianiralux@yahoo.it

C. Pungetti
e-mail: camilla.pungetti@gmail.com

M. Mosca
e-mail: massimiliano.mosca@fastwebnet.it

V. Guzzanti (ed.), *Pediatric and Adolescent Sports Traumatology*,
DOI: 10.1007/978-88-470-5412-7_18, © Springer-Verlag Italia 2014

of looseness or giving way, without any recent acute inversion episode. Pain is not referred as the principal cause of complain. If present, generally, follows a sprain recurrence, while, patients with pain persisting for more than 6 weeks, should be searched for associated lesions such as fractures of the lateral malleolus, peroneal tendon tears or subluxation and osteochondral lesions of the talus [7]. Failure in identifying associated lesions led to recurrence of symptoms, inappropriate treatment, and prolonged recovery for the patients. Mechanical causes of chronic instability such as tibial varum, calcaneal varus, cavus foot type, forefoot valgus, plantarflexed first metatarsal, or any deformity that increase the supination force through the lateral ankle and foot, should be excluded. Ankle instability can be distinguished into mechanical and functional. Mechanical ankle instability (MAI) is characterized by an abnormal ankle mobility, assessed clinically using manual stress application via the anterior drawer and the talar tilt tests [8, 9]. Functional ankle instability (FAI) was firstly described by Freeman et al. [10] as a subjective feeling of the ankle giving way during either physical activity or during common activities of daily living. Tropp in 1985 described functional instability as a movement that is independent from voluntary control, even if the physiological range of motion (R.O.M.) is not always exceeded. Unfortunately, the relationship between mechanical and functional instabilities is still unclear; Hirai et al. [11] recently stated that severity of FAI is not correlated with severity of MAI. This led to the hypothesis that the symptoms of FAI should not always be attributed to the mechanical laxity assessed clinically, but other factors may be involved, such as adhesion formation causing a decreased mobility of the ankle, peroneal muscle weakness or atrophy, and tibiofibular sprain. Patient's evaluation should focus on previous ankle sprain experienced, the mechanism of injury, level of activity and disability. The evaluation of chronic ankle instability proceeds through the anterior drawer and the talar tilt tests. The anterior drawer test is performed stabilizing the tibia and the fibula

with one hand, with the foot held in 20° of plantar flexion, and then, the talus is drawn forward in the ankle mortise. The test estimates the integrity of the ATFL and the anterior capsule. The test is considered positive when there is more than 10 mm of anterior translation on one side or the side-to-side difference is over 3 mm [12]. Talar tilt test evaluates the integrity of the CFL, while the talus is tilted into adduction and abduction with the foot held in neutral position. A positive result would be 9 degrees of increased inversion on one side or when the side-to-side difference is more than 3 degrees [13]. Radiographic assessment should start obtaining standard weight-bearing antero-posterior, lateral, and oblique views, to evaluate the alignment of the hindfoot and the presence of associated lesions of the adjacent structures. Anterior drawer and talar tilt stress views can be obtained either manually or mechanically with a Telos device. Stress radiographs are not routinely required to establish the diagnosis of mechanical instability, still they can be useful when the clinical presentation is unclear. Ultrasound is to be used for the evaluation of ligament and tendon structures. Non-invasivity of ultrasound makes the procedure particularly suitable for youngers even if lack in the visualization of bone and cartilage and the great variability of results depending on the operator are the major drawbacks. MRI is especially useful to investigate the ligament complex and the osteochondral layer.

18.3   Treatment

Conservative treatment of ankle instability is based on a structured physical therapy program focused on proprioceptive-based rehabilitation of the ankle joint. Active muscle strengthening, specifically on the peroneal muscles, and well-planned proprioceptive exercises help the patients return to normal living and sports activities [14, 15]. At times, a short Achilles tendon may be the cause of dynamic instability derived from an equinus ankle during walking or running; in such cases, stretching exercises several times a day and eccentric exercises may have a key role in symptoms resolution and return to sports [16, 17]. Six to 12 weeks after a supervised rehabilitation program, patients should reach the maximum benefit. Patients in whom symptoms persist or who have associated injuries causing morbidity, should be considered candidates for surgery. Isolated mechanical instability without giving-way episodes is not in itself an indication of surgery; hence, the surgical treatment is valued when patients are not willing to accept the recurrence of spraining episodes or subjective feelings of giving way. The coexistence of subtalar instability should be investigated in the surgical planning, because it may affect operative decision making [18, 19]. Surgical treatment in skeletally immature patients may be more technically demanding with respect to their adult counterparts because of concern regarding future skeletal growth. Each patient must be assessed individually to arrive at the decision for surgical reconstruction based on the child's activity level, the parent's expectations, and the child's potential for further growth. Aim of the operative treatment is to restore the native anatomy of the ligaments injured, focusing especially on the length, direction, and tightness of the ligaments that have to be reconstructed. Despite a peak incidence of ankle sprains in the adolescent population, few studies address the chronic instability in this age group [20]. More than 80 different surgical procedures have been described in literature for managing chronic ankle instability. Operative techniques can be distinguished into anatomic and non-anatomic. Anatomic repairs consist of direct repair of injured ligaments with the use of local tissue, free tendon graft, or a combination of these. The well-known advantages of anatomic procedure are the simplicity of the procedure, the restoration of the physiological joint mechanics and anatomy, and the preservation of the subtalar mobility. The main disadvantages of anatomic repair are the inability to achieve a reliable ankle stability with poor or lax ligamentous structures, and failure to address subtalar instability [21–23]. Anatomic reconstruction should be the primary choice for

the surgical treatment of chronic ankle instability in young patient and more widely in athletes. A Brostrom modified technique is one of the most popular techniques used when local tissues are sufficient to perform the reconstruction. When local tissues are weak and of low quality, the anatomic reconstruction may be performed using an autologous graft of plantar gracilis tendon, or allograft (posterior tibialis tendon) from cadavers. The author's preferred technique consists in a Brostrom modified reconstruction using a regional periosteal flap.

Surgical technique: patients' preferred position is in semilateral decubitus, under spinal anesthesia and tourniquet control. The skin incision is made just anterior to the distal fibula and curves posteriorly to the tip of the lateral malleolus, taking care to preserve the integrity of the superficial peroneal nerve. The inferior extensor retinaculum is retracted anteriorly to identify the joint capsule and the torn ends of the ATFL. A periosteal flap is elevated proximally from the distal lateral malleolus surface for about 1 cm long. With the ankle at a slight everted and dorsiflexed position (about 5 degrees), repair of the ATFL is performed by pulling and reattaching the distal stump of the ATFL to the lateral malleolus using reabsorbable suture threads in transosseus fashion. The periosteal flap created on the lateral malleolus is plicated in a "vest over pant" fashion over the newly sutured ATFL (Fig. 18.1). In case of reconstruction of the CFL, the incision is made distally and posteriorly while preserving the sural nerve and the lesser saphenous vein. Then, the peroneus brevis tendon is retracted in order to identify the CFL. Repair of the CFL is done with the ankle in neutral position, by pulling proximally the distal stump of the torn CFL, and fixing it to the lateral malleolus using the same reabsorbable suture threads, as close to the anatomic origin of the CFL as possible. The reconstruction may be finally reinforced by suturing the periosteal flap in "vest over pant" fashion (Fig. 18.2).

In selected cases with long-standing ankle instability resulting in lack and poor tissue quality, or in patients with generalized

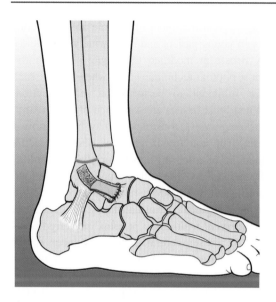

Fig. 18.1 Anatomic repair of the ATFL and the periosteal flap plicated in a "vest over pant" fashion

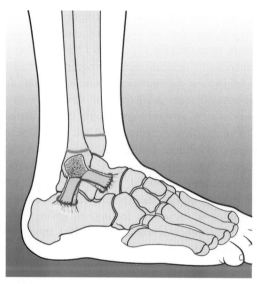

Fig. 18.2 Anatomic repair both of the ATFL and CFL, reinforced with a periosteal flap sutured in a "vest over pant" fashion

ligamentous laxity, the reconstruction of the anterior talo-fibular ligament, in association or not the calcaneo-fibular ligament, may be performed using an autologous tendon or a tendon allograft from a donor. For this purpose, the plantar gracilis, previously isolated or the allograft tendon, is firstly passed into the heel, from medial to lateral, then routed through the fibula from posterior to anterior, and secured to the talus. In association with the reconstruction of the lateral ligament complex, care should be taken to correct any obvious predisposing factor. In particular, a cavo-varus foot may predispose to repetitive ankle sprain episodes and may easily be corrected through a calcaneal osteotomy. Brostrom in 1966 firstly reported the results obtained on a series of 60 patients affected by chronic ankle instability [21]. The Brostrom technique involved mid-substance imbrication and suture of the rupture ligament ends. Subsequently, Gould et al. augmented the Brostrom procedure with the mobilized lateral portion of the extensor retinaculum, which was attached to the fibula after imbrication of the ATFL and the CFL [24]. Karlsson et al. reported satisfactory results in more than 150 patients treated with anatomic repair for lateral chronic ankle instability. The authors stated that frequently the ATFL and CFL were found to be elongated and worn during surgical procedure; thus they recommended shortening the ligaments and reattaching them to the fibula at their anatomic origins through drill holes [25]. More recently, Xinning et al. reported a series of over 50 high-demand athletes aged from 16 to 26 years, in whom ligaments were repaired with a variant of the Gould modified Brostrom procedure with suture anchors placed at the anatomic footprint of both the ATFL and CFL. Results were widely satisfactory and 94 % of the patients returned to the preinjury level of competition within 2 years [26]. Non-anatomic techniques rely on tenodesis in order to substitute the injured ligaments and to restrict the pathological ankle mobility. These are, in our experience, scarcely tolerated in younger athletes due for the need of bony tunnels in growing epiphysis and the high frequency of restricted subtalar motion and arthritis at long-term follow-up and should be considered, most of all, for severe chronic instability in syndromes [27–29]. The predominant procedures reported in literature are those described by Chrisman and Snook [30], Watson-Jones [31] and Evans [32].

The Chrisman-Snook procedure is the most frequently described in children. The original technique relies on a split of peroneus brevis tendon [30]. The proximal part of the graft is passed from anterior to posterior through the fibula and then down into the calcaneus, where the split tendon is passed through an oblique drill hole from posterior to anterior, reconstructing ATFL and CFL (Fig. 18.3). Recently, Marsh et al. [33] reported their experience on a case series of 42 patients, aged from 8 to 17 years, treated with a modified Chrisman-Snook repair. The procedure was modified practicing a significantly smaller incision (a 5-cm-only incision immediately posterior to the lateral malleolus), and positioning the graft more distally in the fibula at the anatomic origin of the ATFL, to improve graft isometry. In case of skeletally immature child, the drill is placed distal to the fibular physis, while in the skeletally mature child 1 cm above the tip of the fibula. Results were satisfactory in the 95 % of the cases, and only one was unstable at the mean follow-up of 6.5 years. All the patients returned to their usual preoperative level of function, including sports, and the authors concluded that this technique is an excellent mean of treating children with chronic ankle instability who have failed to respond to conservative treatment. Weiner et al. [34] described a modified Chrisman-Snook procedure, where the anterior half of the peroneus brevis tendon was routed subperiostally along the lateral wall of the calcaneus, instead of directly drilling a tunnel through the calcaneus, during its course back to the distal anatomic attachment on the fifth metatarsal. Hundred surgeries were performed on 66 children, with good overall satisfaction. 53 patients with at least 2 years of follow-up were able to return to full activities of their choice and were pain free or had only occasional discomfort.

Evans procedure [32] involved the entire peroneus brevis tendon, which is passed from anterior-inferior to posterior-superior through an oblique drill hole in the distal fibula and then reattached to the proximal end with the foot held in slight eversion (Fig. 18.4) Barnum et al. [35] published long-term results (average 12.6 years) on 20 young patients (mean age 12.6 years) that underwent an Evans procedure for chronic lateral ankle instability. Overall functional results were satisfactory in 85 % of patients at the last follow-up, with 6 of 12 competitive athletes

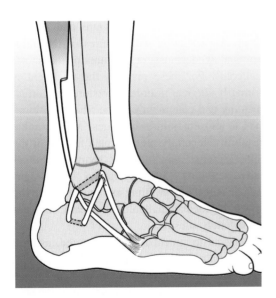

Fig. 18.3 Non-anatomic reconstruction of the ATFL and CFL described by Chrisman-Snook

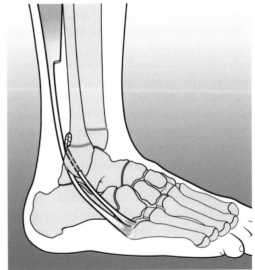

Fig. 18.4 Evans procedure

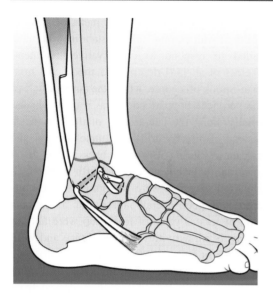

Fig. 18.5 Non-anatomic reconstruction of the ATFL according to Watson-Jones

returning to preinjury level of activity, compared with seven of eight recreational athletes. The authors stated that the moderate-activity-level athlete is eligible to undergone an Evans procedure, while in the elite athlete, an anatomic reconstruction should be firstly advised. Nevertheless, despite very promising early results reported in literature, in the mid-long-term follow-up, residual anterior talar instability and restricted subtalar motion were described [36].

The original Watson-Jones technique [31] detached the entire peroneus brevis tendon proximally, then routed it through the fibula from posterior to anterior and secured it to the talar neck through drill holes (Fig. 18.5). Initially, good to excellent results were reported in literature; Sugimoto et al. reported high rate of satisfactory results at 10–18 years of follow-up [37]. Nevertheless, major drawbacks of Watson-Jones tenodesis are the failure to reconstruct the CFL associated with a restricted subtalar motion, likely because of its non-anatomic nature [29]. Recently, Morelli et al. [38] reported mid- to long-term results (mean follow-up 10 years) on a series of 28 young athletes (mean age 22.7 years), who underwent non-anatomic

reconstruction with a modified Watson-Jones tenodesis according to Lemberger and Kramer. The peroneus brevis tendon was longitudinally dissected in half from its muscolotendineous junction; then, two drill holes were performed, one with an oblique orientation from posterior to anterior in the peroneal bone, the other with a vertical direction, starting from the neck of the talus toward the sinus tarsi. The peroneus brevis was passed firstly through the peroneal hole, then through the talar one, and finally fixed to the calcaneum periosteum. The authors concluded that the technique provided satisfactory clinical and radiological mid- to long-term results, which tend to be persistent over time.

Less frequently, sport injuries may involve the medial ligament complex.

The deltoid ligament is an important medial stabilizer of the ankle. This strong ligament is composed by two layers (superficial and deep) separated by fat pad. The superficial layer is composed by four fascicles, but only two of them are constantly present while the deep layer is composed by two components (the deep posterior tibiotalar ligament and the deep anterior tibiotalar ligament) [39]. The predominant mechanism of injury is a trauma when the foot is everted and externally rotated. Isolated ruptures of the deltoid ligament are rare and usually occur in association with injuries of the tibioperoneal syndesmosis or fractures of the lateral malleolus. For these reasons, the treatment is primarily surgical in order to restore the correct anatomy and congruency of the tibio-talar joint, thus to prevent joint's damages. Medial ankle instability generally presents as a feeling of the ankle "giving way," during sports and other daily activities [39]. Typically, early signs include soft tissue swelling and tenderness at the tip of the medial malleolus, but pain does not immediately subside.

Surgical treatment is often required, using a direct repair of the injured ligament. The direct repair is performed with the Du-Vries technique [40], which involves a cross-incision of the scar tissue and then the suture of the edges.

18.4 Summary

Chronic ankle ligamentous instability is not uncommonly encountered in children and adolescent. It may occur as a consequence of repetitive ankle sprains or after an acute injury which predispose the development of secondary degenerative changes in the ankle joint. Nevertheless, in children and adolescent, chronic ankle instability is seen most commonly in association with generalized ligamentous laxity where ankle sprains occur even with minor ankle twisting. With an increasing number of children involved in sports activities, more and more young athletes are presenting clinically with chronic symptoms due to the inadequate recuperation time and improper treatment. Only few studies, nevertheless, address the course and outcomes of children and adolescents.

There is no clear consensus on which type of procedure gives the best results, especially in the young age. To our knowledge, there are no long-term follow-up studies reporting anatomic repair in the pediatric population. Still we think that this technique should be preferred, when possible, because of lower invasiveness and capability to restore the correct anatomy of ligaments themselves. Some studies are available addressing non-anatomic reconstruction in youngers and reporting satisfactory results, even if the majority of the studies consider populations affected by different syndromes and with various grade of activity level. The need of bony tunnels in a growing epiphysis, alteration in ankle biomechanics and the high frequency of restricted subtalar motion are major drawbacks of these techniques that are to be recommended for failure of anatomic repair or either in generalized ligamentous laxity.

References

1. Fernandez WG, Yard EE, Comstock RD (2007) Epidemiology of lower extremity injuries among U.S. high school athletes. Acad Emerg Med 14(7):641–645. Epub 2007 May 18
2. Maehlum S, Daljord OA (1984) Acute sports injuries in Oslo: a one-year study. Br J Sports Med 18(3): 181–185
3. Bulucu C, Thomas KA, Halvorson TL, Cook SD (1991) Biomechanical evaluation of the anterior drawer test: the contribution of the lateral ankle ligaments. Foot Ankle 11(6):389–393
4. Stephens MM, Sammarco GJ (1992) The stabilizing role of the lateral ligament complex around the ankle and subtalar joints. Foot Ankle 13(3):130–136
5. McManama GB Jr (1988) Ankle injuries in the young athlete. Clin Sports Med 7:547–562
6. Larsen E (1988) Tendon transfers for lateral ankle and subtalar joint instability. Acta Orthop Scand 59:168–172
7. DiGiovanni BF, Fraga CJ, Cohen BE, Shereff MJ (2000) Associated injuries found in chronic lateral ankle instability. Foot Ankle Int 21(10):809–815
8. Safran MR, Bendetti RS, Bartolozzi AR III, Mandelbaum BR (1999) Lateral ankle sprains: a comprehensive review part 1: etiology, pathoanatomy, istopathogenesis, and diagnosis. Med Sci Sports 31(7):S429–S437
9. Chandnani VP, Harper MT, Ficke JR, Gagliardi JA, Rolling L, Christensen KP, Hansen MF (1994) Chronic ankle instability: evaluation with MR arthrography, MR imaging, and stress radiography. Radiology 192(1):189–194
10. Freeman MA (1965) Instability of the foot after injuries to the lateral ligament of the ankle. J Bone Joint Surg Br 47:669–677
11. Hirai D, Docherty CL, Schrader J (2009) Severity of functional and mechanical ankle instability in an active population. Foot Ankle Int 30(11):1071–1077
12. Karlsson J, Lansinger O (1992) Lateral instability of the ankle joint. Clin Orthop Relat Res (276):253–261
13. Peters JW, Trevino SG, Renstrom PA (1991) Chronic lateral ankle instability. Foot Ankle 12(3):182–191
14. Urgüden M, Kızılay F, Sekban H, Samancı N, Ozkaynak S, Ozdemir H (2010) Evaluation of the lateral instability of the ankle by inversion simulation device and assessment of the rehabilitation program. Acta Orthop Traumatol Turc 44(5):365–377
15. Van Dijk CN (2002) Management of the sprained ankle. Br J Sports Med 36(2):83–84
16. Ajis A, Maffuli N (2006) Conservative management of chronic ankle instability. Foot Ankle Clin 11:531–537
17. Mattacola CG, Dwyer MK (2002) Rehabilitation of the ankle after acute sprain or chronic instability. J Athl Train 27:413–429
18. Clanton TO, Berson L (1999) Subtalar joint athletic injuries. Foot Ankle Clin 4:729–743
19. Kato T (1995) The diagnosis and treatment of instability of the subtalar joint. J Bone Joint Surg 77-B:400–406
20. Letts M, Davidson D, Mukhtar I (2003) Surgical management of chronic lateral ankle instability in adolescents. J Pediatr Orthop 23(3):392–397

21. Bröstrom L (1966) Sprained ankles VI. Surgical treatment of "chronic" ligament ruptures. Acta Chir Scand 132:551–565

22. Rosenbaum D, Becker HP, Wilke HJ et al (1998) Tenodeses destroy the kinematic coupling of the ankle joint complex. A three-dimensional in vitro analysis of joint movement. J Bone Joint Surg Br 80:162–168

23. Cheng M, Tho KS (2002) Chrisman-Snook ankle ligament reconstruction outcomes: a local experience. Singapore Med J 43(12):605–609

24. Gould N, Seligson D, Gassman J (1980) Early and late repair of lateral ligament of the ankle. Foot Ankle 1(2):84–89

25. Karlsson J, Bergsten T, Lansinger O, Peterson L (1988) Reconstruction of the lateral ligaments of the ankle for chronic lateral instability. J Bone Joint Surg Am 70(4):581–588

26. Li X, Killie H, Guerrero P, Busconi BD (2009) Anatomical reconstruction for chronic lateral ankle instability in the high-demand athlete: functional outcomes after the modified Broström repair using suture anchors. Am J Sports Med 37(3):488–494

27. Coughlin MJ, Schenck RC, Grebing BR, Gehron T (2004) Comprehensive reconstruction of the lateral ankle for chronic instability using a free gracilis graft. Foot Ankle Int 25:231–241

28. Pagenstert G, Valderrabano V, Hintermann B (2005) Lateral ankle ligament reconstruction with free plantaris tendon graft. Tech Foot Ankle Surg 4:104–112

29. Liu SH, Baker CL (1994) Comparison of lateral ankle ligamentous reconstruction procedures. Am J Sports Med 22:313–317

30. Chrisman OD, Snook GA (1969) Reconstruction of lateral ligament tears of the ankle: an experimental study and clinical evaluation of seven patients treated by a new modification of the Elmslie procedure. J. Bone Joint Surg 51-A:904–912

31. Watson-Jones R (1952) Recurrent forward dislocation of the ankle joint. J Bone Joint Surg 34-B:519

32. Evans DL (1953) Recurrent instability of the ankle-a method of surgical treatment. Proc R Soc Med 46:343–344

33. Marsh JS, Daigneault JP, Polzhofer GK (2006) Treatment of ankle instability in children and adolescents with a modified Chrisman-Snook repair: a clinical and patient-based outcome study. J Pediatr Orthop 26(1):94–99

34. Yang J Jr, Morscher MA, Weiner DS (2010) Modified Chrisman-Snook repair for the treatment of chronic ankle ligamentous instability in children and adolescents. J Child Orthop 4(6):561–570

35. Barnum MJ, Ehrlich MG, Zaleske DJ (1998) Long-term patient-oriented outcome study of a modified Evans procedure. J Pediatr Orthop 18(6):783–788

36. Orava S, Jaroma H, Weitz H, Loikkanen T, Suvela M (1983) Radiographic instability of the ankle joint after Evans' repair. Acta Orthop Scand 54:734–738

37. Sugimoto K, Takakura Y, Akiyama K, Kamei S, Kitada C, Kumai T (1998) Long-term results of Watson-Jones tenodesis of the ankle. Clinical and radiographic findings after ten to 18 years of follow-up. J Bone Joint Surg Am 80(11):1587–1596

38. Morelli F, Perugia D, Vadalà A, Serlorenzi P, Ferretti A (2011) Modified Watson-Jones technique for chronic lateral ankle instability in athletes: clinical and radiological mid- to long-term follow-up. Foot Ankle Surg 17(4):247–251

39. Hintermann B, Knupp M, Pagenstert GI (2006) Deltoid ligament injuries: diagnosis and management. Foot Ankle Clin 11(3):625–637

40. Du Vries (1978) Surgery of the foot. St. Louis CV Mosby Company

Ankle and Foot: Foot Abnormalities and Pathologies

19

Sandro Giannini, Roberto E. Buda, Alessandro Parma,
Laura Ramponi, Antonio Mazzotti and Francesca Vannini

Children and adolescents start sports at earlier ages and with higher intensity. In the USA, more than half of people between 8 and 16 years old are engaged in some kind of sport during the school years [1]. In Italy, 22 % of children between 6 and 10 years of age play sport for less than one hour in the week, and at 13 years of age, 51 % of boys and 34 % of girls are engaged in some kind of sport. Foot and ankle abnormalities are common in children under 10 years old and may result in impairment while starting a sports activity. Pathologies that can affect young athlete include flatfoot, tarsal coalition, cavus foot, juvenile hallux valgus, ankle impingement, os trigonum, Haglund's disease, and osteochondroses [2].

S. Giannini (✉) · R. E. Buda · A. Parma ·
L. Ramponi · A. Mazzotti · F. Vannini
First Clinic of Orthopedics and Traumatology,
Rizzoli Orthopedic Institute, University of Bologna,
Via Pupilli 1, 40136 Bologna, Italy
e-mail: sandro.giannini@ior.it

R. E. Buda
e-mail: roberto.buda@ior.it

A. Parma
e-mail: alessandro.parmaz@libero.it

L. Ramponi
e-mail: laura.ramponi@gmail.com

A. Mazzotti
e-mail: antonio.mazzotti2@studio.unibo.it

F. Vannini
e-mail: france_vannini@yahoo.it

19.1 Flatfoot

Flatfoot is a common disorder characterized by morphological reduction in plantar arch and valgus hind foot. Functionally, the subtalar joint does not alternate the physiologic movements of pronation during the stance phase and supination during the propulsive phase. A state of persistent or prevailing pronation is instead maintained during gait with consequent loss of propulsive efficacy and overload of ipsilateral foot joints.

Flatfoot may be an isolated pathology or part of a larger clinical entity like collagen disorders, generalized ligamentous laxity, genetic conditions, and neuromuscular abnormalities. As reported by Harris [3], pediatric flatfoot can be divided into flexible and rigid categories, symptomatic and asymptomatic. Most flatfeet are flexible physiologic and asymptomatic. Rigid flatfoot is often associated with underlying pathology as congenital vertical talus or tarsal coalition and is characterized by a deformity non-reducible manually.

At 10 years of age, children with flatfoot are 4 % but only 10 % of these have a functional flatfoot which needs treatments in order to reduce pain and prevent disability in adulthood like hallux valgus, metatarsalgia, Morton's neuroma, and posterior tibialis tendon dysfunction.

The diagnosis of flexible flatfoot is based on clinical and radiographic examinations.

V. Guzzanti (ed.), *Pediatric and Adolescent Sports Traumatology*,
DOI: 10.1007/978-88-470-5412-7_19, © Springer-Verlag Italia 2014

The young patient is usually referred to orthopedic control because of foot morphology and discomfort during activity.

The most common symptoms are pain in foot sole and medial hind foot, leg and knee with prevalence in girls and in patients with increased BMI [4]. Increased heel valgus at rest more or less reducible during the tiptoe standing test, footprint enlargement at rest and during the Jack test, restriction of dorsiflexion of the ankle joint after manual correction of the deformity are evident during examination.

Radiographs of the flexible flatfoot are not necessary for diagnosis, but they may be helpful in case of uncharacteristic pain, decreased flexibility, and for surgical planning.

Weight-bearing anteroposterior (AP) and lateral views are generally sufficient to evaluate the flexible flatfoot. The lateral radiograph reveals alteration in talocalcaneal and intermetatarsal angle and Meary's line interruption. Meary's line is formed by the lines drawn through the mid-axis of the talus and the mid-axis of the first metatarsal on a standing lateral radiograph.

Though there is no disadvantage in sport performance originating from flexible flatfoot and no significant correlations between the arch height and motor skills [5], about 1/3 patients with flatfeet have complain during sports practice, and in a large part of patients, the sport practice is limited to swimming or lower impact activities [4].

From 4 to 6 years of age, a conservative treatment is indicated: stretching exercises and insoles. From 6 to 8 years of age, orthoses loose their corrective function. So that it is advisable to permit the young athlete every activity without insoles in order to understand if the foot is somehow symptomatic deserving further treatment.

Eight to twelve years is considered the most suitable age if surgical correction is needed. The aim of surgical treatment is to restore the normal relationship between the talus and calcaneus through either arthroereisis, osteotomy, or arthrodesis. Arthroereisis is the principal option for children since permits a foot correction

without osteotomies nor arthrodesis, relying basically on skeletal growth [6]. Arthroereisis is performed by inserting a screw (calcaneo-stop) into calcaneus or an endorthesis into sinus tarsi in order to correct the subtalar pronation and permit a remodeling of the foot over time. A major improvement in the technique has been given by the introduction of bioreabsorbable materials for the implants, such as poly-L-lactic acid (PLLA), which are degraded in 4 years without the need of a second surgery for device removal [7] (Fig. 19.1).

Achilles tendon lengthening may be performed subcutaneously as an associated procedure to arthroereisis if 90° dorsiflexion of the foot is not obtained once the valgus of the hind foot is corrected. Other accessory procedures include medial procedure for prominent navicular bone or accessory navicular. During this procedure, the accessory navicular is removed, or the prominent navicular is tangentially resected and the tibialis posterior is sutured back in place having care to restore the correct tension.

Grice extra-articular subtalar arthrodesis is considered to be a valid surgical method which improves foot alignment in patients with severe ligamentous laxity and can achieve significant correction. This procedure relies on a bone autograft inserted into the sinus tarsi to create an "extra-articular arthrodesis" and thus correcting the valgus hind foot [8].

If the skeletal maturity is reached, calcaneal osteotomy is to be preferred. This procedure consists in an oblique osteotomy of the posterior calcaneus in which the posterior fragment is displaced medially to correct the apparent heel valgus. This procedure does not actually correct the malalignment of the subtalar joint, but merely creates a compensating deformity to improve the valgus angulation of the heel [9].

19.2 Tarsal Coalition

Tarsal coalition is a congenital union of two or more tarsal bone fibrous, cartilaginous, or osseous in nature which is cause of a rigid flatfoot deformity.

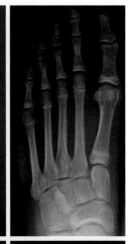
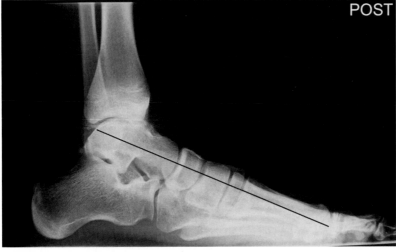
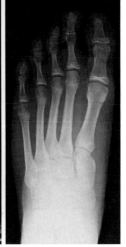

Fig. 19.1 Weight-bearing lateral and dorsoplantar X-ray view of foot in 11-year-old boy, *pre*- and *post*-surgery. Before subtalar arthroereisis with bioreabsorbable implant, Meary's line is interrupted. After surgery, Meary's line is continued and foot is corrected

Synostosis affects 1 % of population and is believed to result from a failure of embryonic mesenchymal differentiation and segmentation. Talocalcaneal and calcaneonavicular synostoses are the most common coalitions and in 50 % of cases are bilateral, while calcaneocuboid and talonavicular are rare [10].

Symptoms are not always evident in children, and in adults tarsal coalition may become symptomatic after trauma. The onset of symptoms usually coincides with the ossification of the coalition that limits the residual subtalar motion.

Clinically, the degree of deformity is variable, and pain may range from vague and insidious at sinus tarsi or below lateral malleolus during physical activity, to persistent pain. Limitation of inversion–eversion movement of the subtalar joint and/or midtarsal is evident. A history of frequent ankle sprain may be reported.

Standard RX projections united to oblique are the first step for the diagnosis of synostosis, in particular for the calcaneonavicular coalition but may not be diriment.

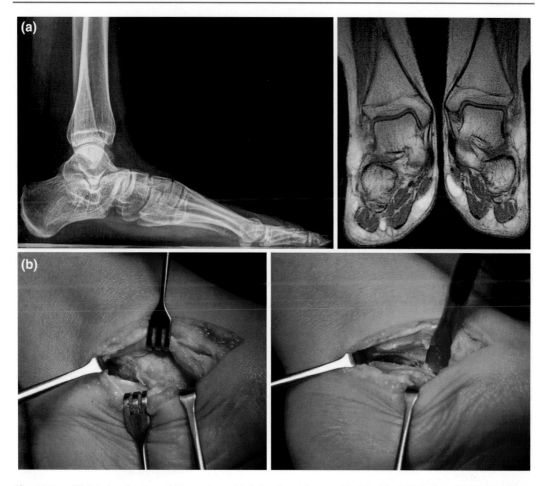

Fig. 19.2 **a** Weight-bearing lateral X-ray view of *left* foot in a 10-year-old girl with rigid flatfeet. RMN view shows bilateral talocalcaneal coalition. **b** Intraoperative views of talocalcaneal coalition and its excision

Full-length, weight-bearing anteroposterior and lateral radiographs of the foot may show signs of coalition. Lateral X-ray may show the "anteater nose" sign (extensions of the anterior process of the calcaneus toward its junction with the navicular) in the presence of calcaneonavicular coalition or "C" sign (continuous circular density formed by the outline of the talar dome and the inferior outline of the sustentaculum tali) in the presence of talocalcaneal coalition. This last coalition is most commonly found at the middle facet [11].

A 45° medial oblique view is useful for identifying calcaneonavicular coalition.

CT or MRI is usually necessary to confirm the diagnosis: both are excellent in recognizing the coalition compared to radiography and allow to describe size and location of the lesion (Fig. 19.2a).

As larger parts of coalition are asymptomatic, a conservative treatment may be effective, using orthoses with shell and medial heel wedge, a cast in severe cases with peroneal spasm [12].

If the coalition results in a recurrent symptomatic flatfoot, surgery is required.

Surgical treatment depends on the type of coalition and the status of joint.

Talocalcaneal coalitions, in skeletally immature individuals, are usually managed by coalition excision (Fig. 19.2b). Subtalar arthroereisis by implanting a bioreabsorbable device after removal of the tarsal coalition, in the same surgical session, is an effective procedure for restoring the alignment of the hind foot and prevents coalition recurrence. In patients reached skeletal maturity, or when the conditions of the subtalar joint are too compromised, due to coalition size or arthritis, arthrodesis is to be performed [11].

Calcaneonavicular coalitions are also managed by coalition resection. However, a high rate of coalition recurrence and progressive radiographic evidence of transverse tarsal joint arthrosis have been reported. Some form of interposition is recommended in literature at the site of resection, and the most commonly used is extensor digitorum brevis muscle [12, 13]. Otherwise, also in this type of coalition, an arthroereisis by a reabsorbable device is capable to correct the deformity and have a positive impact on the recurrence, which if eventually happens, will happen in a good foot position with reduced or no impairment.

19.3 Cavus Foot

Cavus foot is a complex deformity that can be morphologically defined as a dorsiflexed and varus hind foot, a plantar flexed forefoot, and subsequent elevation of the plantar arch in weight bearing.

The difference in height between the forefoot and the hind foot and the persistent supination of the foot during gait are primarily responsible for functional consequences that produce instability, soft tissue overloading, stretching, adaptive secondary joint positions, and footwear problems [14].

The incidence in population is 1/1000 and from clinical observation is common in population who plays sports. The deformity tends to develop by growth after the three years of age.

The etiology of the deformity can be generally divided into 5 major groups: neuromuscular, congenital, post-traumatic, idiopathic, and miscellaneous [15].

The neuromuscular disorders that can lead to pes cavus are varied and include Charcot–Marie–Tooth disease, Duchenne's muscular dystrophy, poliomyelitis, and cerebral palsy.

Typical congenital cavus foot deformities are the residual of club foot, arthrogryposis or less frequently, the presence of tarsal coalition, and they are quite rare. Traumatic etiologies can include fractures, tendon lesions, or foot and leg compartmental syndrome.

In the miscellaneous group, we can include a number of endocrine, rheumatic, or iatrogenic problems, such as excessive lengthening or failed repair of Achilles tendon rupture [16].

Idiopathic cavus foot can be functionally defined as a foot in a persistent or prevalent state of supination.

Based on the location of deformity, cavus foot can be divided into anterior, posterior, and cavovarus. Anterior cavus foot is characterized by flexion of forefoot, posterior cavus foot from the vertical heel, and cavovarus is a result of these two conditions together. In detail, the cavovarus foot is a three-dimensional deformity characterized by the fixed cavus deformity of the first ray with internal rotation of the foot, varus deviation of the heel, and forefoot pronation [17].

During the cycle of gait, cavus foot keeps a state of prevalent supination in correspondence of the subtalar joint.

The site of the deformity (forefoot or hind foot) and the persistent supination of the foot are responsible for functional consequences and the extremely variety of clinical presentation of this deformity. Frequent symptomatologies are ankle instability, soft tissue overloading, anterior impingement, toes deformity, plantar fasciitis, Achilles tendinopathies, and plantar hyperkeratosis leading to footwear difficulties.

Depending on the degree of deformity and reducibility of the deformity itself, sports activity is more or less impaired. Because running requires the foot to accept 2.5 times the body weight at heel strike, the cavovarus deformity causes less stress dissipation and increases lack of shock absorption. So, runners with a cavus foot configuration can have additional problems such as plantar fasciitis, metatarsalgia, stress fracture, tendinitis, medial longitudinal arch pain ankle instability, and recurrent sprain [18].

At RX, lateral view is characterized by accentuation of the arch and the angle of arc decreased.

The choice among available surgical procedures is dictated by the age of the patient, the flexibility, and cause of the deformity.

Conservative treatment consists of stretching exercises and insoles.

Surgical treatment has to be carefully planned case by case and may consist of soft tissues and bony procedures. Among soft tissue procedures are widely used Steindler's plantar fasciotomy and Achilles tendon lengthening. Among bony procedures, is to be noticed the Jones procedure, in association or not with first metatarsus osteotomy, consists in transposition of the tendon of the flexor hallucis longus on the first metatarsus to facilitate dorsiflexion of the first metatarsal and correct deformity cock-up of metatarsophalangeal joint. Other tendon transpositions include tibialis anterior, tibialis posterior, and long hallux extensor in patients with muscular or neurological deficit [19].

Bony procedures are usually performed in mature feet because soft tissue procedures do not provide a complete correction of the deformity. Calcaneal osteotomy, tarsectomy, subtalar arthrodesis, midtarsal arthrodesis, and interphalangeal arthrodesis are among the different arthrodeses used.

19.4   Juvenile Hallux Valgus

Juvenile hallux valgus deformity is described as valgus deviation of the great toe proximal phalanx and varus deviation of the great toe metatarsal, occurring in patients who are skeletally immature. The incidence, etiology, risk factors, and natural history of juvenile hallux valgus (JHV) have not been completely defined. The strong preponderance of girls with JHV (surgical series report 84–100 % girls) and the presence of a positive family history in most cases (72 %) suggest a hereditary component to the etiology of JHV [20].

Etiology includes also ligamentous laxity, forefoot deformities, including lesser toes deformity or hind foot deformities such as flatfoot which is a strong predisposing condition.

In sportive people, hallux valgus may be correlated with hyperextension, acute luxation or subluxation of the first metatarsophalangeal joint, or chronic condition of overuse like flatfoot with increment of stress acting on the hallux, squatting, and abduction stress. Athletes most frequently involved in hallux valgus are dancers, fencers, and American football, soccer, and golf players [19].

With respect to the adult hallux valgus, in younger, the deviation is less pronounced and the medial eminence is smaller. The large part of patients is asymptomatic, and the hallux valgus is often an incidental finding but sometimes it can be painful, exacerbated with shoe wear. The probability of progression of deformity is assumed because of remaining skeletal growth but is not actually known because no study to date has documented the progression of JHV without treatment. At radiographs, it is possible to measure intermetatarsal angle, hallux valgus angle, proximal metatarsal articular angle, and metatarsal length ratio.

The first approach of treatment is conservative with comfortable shoes, orthotics, bunion pads, and physical therapy. Usually, the advice is to postpone surgical correction until skeletal maturity to minimize the risk of recurrent deformity. If pain persists, surgery becomes necessary. Although several techniques have been described to correct this deformity in adults, limitations exist for adolescents because of the presence of open growth plates and high recurrence rates. Procedures include soft tissue balancing or skeletal realignment.

Distal first metatarsal osteotomy fixed with Kirschner wire (SERI) is a valid technique for realignment of the hallux valgus without interesting of growth cartilage (Fig. 19.3) and can be associated with Akin procedure if interphalangeal deformity is also present or in

Fig. 19.3 Weight-bearing dorsoplantar X-ray view of foot in 10-year-old girl, *pre-* and *post-*distal first metatarsal osteotomy

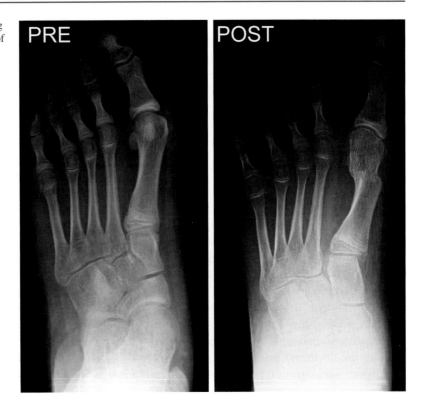

hypermetric toe. Other techniques include lateral hemiepiphysiodesis of the great toe metatarsal physis, Chevron osteotomy for mild deformities, distal soft tissue procedure with proximal first metatarsal osteotomy for moderate and severe deformities with MTP subluxation, and double osteotomy (extra-articular correction) for moderate and severe deformities with an increased distal metatarsal articular angle [20].

19.5   Ankle Impingement

Ankle impingement is infrequent in children and still is one of the most common causes of chronic ankle pain in young athlete. It is the result of a conflict between bony or soft tissue structures during the normal range of motion of the ankle. The etiology and the pathologic anatomy are heterogeneous.

19.5.1 Anterior Ankle Impingement

Can be bony or soft tissue related. It appears as an anterior pain exacerbated by forced dorsiflexion.

An anterior bony impingement may be present in dancers or soccer players which perform repetitive movements in dorsiflexion, with compression and damage of the anterior capsular structures and joints. Dancers try to compensate by overpronating, leading to other injuries [21].

A soft tissue impingement generally occurs as a result of synovitis or capsulitis: It develops as a consequence of inversion ankle sprain or repetitive microtrauma. In young gymnasts, it may occur as result of repeated extreme dorsiflexion under load.

On examination, it is possible to find pain and tenderness to palpation in the anterior region of the ankle, exacerbated by the simultaneous movement of dorsiflexion. The Achilles tendon can be shortened.

A bony impingement instead is a rare occurrence in younger's, since is related to an early stage of arthritis. Still, professional athletes may be affected by bony impingement even at young age.

Plain ankle X-rays can show the bony impingement, while MRI is capable to evidentiate also the soft tissue and cartilage pathology being usually diagnostic.

Conservative treatment includes rest, heel lifts, ice, non-steroidal anti-inflammatory, and stretching exercises.

In case of conservative treatment failure, arthroscopic excision of the lesion with a partial synovectomy is indicated [22]. Surgical treatment should be followed by stretching exercises to prevent recurrence.

A "meniscoid lesion" can occur due to repeated ankle sprain: In these cases, a meniscus-like reactive fibrous tissue may develop between the fibula and the talus and because of pain. The young sportive patient presents pain and swelling on the anterior aspect of the fibula, sometimes with a snap when testing inversion stability. The diagnosis is completed by MRI. The arthroscopic treatment of the lesion is usually resolving [23].

Hypertrophy of the distal anterior talofibular ligament is another cause of pain impingement related. Usually, it is a result of repeated trauma. Clinically, the young complains pain on the syndesmosis, dramatically increased by forced dorsiflexion. It is necessary to exclude an osteochondritis dissecans with MRI. The treatment, also in this case, is arthroscopic and provides for the debridement of the lesion.

19.5.2 Posterior Ankle Impingement

Posterior impingement of the ankle [24] is a common syndrome consisting in posterior ankle pain exacerbated by forced plantarflexion. Bony structures involved in posterior bony impingement of the ankle lie in the tibiocalcaneal interval: these structures are the posterior tibial malleolus, the posterolateral talar process (Stieda's process), the os trigonum, the posterior subtalar joint, and the posterior process of the calcaneus.

Posterior ankle impingement is more frequent in athletes participating in sports involving repeated plantarflexion with compressing the posterior structures of the ankle [23, 25], especially in young female dancers, ice skaters, soccer players, or gymnasts.

On physical examination, patient has pain in palpation of the posterior ankle, dramatically increased with forced plantarflexion. Plain radiographs of the ankle, possibly with oblique views, may be taken to check for a bone etiology (i.e., os trigonum) [23]. Soft tissue etiology includes flexor hallux long irritation, thickened or invaginated posterior capsule, synovitis, and posterior impingement by anomalous muscles [25].

19.6 Os Trigonum

The posterior region of the talus often shows a core of separate ossification that appears at 8–10 years of age in females and 11–13 years in males. Fusion usually occurs one year after its appearance [24], but if fusion does not occur, os trigonum is formed. Approximately 10 % of the general population presents os trigonum, often unilateral [24, 26], and usually, it is asymptomatic. Os trigonum can be congenital or acquired. The congenital one appears when separation of the nucleus of ossification of the lateral tubercle of the talus is maintained, secondary to microtrauma during growth. It is acquired when it occurs secondary to a fracture of the posterolateral process unconsolidated [24].

In some cases, it may become symptomatic in young athletes who engaged in forced plantarflexion, as dancers, gymnasts, and soccer players [24, 26–28].

Clinical presentation usually consists in pain in the posterolateral side of the ankle, behind the peroneal tendons [24], exacerbated by forced plantarflexion. An anteromedial pain can be associated if tendinitis of the flexor hallucis longus occurs [24, 27].

Radiographic diagnosis includes standard X-rays and lateral projection in plantarflexion.

Differential diagnosis should exclude Achilles tendonitis, flexor hallucis longus, and peroneal tendinitis.

Conservative treatment consists in rest, anti-inflammatory, discharge of plantarflexion, orthopedics cast, and infiltrative therapy [24, 27]. However, symptoms often recur when the subject returns to play sports, especially in dancers. In these cases, surgical treatment (endoscopic and open) is indicated to remove os trigonum. The open lateral approach is considered safer, and the medial approach may be indicated in case of concomitant tendinitis of the flexor hallucis longus.

19.7 Haglund's Disease

Haglund's disease is an alteration of the morphology of the calcaneus, described for the first time in 1928 by Patrick Haglund and characterized by the prominence of the posterosuperior margin of the calcaneal tuberosity [29].

Haglund's disease is not rare in adolescent females due to the use of rigid rear shoes, while in sport it is more frequent in young males and female runners, ice skaters, and soccer players.

On physical examination, the prominence is usually located to the lateral side of the heel.

Sometimes it can be observed an associated retrocalcaneal bursitis or Achilles tendonitis with thickening of the overlying skin and may be associated with varus hind foot.

Goal of the treatments is to reduce friction between shoe and prominence by padding the prominence and using a higher heel to download the region.

Conservative treatment also includes physical therapy and stretching of the Achilles tendon in association with non-steroidal anti-inflammatory. If the problem persists, open or endoscopic resection of the lesion is indicated [29].

19.8 Osteochondrosis of the Foot

Osteochondrosis is defined as deviations from the normal process of bone growth, non-inflammatory, or infectious. They appear as an abnormal ossification process, accompanied by a specific set of symptoms [30] in order to differentiate from normal variants of ossification.

In foot, the following diseases occur:
1. Sever's disease or osteochondrosis of the calcaneus
2. Kohler's disease or osteochondrosis of the tarsal navicular
3. Freiberg's disease or osteochondrosis of the head of the second metatarsal or Kohler's disease II
4. Iselin's disease or osteochondrosis of the base of the fifth metatarsal

The cause is still under investigation. However, it is believed that vascular disorders in combination with repeated microtrauma are at the base of the pathology. Hereditary and endocrine theories have also been proposed. Males are most frequently affected.

The main feature is an alteration degenerative–necrotic core of epiphyseal ossification followed by reparative processes that may hesitate in an anatomical deformity.

In the foot, the role of biomechanical factors as pathogenetic elements or aggravation is important: Forces that develop on the plantar structures are related both to load and direct reaction of the ground and to the tension that develops through tendons and ligaments on apophysis.

High stresses are transferred to foot's different bone structures, during gait or running, according to the performance helix breech: The calcaneal region will be severely stressed in the initial phase of step (heel strike), and thereafter at the end of the contact phase, the scaphoid is stressed while occurs the pronation of the subtalar joint. Finally shortly before the transfer of weight on the first finger, this is concentrated in a combination of vertical and horizontal forces on the condyle of the second metatarsal.

Sports increase quality and quantity of stress over structures, so it is possible to highlight the connection between sports and osteochondrosis in foot.

1. *Sever's disease (osteochondrosis of lower posterior calcaneal apophysis)*

Sever's disease is an avascular necrosis interesting calcaneal apophysis with pain in the posterior surface of the calcaneus [31] (Fig. 19.4). It is a non-articular osteochondrosis in the tendon insertions, particularly exposed to trauma: The region is subjected to damaging stresses resulting from contact with the ground directly and indirectly by the action of the Achilles tendon and plantar band.

Among the various osteochondrosis of the foot Sever's disease is the one that is more directly connected to sport. It affects mainly robust males engaged in sports as football, basketball, mini-rugby usually aged between 7 and 10 years. The higher prevalence is found among 8–9 years.

It occurs both bilaterally and unilaterally, and length difference should be evaluated in order to justify asymmetrical stresses. In 61 % of cases, this osteochondrosis is bilateral [32].

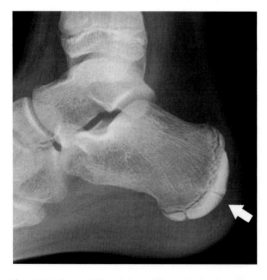

Fig. 19.4 Lateral X-ray view of foot shows osteochondrosis of lower posterior calcaneal apophysis in Sever's disease

Onset of the disorder is influenced by pronated foot and gastrocnemius–soleus complex retraction.

It presents with pain in the heel region usually without clinical local signs and may be accompanied by pain at the insertion of Achilles tendon.

At X-rays, secondary ossification center of the heel makes its appearance in the back around 8 years and undergoes fusion to 14 years [30]. In children between 9 and 11 years old, it is possible to detect a thickened apophysis, sometimes interrupted with or without fragmentation [33]. However, this isolated X-ray aspect is not to be considered specific because it is very common in the development of the calcaneal apophysis.

With ultrasound investigation, it is possible to find an inflammatory, edematous framework of insertion of Achilles and peritendinous tissues.

Treatment is conservative: rest and abstention from sport, discharge heel, and heel soft silicone are indicated. In the acute phase, treatment includes ice and anti-inflammatory therapy and is useful to avoid walking bare feet and stretching of the triceps surae until it becomes asymptomatic [34]. In the long term, it is important to reduce stress controlling the weight.

This osteochondrosis usually solves after a maximum of 8–12 months, depending on the subject and observation of prescriptions. Recurrence of symptoms may occur in subjects which do not suspend the activities or that start again early.

2. *Kohler's disease (osteochondrosis of the tarsal navicular)*

Kohler's disease is an idiopathic ischemic necrosis of the tarsal navicular [35] (Fig. 19.5). It was reported by Kohler (1908) as a thickening and flattening of the bone seen radiographically. Kohler later described the osteochondrosis of the second metatarsal; therefore, the pathology of the scaphoid is also defined Kohler's disease I. It is more frequent in males than females with a ratio of 6:1, and sport is not considered an etiological cause but a cause of aggravation. An etiological factor as a traumatic episode was found in 50 % of cases and is bilateral in 30 %.

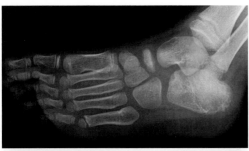

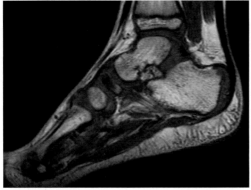

Fig. 19.5 Oblique X-ray view and MRI view show injury to the scaphoid in Kohler's disease

Scaphoid is last bone of the tarsus to appear, and its ossification is late [33]. The process normally is completed between the 4th and 5th year.

The age of greatest incidence of the disease is between 3 and 8 years, coinciding with that of the proximal femoral epiphysis involvement. As tarsal navicular is positioned at the apex of arch, it is supposed to be strongly stressed when it was still in cartilage phase.

Frequently, Kohler's disease is associated with flatfoot, and clinically, it shows antalgic lameness, swelling, and medial edema [36].

Radiographic diagnosis is simple: It presents a thickening and thinning of the core of scaphoid. X-rays may be non-diriment in case of young children, when the core is not yet present. The densification of the nucleus is followed by fragmentation, and generally, it is followed by an almost normal bone morphology. Nevertheless, in rare cases, it may remain a flattening of the scaphoid with osteophytosis of talonavicular joint.

The treatment is conservative: reduction in weights, abstention from sports, orthoses with plantar support of the medial longitudinal arch for unloading the medial arch and for the pronation control. In severe cases, a plaster cast is needed in order to reduce recovery time [36].

The healing process is completed in 9–12 months, and recovery is faster in children.

Sport must be suspended in the acute phase except for swimming and may be resumed gradually in association with the use of orthotics.

3. *Freiberg's disease (osteochondrosis of the head of the second metatarsal)*

Also referred to as Kohler disease II, Freiberg's disease is an avascular necrosis of second metatarsal epiphysis.

The osteochondrosis of the head of the second metatarsal is due to a suffering of the epiphyseal nucleus, which affects therefore the metatarsophalangeal joint. Described by Freiberg in 1914 [37] can occur more rarely at the level of the third, fourth, or fifth metatarsal.

Usually, it occurs in childhood or adolescence around 13 years old and often regard females, in particular girls who practice dance or volleyball. The suffering epiphyseal develops in response to a solicitation of the metatarsal head which, during growth, changes its mechanical properties.

The joint is stressed in the propulsive phase of the step, and the disease appears to be related to sports repeated traumatism that is developed, especially in the presence of flatfoot and insufficiency of the first metatarsal [34].

Clinically, Freiberg's disease is characterized by unilateral pain in correspondence with the metatarsal head.

At X-ray examination, the metatarsal head shows a progression from osteosclerosis to osteolysis with a lacunar appearance and a dome-shaped deformity of the head. In the joints, a lesion of the cartilage or subchondral bone appears.

Conservative treatment provides for rest and use of orthotic plantar to control the pronation with bar or olive for unloading metatarsal. In severe forms, it is appropriate to use a cast.

In adulthood may manifest osteoarthritis of the second metatarsal joint with typical deformity in the shape of Burmese pagoda. Surgical treatment is indicated in these cases for joint debridement, removal of any residual lost body up to resection of the head or osteochondral transplantation [38].

4. *Iselin's disease (osteochondrosis of the base of the fifth metatarsal)*

Iselin's disease is an apofisite caused by traction on the tuberosity of the fifth metatarsal, and it is very rare. It occurs in late childhood–adolescence in subjects who play sports [39].

The secondary ossification center appears as a small shell-shaped oblique at the level of the tuberosity, which is part of the tendon of the peroneus brevis. The nucleus appears late in an average of 9 years in females and 12 years in males and ends its maturation at 11 and 14 years, respectively.

Patients affect by Iselin's disease are usually athletes involved in sports that include running and jumping, and generally, there is a real trauma. The movement in eversion against resistance generally evokes pain. The differential diagnosis should be placed with fracture of the base of the fifth metatarsal. The oblique X-ray is the one that best shows the apophyses.

Treatment is conservative and includes immobilization in the acute phase, no weight bearing, and then stretching and strengthening of the peroneal muscles [39].

References

1. Stanitski C (1988) Management of sports injuries in children and adolescents. Orthop Clin North Am 19:689–698
2. Omey ML, Micheli LJ (1999) Foot and ankle problems in the young athlete. Med Sci Sports Exerc, 31(7):S470–S486 (Suppl.)
3. Harris EJ, Vanore JV, Thomas JL et al. (2004) Diagnosis and treatment of pediatric flatfoot. J Foot Ankle Surg, 43(6):341–73
4. Benedetti MG, Ceccarelli F, Berti L, Luciani D, Catani F, Boschi M, Giannini S (2011) Diagnosis of flexible flatfoot in children: a systematic clinical approach. Orthopedics 34(2):94. doi: 10.3928/01477447-20101221-04
5. Tudor A, Ruzic L, Sestan B, Sirola L, Prpic T (2009) Flat-footedness is not a disadvantage for athletic performance in children aged 11–15 years. Pediatrics, 123(3):e386–92
6. Giannini S, Ceccarelli F, Benedetti MG, Catani F (2001) Surgical Treatment of Flexible Flatfoot in Children : A Four-Year Follow-up Study. J Bone Joint Surg Am, Nov 01;83(2 suppl 2):S73-79
7. Giannini S, Girolami M, Ceccarelli F (1985) The surgical treatment of infantile flat foot, a new expanding endo-orthotic implant. Ital J Orthop Traumatol 11:315–322
8. Mazis GA, Sakellariou VI et al. (2012) Results of extra-articular subtalar arthrodesis in children with cerebral palsy. Foot Ankle Int, 33(6):469–74
9. Mosca VS (2010) Flexible flatfoot in children and adolescents. J Child Orthop 4:107–121. doi: 10.1007/s11832-010-0239-9
10. Ehlrich MG, Elmer EB (1991) Tarsal coalition. In: Jhass M (ed.) Disorder of the foot and ankle W.B. Saunders, Philadephia, 021–028
11. Giannini S, Ceccarelli F, Vannini F, Baldi E (2003) Operative treatment of flatfoot with talocalcaneal coalition. Clin Orthop 411:178–187
12. Lamley F, Berlet G et al. (2006) Current concepts review: tarsal coalition foot ankle int, 27(12):1163–9
13. Swiontkowski MF, Scranton PE, Hansen S (1983) Tarsal coalitions: longterm results of surgical treatment. J Pediatr Orthop 3:287–292
14. Giannini S, Ceccarelli F, Mosca M (1995) La nostra esperienza nel trattamento del piede cavo essenziale mediante osteotomia del cuboide e resezione-artrodesi della scafo-cuneiforme. In: Mori F, Giannini S (eds) Progressi in Medicina e Chirurgia del Piede, vol 4. Aulo Gaggi Editore, Bologna, pp 179–193
15. Ibrhaim K (1990) Pes cavus. In: Evarts CH (ed.) Surgery of the muscoloskeletal system Churchill Livinstone, New York
16. Fortems Y (1993) Development of cavus foot deformity in failed repair of the Achilles tendon. Arch Orthop Trauma Surg 112:121–123
17. Wicart P (2012) Cavus foot, from neonates to adolescents. Orthop Traumatol Surg Res, 98(7):813–28. doi:10.1016/j.otsr.2012.09.003. Epub 2012 Oct 23
18. Lutter LD (1981) Cavus foot in runners. Foot Ankle 1:225–228
19. Coughlin MJ, Mann RA (eds) (1999) Surgery of the Foot and Ankle, 7th edn. St. Louis, Mosby
20. Coughlin MJ, Mann RA (1995) Juvenile hallux valgus: etiology and treatment. Foot Ankle Int, 16(11):682–697
21. Khan K, Brown J, Way S et al (1995) Overuse injuries in classical ballet. Sports Med 19:341–357
22. Thein R, Eichenblat M (1992) Arthroscopic treatment of sports-related synovitis of the ankle. Am J Sports Med 20:496–498
23. McCarroll J, Schrader JW, Shelbourne KD, Rettig AC, Bisesi MA (1987) Meniscoid lesions of the

ankle in soccer players. Am J Sports Med 15:255–257

24. Brodsky AE, Khalil MA (1986) Talar compression syndrome. Am J Sports Med 14:472–476

25. Hamilton WG, Geppert MJ, Thompson FM (1996) Pain in the posterior aspect of the ankle in dancers. J Bone Joint Surg 78A:1491–1500

26. Keene JS, Lange RH (1986) Diagnostic dilemmas in foot and ankle injuries. JAMA 256:247–251

27. Hedrick MR, McBryde AM (1994) Posterior ankle impingement. Foot Ankle 15:2–8

28. Wredmark T, Carlstedt CA, Bauer H, Saartok T (1991) Os trigonum syndrome: a clinical entity in ballet dancers. Foot Ankle 11:404–406

29. Stephens MM (1994) Haglund's deformity and retrocalcaneal bursitis. Orthop Clin North Am 25:41–46

30. Kanz JF (1980) Non-articular osteochondrosis. Clinical Orthopaedics 150:70

31. Sever JC (1912) Apophysitis of the os calcis. New York Med. 95, 1025

32. Micheli LJ, Ireland ML (1987) Prevention and management of calcaneal apophysitis in children: an overuse syndrome. J Pediatr Orthop 7:34–38

33. Zimmer EA (1986) Limiti del normale ed inizio del patologico nella diagnostica radiologica dello scheletro. Ambrosiana Ed, Milano

34. McManama GB Jr (1988) Ankle injuries in the young athlete. Clin Sports Med 7:547

35. Yale I (1953) Kohler's disease of the tarsal navicular. J Natl Assoc Chirop, 43(12):33–5

36. Williams GA, Cowell HR (1981) Kohler's disease of the tarsal navicular. Clinical Orthopaedics 158:53

37. Freiberg AH (1914) Infraction of the second metatarsal bone. Surgery, Gynecology and Obstetrics, 19, 191

38. Miyamoto W, Takao M, Uchio Y, Kono T, Ochi M (2008) Late-stage Freiberg disease treated by osteochondral plug transplantation: a case series. Foot Ankle Int, 29(9):950–5

39. Canale TS, Williams KD (1992) Iselin's disease. J Pediatr Orthop 12(1):90–93

Orthopedic Diseases: Non-Sports-Related Pathologies in Young Athletes

20

Sean P. Kearney and John P. Dormans

Although injuries are primarily responsible for presenting conditions in young athletes, this population is not immune to non-sports-related orthopedic pathologies . These disorders are often preexisting, but minor trauma or injury may direct attention to the condition. Several orthopedic conditions should be considered when evaluating the young athlete. Some of the more common conditions include slipped capital femoral epiphysis (SCFE), Legg–Calvè–Perthes disease (LCPD), bone and soft tissue tumors, and juvenile idiopathic arthritis (JIA).

20.1 Slipped Capital Femoral Epiphysis

SCFE is a common pediatric hip disorder where the femoral epiphysis displaces from the metaphysis through the proximal physis. Incidence ranges from 0.2 per 100,000 in Japan to 10 per 100,000 in the United States [1]. The etiology is not completely understood. Several

biomechanical and biochemical factors have been proposed, including obesity, femoral retroversion, increased pelvic obliquity, and decreased structural support of the physeal region [2]. SCFE classically occurs in overweight or obese adolescent males and should particularly be considered in young athletes participating in sports like American football. Obesity increases the shear stress across the physis and is associated with increased femoral retroversion. Shear forces across the physis continue to increase as femoral retroversion increases. During adolescence, hormones may weaken the physis by increasing its growth rate. Testosterone, in particular, weakens the physis and is thought to explain the male predominance [3].

In the early stages, common presenting symptoms include weakness in the affected lower extremity, limping, or exertional groin, thigh or knee pain. Onset is often insidious and can be present for several weeks or even months. Knee or lower thigh pain is the initial symptom in up to 46 % of patients with SCFE [4], making hip evaluation mandatory in the young athlete with knee or thigh pain. Physical examination demonstrates decreased hip range of motion, particularly with internal rotation. Anterior–posterior (AP) and frog-leg lateral pelvis radiographs confirm the diagnosis. On a normal AP radiograph, a line drawn from the anterosuperior aspect of the femoral neck, termed Klein's line, should intersect the epiphysis. In SCFE, Klein's line is flush with or fails to intersect the epiphysis altogether (Fig. 20.1) [2].

S. P. Kearney · J. P. Dormans (✉)
Orthopedic Surgery, Children's Hospital of Philadelphia, 34th and Civic Center Blvd, Philadelphia, Pennsylvania 19104, USA
e-mail: Dormans@email.chop.edu

S. P. Kearney
e-mail: Spkearney1@gmail.com

V. Guzzanti (ed.), *Pediatric and Adolescent Sports Traumatology*,
DOI: 10.1007/978-88-470-5412-7_20, © Springer-Verlag Italia 2014

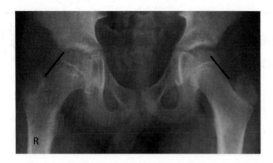

Fig. 20.1 Anterior–posterior pelvis radiograph showing Klein's line intersecting the epiphysis of the normal (*left*) hip, but flush with the epiphysis of the affected hip (*right*) with a slipped capital femoral epiphysis

Once SCFE is diagnosed, operative treatment is indicated. Many procedures have been advocated, depending on slip severity, ranging from in situ screw fixation to open surgical hip dislocation with repositioning of the epiphysis. The common goal of treatment is to prevent further displacement and limit the risk of femoral head osteonecrosis [2] and, in skeletally immature patients, avoid premature proximal femoral physeal arrest [5–7].

20.2 Legg–Calvè–Perthes Disease

LCPD is a hip disorder of unknown etiology presenting in childhood, most commonly between the ages 5 and 8 years. The male-to-female ratio is 5:1, and bilateral involvement is 10–15 % [8].

The child typically presents with insidious onset hip pain, limp, and/or limited hip range of motion. Physical examination may demonstrate a Trendelenburg sign. Depending on the stage of disease, hip range of motion varies. Loss of abduction and internal rotation is seen early, whereas global loss of motion can occur in the later stages [8].

Current clinical and experimental evidence suggests that lack of femoral head blood supply leads to deformity, causing hip pain [8]. Depending on the stage of disease, hip radiographs will show characteristic features. In the initial stage, radiographs show increased radiodensity of the femoral head. In the fragmentation stage, femoral head deformity develops and progresses for approximately one year. During the reossification stage, typically lasting 3–5 years, femoral head deformity can improve, worsen, or remain unchanged. Finally, in the healed stage, the femoral head deformity remains constant (Fig. 20.2) [9].

Management of LCPD is controversial and is based primarily on age at presentation and severity of femoral head deformity. Current research supports non-surgical treatment for patients aged <6 years. Optimal treatment for patients presenting after age of 6 years is not clear [10, 11]. Non-operative treatment can range from no treatment to symptomatic treatment with anti-inflammatory medications, physical therapy, casting, or bracing. Surgical management can involve adductor tenotomy and femoral and/or pelvic osteotomies, all with the common goal of femoral head containment in the acetabulum.

20.3 Benign and Malignant Bone Tumors

Several different benign and malignant bone tumors can present in the young athlete. Compared to traumatic sports injures, musculoskeletal tumors are far less likely to be the cause of an athlete's symptoms. The true incidence of benign bone tumors in children and adolescents is unknown, as many are asymptomatic and are never discovered [12]. Malignant bone tumors are uncommon. Osteosarcoma is the most common bone sarcoma and affects approximately 560 children and adolescents annually in the United States [13]. Ewing's sarcoma is the second most common malignant bone tumor in children and adolescents, with an annual peak incidence of 5 per million in adolescents (Fig. 20.3) [14, 15]. Regardless of their relative infrequency, musculoskeletal tumors should always be part of the differential diagnosis when evaluating a young athlete. Tumors misdiagnosed as athletic injuries have been reported, and inappropriate invasive procedures can result in extension of the tumor, necessitating more

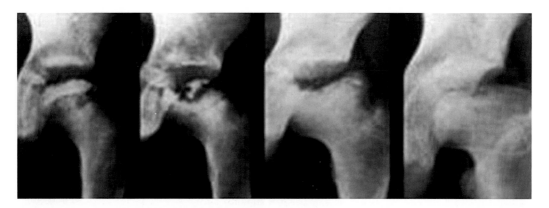

Fig. 20.2 Anterior–posterior hip radiographs demonstrating the four successive stages of Legg–Calve–Perthes disease: initial, fragmentation, reossification, and healed

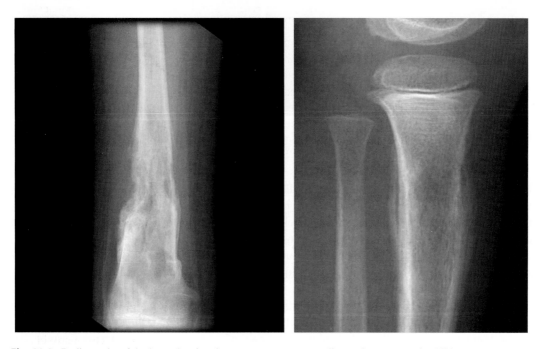

Fig. 20.3 Radiographs of the knee showing the two most common malignant bone tumors in children: osteosarcoma (*left*) and Ewing's sarcoma (*right*)

extensive treatment in some cases [16]. Maintaining a high index of suspicion, particularly in a young athlete presenting with unexplained musculoskeletal pain, can prevent misdiagnosis of a tumor.

Most benign tumors have distinct clinical and radiographic characteristics that often allow diagnosis without biopsy. Some benign tumors, like fibrous cortical defects and enchondromas, appear as incidental findings in the young athlete being evaluated for a sports injury (Fig. 20.4). Other benign and malignant tumors are associated with symptoms and prompt a young athlete to seek medical evaluation. For instance, benign tumors, like osteoid osteomas and aneurysmal bone cysts, are associated with pain, often independent of activity (Fig. 20.5). Slow-growing masses, like osteochondromas, can become

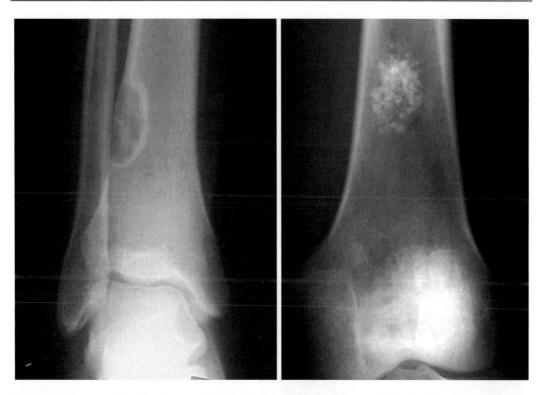

Fig. 20.4 Fibrous cortical defect in the tibia (*left*) and enchondroma in the femur (*right*) are examples of benign bone tumors that may be asymptomatic and are often discovered incidentally

bothersome to athletes who may repeatedly traumatize the area or irritate underlying structures like tendons, muscles, vessels, or nerves, depending on tumor location (Fig. 20.6). Malignant tumors, like osteosarcoma and Ewing's sarcoma, can present with a wide spectrum of symptoms from mild pain to a dramatic painful mass associated with systemic symptoms. Pathologic fractures from relatively minor trauma can occur through benign and malignant bone tumors, like unicameral bone cysts or osteosarcomas (Fig. 20.7).

When unexplained musculoskeletal pain is the presenting symptom in the young athlete, benign and malignant tumors should be included in the differential diagnosis. It is important to elicit the nature and location of the pain, duration, timing, aggravating and alleviating factors, and any associated symptoms. This information is invaluable. For instance, an athlete presenting with weeks to months of dull aching pain that is worse at night and alleviated with aspirin and

non-steroidal anti-inflammatory medications is essentially diagnostic of osteoid osteoma. Alternatively, malignant tumors should be suspected in an athlete presenting with a constantly painful, enlarging soft tissue mass with associated fatigue, weight loss, fever, and night pain [13].

A careful physical examination should accompany the history. Observing and palpating the symptomatic area can identify masses, and if present, important characteristics must be appreciated. Masses can be firm, soft, or both. They can be well or poorly defined and either fixed to or mobile relative to surrounding structures. They can be painful, painless, or irritating to surrounding structures. Like a detailed history, a meticulous physical examination can provide valuable clues to the diagnosis. For instance, an osteochondroma should be suspected in an athlete with a firm, well-defined, pedunculated bony mass that is fixed to the surrounding bone. Once a mass is identified, complete evaluation for other masses is necessary.

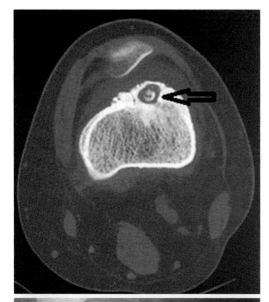

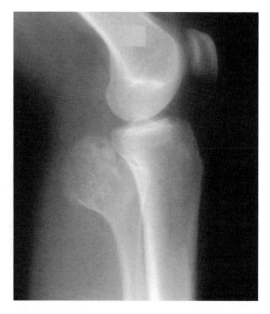

Fig. 20.6 Radiograph of an osteochondroma, a benign bone tumor that can irritate surrounding structures, such as nerves, tendons, or muscles based on location, in this case about the knee

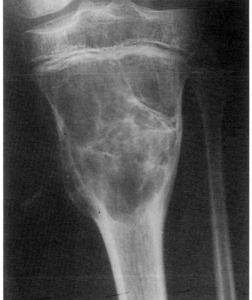

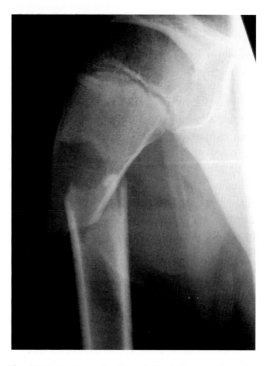

Fig. 20.5 Computed tomography (*CT*) scan of an osteoid osteoma (*top*) and radiograph of an aneurysmal bone cyst (*bottom*), both about the knee, are examples of benign bone tumors that are symptomatic and independent of activity

Fig. 20.7 Radiograph of a pathologic fracture through a proximal humerus unicameral bone cyst

Fig. 20.8 Radiographs demonstrating typical locations of benign bone tumors: unicameral bone cyst in the proximal humerus (*top*), non-ossifying fibroma in the proximal tibia (*middle*), and osteoblastoma in the posterior elements of the spine (*bottom*)

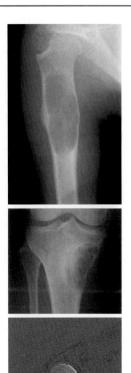

bones, like unicameral bone cysts (proximal humerus and femur), non-ossifying fibromas (distal femur and proximal tibia), and osteoblastoma (posterior spinal elements) [17] (Fig. 20.8). Regional location in the bone is also important. Most benign bone tumors are located in the metaphysis of the long bones, with few occurring in the epiphyseal or diaphyseal regions. The appearance of the tumor in the bone can offer diagnostic clues. Tumors can be cortically based (osteochondroma, osteoid osteoma), central in the medullary canal (enchondroma, unicameral bone cyst), or eccentric in the medullary canal (non-ossifying fibroma, aneurysmal bone cyst). The effect of the tumor on bone can be described as geographic, moth-eaten, or permeative, in increasing magnitude of bony destruction [18]. Malignant tumors are usually very destructive (permeative) bony lesions, while benign tumors are usually minimally or not destructive (geographic) or moderately destructive (moth-eaten). The effect of bone on the tumor is also important and is typically based on presence or absence of sclerotic margins. Tumors that exhibit sclerotic margins (fibrous cortical defect) are indolent, where the bone has time to react to tumor growth. On the contrary, tumors with no sclerotic margins (aneurysmal bone cyst, most malignant tumors) suggest increasing growth rate, where the bone cannot respond to the tumor destruction.

While initial treatment for suspected malignant tumors requires expedited workup and biopsy, treatment for benign tumors varies widely. Some tumors, like fibrous cortical defects, usually require no treatment and resolve spontaneously. Others, like aneurysmal bone cysts and osteoblastoma, often require surgical treatment and are prone to recurrence. Still others, like osteoid osteoma, follow an unpredictable course, where operative intervention may or may not be necessary. Size and location of the tumor are also important in treatment decisions. A large unicameral bone cyst or non-ossifying fibroma may pose a risk of pathologic fracture in a young athlete, making operative treatment a strong consideration.

Plain radiographs consisting of two orthogonal views centered over the lesion of interest are always the first and are often the most helpful imaging study in evaluating benign and malignant bone tumors. In many benign bone tumors, plain radiographs, along with a careful history and physical examination, are the only imaging studies needed. Other imaging studies, such as computed tomography (CT), magnetic resonance imaging (MRI), and/or technetium bone scanning, may be helpful for staging and treatment purposes, but these modalities are rarely needed to make the diagnosis.

As in their clinical presentation, benign and malignant bone tumors often exhibit characteristic radiographic findings. Specific characteristics include tumor size, shape, location, and appearance of the bone and surrounding soft tissues. Some tumors have a predilection for specific

20.4 Benign and Malignant Soft Tissue Tumors

Like bone tumors, soft tissue tumors comprise a heterogeneous group of lesions in children and adolescents. Approximately 600 soft tissue sarcomas are diagnosed annually in children under 18 years old in the United States [19, 20]. Most soft tissue sarcomas in children are vascular, neurogenic, myogenic, fibroblastic, or myofibroblastic [21, 22].

Clinically, the child typically presents with a palpable mass. Often, a recent trauma brings attention to the mass. Symptoms, such as pain, joint contracture, or impaired function, may be associated with the mass. It is important to ascertain the nature and location of the symptoms as well as aggravating and alleviating factors. For instance, a child with a hemangioma may have increasing pain when the involved extremity is in a dependent position, but pain dissipates when the extremity is elevated [23].

Physical examination should focus on the characteristics of the mass including size, consistency, depth, and mobility. Some common lesions can be diagnosed on physical examination and often do not require imaging. For instance, superficial lipomas are doughy, well-defined, non-tender masses that generally do not increase in size. Ganglia are non-tender, firm, but compressible masses that transilluminate and are associated with a joint, commonly in the hand and wrist. Masses that are greater than 5 cm in diameter, firm, and deep to the fascia are concerning for malignancy [23]. Rhabdomyosarcoma is the most common soft tissue malignancy in children and exhibits the aforementioned characteristics [24]. Other deep soft tissue tumors to consider include synovial cell sarcoma, fibrous and neurogenic tumors, and desmoid tumors. Joint range of motion should be examined as some lesions (e.g., desmoid tumors) may cause flexion contractures. Additionally, the lymph system in an affected extremity should be examined for enlarged or tender nodes if a soft tissue malignancy is suspected since nodal metastasis

can occur in rhabdomyosarcoma, synovial sarcoma, and epithelial sarcoma [23].

Plain radiographs and MRI are the most commonly used imaging studies to define soft tissue masses. CT scan and ultrasound may also be helpful. Two orthogonal plain radiographs of the affected area are recommended initially and can provide important clues, such as presence of mature trabecular bone in myositis ossificans or phlebolith in hemangiomas. Tumor erosion into bone can also be appreciated on radiographs. MRI is the most useful imaging modality for soft tissue tumors and is recommended for all deep lesions. Tumor size, location, density, and involvement of any surrounding structures (e.g., neurovascular) are apparent. MRI is not only useful in diagnosing soft tissue tumors, but also provides valuable treatment planning information.

Biopsy is required for all soft tissue tumors that cannot be accurately diagnosed after appropriate clinical examination and imaging studies are complete. Based on biopsy results, a treatment plan is formulated. Like with bone tumors, treatment varies widely based on the natural history, potential for local recurrence, and presence of or potential to metastasize. For example, asymptomatic hemangiomas can be observed, whereas malignant soft tissue sarcomas often require wide surgical resection combined with chemotherapy or radiation [23].

20.5 Juvenile Idiopathic Arthritis

JIA is a group of conditions characterized by the onset of chronic arthritis in childhood. Diagnosis requires the onset of arthritis by age of 16 years, involvement of at least one joint for ≥6 weeks, and the exclusion of other causes of arthritis [25]. JIA can affect young athletes and should be considered in patients presenting with joint stiffness and swelling.

Oligoarticular JIA is the most common variant of chronic childhood arthritis and involves 4 joints or fewer. Females are affected 5:1 over males, and age at onset is between 1 and 3 years [26]. Onset is insidious, and symptoms include morning stiffness and swelling in the involved joints and limp, but continued ability to bear weight. A minor trauma may bring attention to a swollen joint that is often painless. In fact, musculoskeletal pain is not usually a presenting symptom of JIA [27]. One joint is involved in half of all patients with oligoarticular JIA, with the knee and ankle most commonly affected. Uveitis may be present and is usually chronic, bilateral, and asymptomatic [28]. It is important to refer these patients for eye examination, as 20–30 % of patients may experience vision loss [29].

Polyarticular JIA involves at least 5 joints during the first 6 months of the condition. Approximately 40 % of patients with oligoarticular JIA progress to the polyarticular form [30]. Female-to-male ratio is 3:1, and age at onset is typically 1–4 years. Those presenting at 6 years or older tend to demonstrate a disease pattern similar to rheumatoid arthritis in adults [31]. Like the oligoarticular form, symptoms involve stiffness and swelling, but not typically pain of the involved joints. If significant joint pain exists or extra-articular systemic symptoms are present, systemic collagen vascular diseases should be considered [29].

When JIA is suspected, all joints should be examined, not just the presenting joint(s). The differential diagnosis is influenced by the number and location of the involved joints. Swelling, range of motion, pain with motion, and tenderness should be assessed. It is also important to examine the cervical spine and assess gait. Findings inconsistent with JIA include severe joint pain or tenderness, refusal to bear weight, joint erythema, migratory pattern, isolated hip involvement, and pain worse at night or with activity. If these findings exist, other conditions should be considered, such as septic or reactive arthritis, benign or malignant tumors, or acute rheumatic fever [29].

While no laboratory test can conclusively diagnose JIA, recommended tests include complete blood count with differential, erythrocyte sedimentation rate, C-reactive protein, urinalysis, serum creatinine, albumin, liver function tests, creatine phosphokinase, and aldolase. Oligoarticular JIA is not commonly associated with systemic inflammation, while the polyarticular form demonstrates mild-to-moderate systemic inflammation. Rheumatoid factor, antinuclear antibody , and HLA B-27 are often not useful in diagnosing JIA [32, 33].

Initial treatment for most forms of JIA is nonsteroidal anti-inflammatory [35]. Aspirin is rarely prescribed [36]. Referral to a pediatric rheumatologist is advised in young athletes with suspected JIA.

References

1. Loder RT (1996) The demographics of slipped capital femoral epiphysis: an international multicenter study. Clin Orthop Relat Res 322:8–27
2. Aronsson DD, Loder RT, Breur GJ et al (2006) Slipped capital femoral epiphysis: current concepts. J Am Acad Orthop 14:666–679
3. Loder RT, Aronsson DD, Dobbs MB et al (2001) Slipped capital femoral epiphysis. Instr Course Lect 50:555–570
4. Matava MJ, Patton CM, Luhmann S et al (1999) Knee pain as the initial symptom of slipped capital femoral epiphysis: an analysis of initial presentation and treatment. J Pediatr Orthop 19:455–460
5. Guzzanti V, Falciglia F, Stanitski CL (2004) Slipped capital femoral epiphysis in skeletally immature patients. J Bone Joint Surg Br 86(5):731–736
6. Sailhan F, Courvoisier A, Brunet O, Chotel F, Berard J (2011) Continued growth of the hip after fixation of slipped capital femoral epiphysis using a single cannulated screw with a proximal threading. J Child Orthop 5(2):83–88
7. Hansson G, Nathorst-Westfelt J (2012) Management of the contralateral hip in patients with unilateral slipped upper femoral epiphysis: to fix or not to fix–consequences of two strategies. J Bone Joint Surg Br 94(5):596–602
8. Kim HKW (2010) Legg-Calve-Perthes disease. J Am Acad Orthop 18:676–686
9. Waldenstrom H (1922) The definitive forms of coxa plana. Acta Radiol 1:384
10. Herring JA, Kim HT, Browne R (2004) Legg-Calve-Perthes disease: Part II. Prospective multicenter study of the effect of treatment on outcome. J Bone Joint Surg Am 86:2121–2134
11. Wiig O, Terjesen T, Svenningsen S (2008) Prognostic factors and outcome of treatment in Perthes' disease: a prospective study of 368 patients with five-year follow-up. J Bone Joint Surg Br 90:1364–1371

12. Aboulafia AJ, Kennon RE, Jelinek JS (1999) Benign bone tumors of childhood. J Am Acad Orthop Surg 7:377–388

13. Messerschmitt PJ, Garcia RM, Abdul-Karim FW et al (2009) Osteosarcoma. J Am Acad Orthop Surg 17:515–527

14. Herzog CE (2005) Overview of sarcomas in the adolescent and young adult population. J Pediatr Hematol Oncol 27:215–218

15. Maheshwari AV, Cheng EY (2010) Ewing sarcoma family of tumors. J Am Acad Orthop Surg 18:94–107

16. Muscolo DL, Ayerza MA, Makino A et al (2003) Tumors about the knee misdiagnosed as athletic injuries. J Bone Joint Surg Am 85:1209–1214

17. Garg S, Dormans JD (2005) Tumors and tumor-like conditions of the spine in children. J Am Acad Orthop Surg 13:372–381

18. Madewell JE, Ragsdale BD, Sweet DE (1981) Radiologic and pathologic analysis of solitary bone lesions. Part 1: internal margins. Radiol Clin North Am 19:715–748

19. Gurney JG, Severson RK, Davis S et al (1995) Incidence of cancer in children in the United States: sex, race, and 1 year age-specific rates by histologic type. Cancer 75:2186–2195

20. Miller RW, Young JL Jr, Novakovic B (1995) Childhood cancer. Cancer 75:395–405

21. Kransdorf MJ (1995) Malignant soft-tissue tumors in a large referral population: distribution of diagnoses by age, sex, and location. Am J Roentgenol 164:129–134

22. Kransdorf MJ (1995) Benign soft-tissue tumors in a large referral population: distribution of diagnoses by age, sex, and location. Am J Roentgenol 164:395–402

23. Aflatoon K, Aboulafia AJ, McCarthy EF Jr et al (2003) Pediatric soft-tissue tumors. J Am Acad Orthop Surg 11:332–343

24. Hays DM (1993) Rhabdomyosarcoma. Clin Orthop 289:36–49

25. Cassidy JT, Petty RE (2008) Chronic arthritis in childhood. In: Cassidy JT, Petty RE, Laxer RM, Lindsley CB (eds) Textbook of Pediatric Rheumatology, 5th edn. Elsevier, Philadelphia, pp 206–260

26. Petty RE, Cassidy JT (2008) Oligoarthritis. In: Cassidy JT, Petty RE, Laxer RM, Lindsley CB (eds) Textbook of Pediatric Rheumatology, Ed 5. Elsevier, Philadelphia, pp 274–290

27. McGhee JL, Burks FN, Sheckels JL et al (2002) Identifying children with chronic arthritis based on chief complaints: absence of predictive value for musculoskeletal pain as an indicator of rheumatic disease in children. Pediatrics 110:354–359

28. Guillaume S, Prieur AM, Coste J et al (2000) Long-term outcome and prognosis in oligoarticular-onset juvenile idiopathic arthritis. Arthritis Rheum 43:1858–1865

29. Punaro M (2011) Rheumatologic conditions in children who may present to the orthopaedic surgeon. J Am Acad Orthop Surg 19:163–169

30. Al-Matar MJ, Petty RE, Tucker LB et al (2002) The early pattern of joint involvement predicts disease progression in children with oligoarticular (pauciarticular) juvenile rheumatoid arthritis. Arthritis Rheum 46:2708–2715

31. Weiss JE, Ilowite NT (2005) Juvenile idiopathic arthritis. Pediatr Clin North Am 52:413–444

32. Eichenfield AH, Athreya BH, Doughty RA et al (1986) Utility of rheumatoid factor in the diagnosis of juvenile rheumatoid arthritis. Pediatrics 78:480–484

33. McGhee JL, Kickingbird LM, Jarvis JN (2004) Clinical utility of antinuclear antibody tests in children. BMC Pediatr 4:13

34. Cassidy JT, Petty RE (2008) Juvenile ankylosing spondylitis. In: Cassidy JT, Petty RE, Laxer RM, Lindsley CB (eds) Textbook of Pediatric Rheumatology, 5th edn. Elsevier, Philadelphia, pp 304–323

35. Giannini EH, Cawkwell GD (1995) Drug treatment in children with juvenile rheumatoid arthritis: past, present, and future. Pediatr Clin North Am 42:1099–1125

36. Cron RQ, Sharma S, Sherry DD (1999) Current treatment by United States and Canadian pediatric rheumatologists. J Rheumatol 26:2036–2038

Imaging and Techniques

21

Salvatore Masala, Antonicoli Marco, Giulia Claroni,
Roberto Fiori and Giovanni Simonetti

Over the last decades, diagnostic imaging has become an essential tool for sports traumatology in diagnosis and follow-up in athletes. The modern techniques of conventional radiology, ultrasonography (US), computed tomography (CT), and magnetic resonance imaging (MRI), applied to sports traumatology, can combine high diagnostic power with criteria of radio-protection for pediatric patients (e.g., systems of dose reduction applied to CT). Nowadays, radiologists are able to guarantee accurate diagnosis and follow-up for young athletes undergoing traumatic injuries.

When planning a diagnostic process for pediatric or adolescent patients, a fundamental factor to consider is the great variability that anatomical structures undergo during their growth. Although a traumatic injury may be influenced by many factors, such as age, sex, general physical condition, genetic predisposition, diet, psychological status, and competitive level of sport activity, the rate of physical growth is almost certainly the most important factor in pediatric and adolescent sports medicine.

Several studies reported in the literature have shown that, depending on the physical power muscle, the incidence rate of different pathologies varies throughout the athletes' growth. As a result, a low incidence of muscles and tendons distractive injuries is observed in patients aged less than 10 years; this occurs because younger muscle–tendon units show less muscle strength, thus a reduced muscle power. In teenage athletes, it is possible to observe a higher percentage of torn muscles and/or tendons injuries. Muscular masses with greater power are able to generate energies that can exceed the strength of the muscle–tendon unit itself. After 14 years of age, the incidence rate of traumatic injuries and diseases in young athletes tends to equal that of adult athletes.

In this chapter, we will encounter the role that diagnostic imaging plays in sports traumatology. Several last-generation technologies have been applied to sports traumatology for the evaluation of athletes after traumas and for follow-up. Using diagnostic techniques, physicians are now able to make a statement on a healing process before clinical examination may reveal the same information. Early diagnosis and accurate prognosis are essential when wondering the time that an athlete needs to return to his/her daily and agonistic sport activity. Nowadays, telemedicine represents the greatest expression of diagnostic imaging: sending real-time digital images from a country to another allows to trace the recovery path of athletes from all over the world,

S. Masala (✉) · A. Marco · G. Claroni · R. Fiori ·
G. Simonetti
Department of Diagnostic Imaging, Molecular
Imaging, Interventional Radiology and
Radiotherapy, Foundation Policlinico Tor Vergata,
Viale Oxford 81, 00133 Rome, Italy
e-mail: salva.masala@tiscali.it

permitting a close and comprehensive monitoring of the patient.

This chapter aims to highlight the different diagnostic techniques available for sports traumatology and the role that they play for diagnosis and follow-up of athletes through different ages of growth. The intention is to show the influence of a proper clinical diagnosis, supported by accurate and precise diagnostic examination, on the course of treatment and rehabilitation of the athlete in his/her sport.

21.1 Conventional Radiology

A radiogram is obtained through the X-ray tube that produces X-rays, whose intensity depends on both the number of photons that compose them and their energy properties. The image is determined by X-rays attenuation, and the attenuation itself is influenced by the intensity of the beam and the constitution of crossed matter. In addition, radiological images are determined by differences in tissue density. Currently, digital radiography systems have completely replaced traditional radiography. Although overexposures can still occur, especially in children, the main advantages of digital imaging, i.e., wide dynamic range, post-processing, multiple viewing options, and electronic transfer and archiving possibilities, are clear. The radiological film has been supplanted by techniques of direct and indirect digital radiography [1] Figs. 21.1 and 21.2.

Using conventional radiology, a good visualization of bone tissue is obtainable: for its high concentration of calcium, it is easily distinguishable from cartilaginous tissues, fibrous structures, and surrounding soft tissues. It is also possible to evaluate bone morphology, displaying changes occurring in the shape and/or in the normal structure of the bone [2].

Therefore, radiograms are useful in sports traumatology to study traumatic diseases involving bones and joints, not to forget their applicability to the muscular-skeletal district for the study of bone diseases such as congenital anomalies, malformations, infectious disease like osteomyelitis, in neoplasms and in the

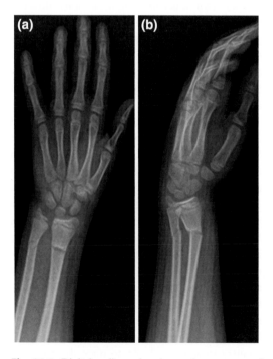

Fig. 21.1 Digital radiography shows the presence of radius and ulna fractures in a young gymnast (**a**) A–P view (**b**) L–L projection

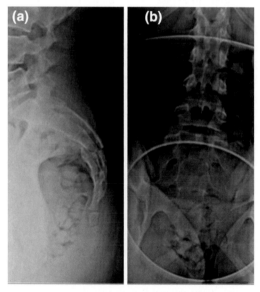

Fig. 21.2 Digital radiography shows the presence of sacrum fracture in a young gymnast (**a**) A–P view (**b**) L–L projection

Fig. 21.3 Slight distraction of the gastrocnemius muscle in a young marathon runner (*a*) B-mode and (*b*) sono elastography of the muscle 3 h after the trauma: the *red* color highlights the inflammatory status of injured tissue (*c*) B-mode ultrasound of muscle injury after 60 days (*d*) and sono elastography: the *green* and *blue* color show the recovering tissue

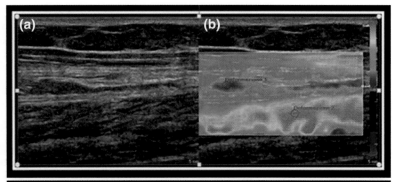

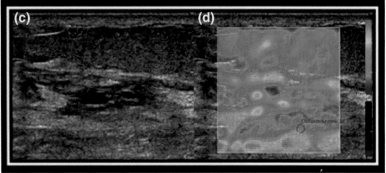

evaluation of metabolic diseases [3, 4]. Thus, conventional radiographic technique is often the first approach for the study of the muscular-skeletal system in cases of traumas causing fractures. In most cases of injuries, it is sufficient to make the diagnosis without the need for further investigations.

When a fracture occurs, radiograms allow the evaluation of the anatomical site of fracture, the extension of the fracture, if it is complete (fully affecting the bone) or incomplete (only affecting cortical bone), also if the joints are involved, and possible fragments. After a first-level radiological evaluation, a treatment planning is often possible. If present, X-rays allow the visualization of the displacement of bones: the radiograms will show if displacement is lateral, when it occurs along the length of the bone, on the major axis of the bone, or around the bone axis. Especially in young athletes, radiograms are useful for the assessment of growth plate fractures after a trauma. The radiographic examination should be easy to interpret when it shows the movement of the ossification nucleus, otherwise it is

necessary to perform a comparative evaluation with contralateral bone, in order to evaluate an increased thickness in the injured side of the epiphyseal line. It is important to confirm the diagnosis in young patients for preventing future deformities and impediments to normal sporting activities [5], Figs. 21.3 and 21.4.

Usually, performing the X-ray examination in the two orthogonal projections, anterior-posterior and lateral projection, including the two joints adjacent to the bone segment of interest, is sufficient to identify a possible subluxation or dislocation associated to the fractures; though, the use of oblique projections allows to show formations and injuries that may overlap in the standard orthogonal projections. Most of the fractures can be diagnosed primarily if good quality radiographs are obtained, but in some particular cases, like scaphoid fractures, a precise diagnosis may be difficult and several common radiograph findings can be misinterpreted and lead to a false-positive diagnosis of a fracture. This is why oblique and specific projections may be required [6].

Fig. 21.4 Contusion
injury of the gluteal muscle
in a player (**a**) 3D
ultrasound (**b**) color-
Doppler ultrasound
(**c**) sono elastography: the
red color highlights the
inflammatory status of
injured tissue

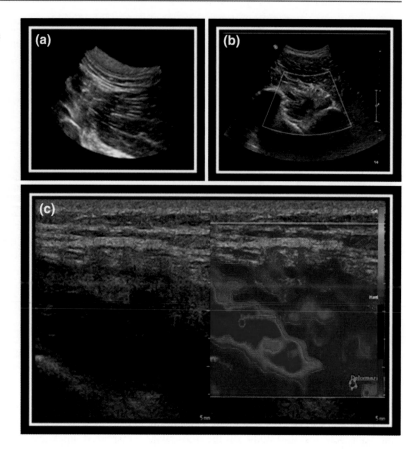

Radiograms of the limbs are indicated for patients who suffered from traumatic injuries when the identification and the characterization of a fracture are needed. Limbs are usually involved in minor traumas of athletes, but in case of major injuries, conventional radiology can represent the first approach to search also for hip fractures. The only AP projection may be diagnostic in the majority of cases, including the pelvis and proximal femurs, in order to distinguish between stable and unstable fractures and to verify a concomitant fracture of the acetabulum [7]. In doubtful cases, a CT scan of the fractured detail may be necessary. Standard radiographic examination also may fail to identify dislocations; dislocations can be concomitant with fractures in various musculoskeletal districts, but they need early diagnosis because they have to be reduced in emergency. Often, the diagnosis is possible with the only AP projection, as it happens with shoulder, elbow, and hip.

In order to evaluate the effects of fractures on soft tissues, ultrasound should be performed, instead.

After diagnosing and treating a fracture, radiological examination is a useful tool to show the formation of primary reparative callus or for surgical follow-up. Periodic examinations are needed to evaluate the process of fracture repair.

In case of dislocation, standard X-ray examination is sufficient to diagnose it only with AP projection, because radiograms can display the spacing of the joint and any signs of complicated dislocation, but a further lateral projection should always be performed. When ligaments and tendons are involved, ultrasounds, computed tomography, and/or magnetic resonance imaging will be necessary [8]. Although conventional radiology represents the basis for patients who suffer from an injury, in some particular districts, such as the knee, X-ray are not diagnostic; as reported in the literature, when comparing results from radiograms with MRI, conventional radiology shows poor diagnostic resolution, resulting completely negative in 98 % of cases when damages on cartilage, menisci, ligaments, and soft tissues need to be diagnosed [9].

21.2 Ultrasonography

In the last decades, the use of ultrasounds (US) in sports medicine has largely spread because of the feasibility of this technique, which has a good cost-effectiveness and is not invasive for the patient. Sonography uses the power of the ultrasound beam to obtain morphological and functional images of the examined anatomical structures [10], allowing an accurate evaluation of the pathology of different tissues (hematomas, torn muscles, tendons injuries, myositis ossificans, muscular fibrosis, cists, etc.), compressions of nervous tissues, and pathologies of vascular structures [11, 12].

Moreover, the ultrasound examination can be largely applied to percutaneous procedures of interventional radiology, as guidance for drainages of superficial and deep hematomas, intra-articular fluid lesions, or local injections of drugs and therapies. Percutaneous procedures of interventional radiology that can be performed on musculoskeletal structures are numerous; among them, the most performed and useful are drainage of hematomas, abscesses, cysts, plus intra-articular injection of anti-inflammatory and corticosteroids, for pathologies that cannot be treated with systemic administration of therapies [13]. The ultrasound beam is generated inside the sonographic probe, letting the visualization of anatomical structures, depending on their diverse acoustic hindrance. Many probes are available and the choice of the probe is based on the power of the US beam; thus, they can be classified as follows: high-frequency probes (10–25 MHz) and low-frequency probes (5–10 MHz). The first ones are dedicated to the evaluation of superficial structures, such as skin, muscles, ligaments, tendons, and joints; low-frequency probes are used to study deep and parenchymal structures.

Ultrasound examination has one great limitation, which is represented by its strict dependence on the operator who performs the exam. This technique is influenced by the ability of the radiologist to choose the best setting for the machine on a specific patient, such as focus, brightness, contrast, probe, and to use probes correctly. Several artifacts may result from an incorrect use of this technique; also two different operators may not obtain similar diagnostic images from the same patient. Ultrasound has a specific indication for the evaluation of injuries affecting the muscles, especially in a range of time from 24–48 h after the trauma [14]. In this specific amount of time after injuries, US allows an accurate visualization, with both morphological and functional characterization, of torn muscles, myositis ossificans, muscular hematomas, cystic lesions, compartmental syndrome, and hernias.

Traumatic pathology of joint ligaments is well visualized with basic morphological scans, evaluating the state of anatomical integrity and the presence of direct and indirect signs of lesion, such as hematomas, edema, or signs of past injuries, such as calcifications [15]. Using US, it is possible to evaluate partial and complete lesions of tendons right after trauma has occurred, especially searching for indirect signs of pathology, as in tendinitis and in tenosynovitis. The assessment of nervous structures is particularly indicated when a nervous dislocation is suspected after a trauma, or for entrapment disorders, or in the presence of neoplasms that can dislocate surrounding nervous structures, such as Morton's neuroma [16]. Sonography is the best diagnostic technique for the evaluation of joints after injuries, in particular for characterizing intra-articular fluids.

Eco-Color-Doppler and power-Doppler are mainly indicated for the visualization of vascular structures, especially when vascular districts are involved in traumatic injuries, congenital diseases, and inflammatory diseases occurring in soft tissues, tendinitis, and tenosynovitis [17]. The power-Doppler methodic is largely used to characterize pathologies affecting joint synovia, mostly in order to distinguish between inflammatory and non-inflammatory diseases [18, 19].

Fig. 21.5 3D-shaded surface-rendering CT reconstruction on different planes (**a, b, c**) highlighting anatomical image of decomposed sacral fracture in a young gymnast

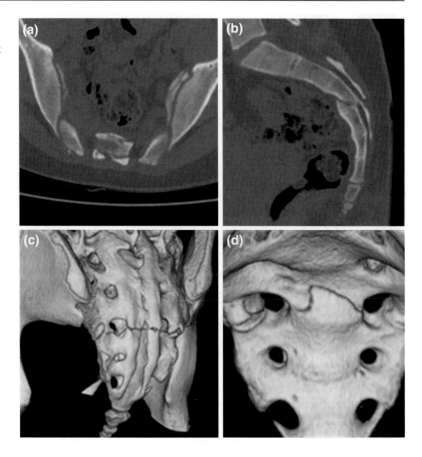

Elasto-sonography is a modern technique of diagnostic imaging that allows to visualize tissues' elasticity on a colorimetric scale, after the examined tissues, such as tendons, have undergone a continuous mechanical stress, performed by ultrasound impulses that come from the probe. Nowadays, this technique is largely used for traumatic and inflammatory diseases affecting musculoskeletal structures during the first hours after trauma; elasto-sonography allows the diagnosis of pathological signs of lesions that cannot be visualized with simple morphological ultrasound. Thus, elasto-sonography can be a very useful tool during follow-up after an injury, because it is possible to follow the changes occurring on affected structures, during the healing process, supporting the diagnosis, and planning the best therapy [20].

Using 3D and 4D probes , US images give morphological and functional accurate information [21], more and more precise and similar to images obtained with computed tomography and magnetic resonance imaging. It has to be mentioned that ultrasound technique is strictly dependent on the operator who performs the exam; this is why operators should be well experienced in sonography, in order to minimize the request for further invasive and expensive examinations when not needed. If used correctly, ultrasound can establish the indication for second-level diagnostic imaging, such as computed tomography and magnetic resonance imaging, in those cases when a deeper understating of the pathology is needed Figs. 21.5 and 21.6.

21.3 Computed Tomography

Computed tomography is a diagnostic tool that uses complex and modern techniques to obtain diagnostic images. It applies the energy coming from X-rays to create high-quality scans, with

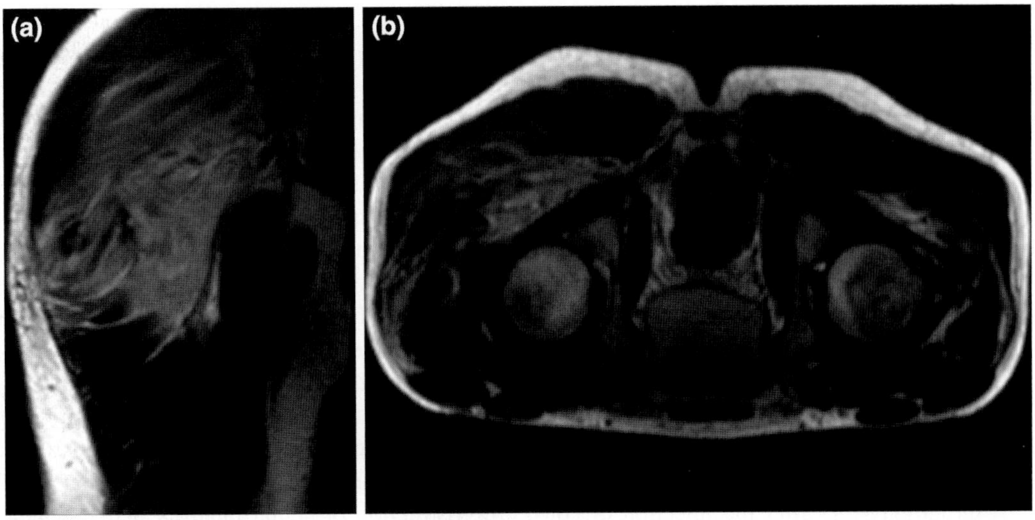

Fig. 21.6 (**a**) coronal (**b**) axial T1-weighted MRI with fat-suppression sequences showing muscle injury of the gluteal muscle after 7 days of blunt trauma: hyper intensity of the signal shows the hemorrhagic component in the injured tissue

maximum spatial resolution and short times of acquisition [22]. In newest CT scanners, named multilayer-multidetector, sophisticated software can measure the attenuation of an X-ray beam coming from the scanner on a spiral trajectory around the patient's body, showing different density of signal in the human body. Attenuated X-rays are supported from a group of detectors that turn data into diagnostic images using computed software. With imaging elaboration software, it is possible to evaluate the anatomical district of interest on multiplanar and tridimensional images, for a better understanding of the pathology. Density of the tissues is expressed as Hounsfield Units (HU), and it is represented on a specific scale of grays: high-density tissues, as bones, appear as barely intense gray, nearly white (hyperdense); low-density structures, as lungs, appear as a more intense gray color (hypodense), while intermediate-density tissues (isodense), are expressed with intermediate grade of gray [23].

The spatial resolution of these machine increases with the dose of X-rays administered to the patient, and this explains why the radiologist needs to know the complete clinical history of the patient in order to avoid a great exposure of the patient to unnecessary exams and unneeded doses of radiation.

In many agonistic sport activities, athletes may be involved in major injuries (e.g., motorcycle accidents, skiing accidents, martial arts, and bike accidents). In emergencies and major traumas, rapid and complete diagnostic evaluation of the patients can be obtained using computed tomography (CT) [24]. CT is particularly indicated in the study of polytrauma patients because it allows to obtain diagnostic images of the whole body in a few seconds and to diagnose all the damages that the trauma has caused. Computed tomography is also useful for the assessment of complex bone fractures, and for pathological fractures, thanks to multiplanar and 3D reconstruction software: with 3D reconstruction, it is now possible to visualize the bone in such an accurate way that conventional radiology does not allow. 3D reconstruction is particularly indicated for stress lesions on tarsal and carpal region, i.e., scaphoid bone and navicular bone; when these structures are involved, especially in athletes that do running, play gymnastics, or martial arts, it is often possible to observe future articular alterations that need to be prevented [25].

The important role of this technique is emphasized in post-surgical evaluation, when evaluating metallic means of synthesis after implantation in the bone; images obtained with conventional radiology and magnetic resonance imaging may result in many artifacts, instead CT allows the use on elaboration filters to reduce artifacts from metallic devices.

The use of organ-hyodate contrast medium gives many advantages that result in high-resolution imaging for the evaluation of splanchnic and vascular pathologies, both in acute and chronic conditions, as post-traumatic aneurisms or thrombosis, and spleen ruptures after traumas [26].

Arthrography-CT, after the injection of contrast medium, allows an excellent evaluation of intra-articular structures, with a specificity of 95 % and sensibility of 99 % in characterizing lesions on cross-ligaments of the knee; thus, it is particularly indicated in pathologies affecting the joints, especially cartilaginous articular structures, as in traumatic pathologies of the shoulder, when focal lesions or degenerative lesions need to be visualized.

Computed tomography shows many advantages if compared to other imaging techniques, including short times to perform the scans, the possibility to study the whole body with one scan, and a good image resolution; also, it is well tolerated by the patients who do not report claustrophobia as it happens often with MRI. There is only one limitation that is the use of X-rays on pediatric patients; though, applying reconstruction algorithms to standard CT scanners a dose reduction of 70 % can be obtained.

21.4   Magnetic Resonance Imaging

Magnetic resonance imaging (MRI) is a diagnostic non-invasive technique that uses high-intensity magnetic fields to obtain diagnostic multiplanar and multifunctional diagnostic images.

During the exam, the patient is placed in the middle of a magnetic field that influences the movements of hydrogen electrons inside the human body, creating a magnetization. Though specific radio-frequency impulses produced by the scanner, the movement of the electrons inside the magnetic field is disturbed and, after analyzing the complex changes occurring to the electrons, it is possible to generate the images [27]. The scanner is made of a magnet, producing the magnetic field, and radiofrequency coils, that are used to generate changes in the movement of electrons, and also of gradient coils that investigate spatial coordinates to create diagnostic images.

Sequences of acquisition protocols are composed by repeated series of radio impulses that allow a better visualization of the lesion, after reconstruction of signal intensity. MRI sequences of acquisition are several: inversion recovery, STIR, turbo spin echo, gradient echo, etc., and they can be T1-weighted sequences or T2-weighted. Each of them has specific physic properties, and they can be used if needed, according to the pathology of interest and the examined district, and if it is more important to study morphology or functionality [28].

MRI guarantees high spatial resolution of images, especially the newest technologies and high-field magnets, and it does not use X-rays, so the patient is not exposed to radiation. This is very useful for pediatric patients, and it can be used to evaluate radiological unknown fractures and impact bone lesions in young athletes. Also, MRI is used for the study of stress fractures of the calcaneus or cuboid that occur often in runners and gymnastic athletes, and for the evaluation of parenchymal lesions in major injuries [29].

MRI plays a primary role in the evaluation of lesion of the joints, tendons, ligaments, menisci, and it is different from other diagnostic techniques because it is very adjustable to the anatomical district of interest. Thanks to its great variability of acquisition, it allows to characterize the study for each patient with specific parameters while performing and to set the precise area of interest and the right sequences while performing.

Concerning   musculoskeletal   pathology involving cartilage, tendons, and bones, MRI is indicated as a second-level diagnostic tool. MRI

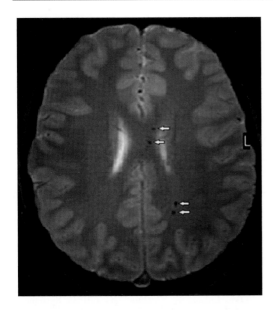

Fig. 21.7 Axial T2 FFE of a young boxer demonstrating the presence of multiple petechial hemorrhages (axonal injury) in the *white* matter and at junctional level of the corpus callosum

is often required after US examination has been performed. The association of these two techniques leads to high spatial resolution images and multiplanar morphological and functional characterization of lesions [30]. MRI is particularly suitable for the evaluation of cruciate ligaments of the knee, both in young and adult patients, reporting values of sensibility of 100 % and specificity of 100 % in diagnosing lesions affecting those ligaments. Values of sensibility and specificity may vary as the amount of time that has passed after the trauma. In recent literature, it has been reported that the use of this diagnostic technique is highly performing in a range of time from 24 to 48 h after a trauma, because there is a better visualization of fluids and edema involving soft tissues in this amount of time. Though, using specific STIR sequences, it is possible to evaluate musculoskeletal traumatic pathology up to 5 days after trauma has occurred, without using invasive methods as

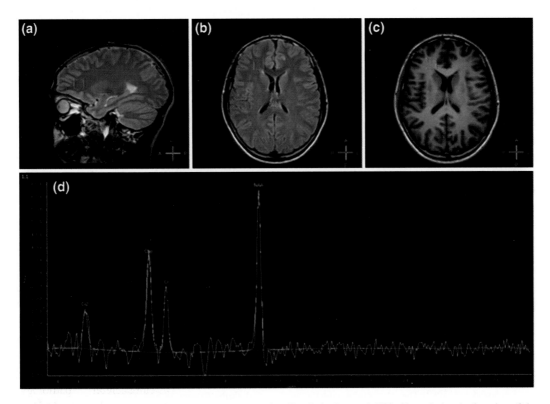

Fig. 21.8 Press (point-resolved spin-echo spectroscopy localized) single voxel (SV). To optimize the location of the voxel at the junction of the frontal cortical lobes, MR images on axial, coronal, and sagittal were used

arthroscopy [31]. MRI is also suggested for the study of pubalgia, because it can distinguish between different tissues, and it can differentiate diverse causes that lead to this affection, i.e., stress fractures frequent in runners, inflammatory states, lesions of the acetabular roof, inguinal hernia, coxa saltans Fig. 21.7.

Moreover, MRI is a great diagnostic tool for the evaluation of articular pathology in shoulder and knee, especially using arthrography-MRI after injection of paramagnetic contrast medium. In pathologies of the shoulder, it reveals data that would be unknown only using other techniques, particularly in rotator cuff's pathology and after surgical evaluation [32].

MRI also plays an important role for the study of the brain and brain stem, associated with CT in emergencies. Several study reported in medical literature show the diagnostic potential of MRI in polytrauma patient, in diagnosis and follow-up, especially for boxers: tractography-MRI has led to assessment of metabolic changes occurring in the brain of athletes after head concussion [33, 34].

MRI is a diagnostic technique that combines the absence of invasiveness for the patient, with high-resolution imaging. Major limitations are represented by long acquisition times, and by the presence of metal objects or devices inside the patients' body, if they are not compatible with magnetic fields; however, recent devices are most likely compatible and rare in young athletes. Claustrophobic patients and very young patients may need to be sedated before undergoing the exam. Since magnetic resonance imaging does not use radiation, it is feasible for young and adolescent patients Fig. 21.8.

References

1. International commission on radiological protection (2004) Managing patient dose in digital radiology, A report of the international commission on radiological protection. Ann ICRP. 34(1):1–73
2. Tehranzadeh J (1987) The spectrum of avulsion and avulsion-like injuries of the musculoskeletal system. Radiographics 7(5):945–974
3. Harper BE, Reveille JD (2009) Spondyloarthritis: clinical suspicion, diagnosis, and sports. Curr Sports Med Rep 8(1):29–34
4. Parikh SN, Allen M, Wall EJ, May MM, Laor T, Zbojniewicz AM, Eismann EA, Myer GD (2012) The reliability to determine "healing" in osteochondritis dissecans from radiographic assessment. J Pediatr Orthop 32(6):e35–e39
5. Park JC, McLaurin TM (2009) Acute syndesmosis injuries associated with ankle fractures: current perspectives in management. Bull NYU Hosp Jt Dis 67(1):39–44
6. Tochigi Y, Suh JS, Amendola A, Pedersen DR, Saltzman CL (2006) Ankle alignment on lateral radiographs. Part 1: sensitivity of measures to perturbations of ankle positioning. Foot Ankle Int 27(2):82–87
7. Potok PS, Hopper KD, Umlauf MJ (1995) Fractures of the acetabulum: imaging, classification, and understanding. Radiographics 15(1):7–23
8. Sierink JC, Saltzherr TP, Reitsma JB, Van Delden OM, Luitse JS, Goslings JC (2012) Systematic review and meta-analysis of immediate total-body computed tomography compared with selective radiological imaging of injured patients. Br J Surg 99(Suppl 1):52–58. doi:10.1002/bjs.7760
9. Nehrer S (2010) Differential diagnostics of the musculoskeletal system in sports medicine. Radiologe 50(5):427–434
10. MiedanyY El (2012) Musculoskeletal US: examining the joints. Br J Nurs 21(6):340–344
11. Cohen M, Vuillemin V, Jacob D (2011) Periarticular diseases of the hip in young adults J Radiol. 92(6): 515–23
12. Yim ES, Corrado G (2012) Ultrasound in sports medicine: relevance of emerging techniques to clinical care of athletes. Sports Med 42(8):665–680
13. Lento PH, Strakowski JA (2010) The use of ultrasound in guiding musculoskeletal interventional procedures. Phys Med Rehabil Clin N Am 21(3):559–583
14. Zamorani MP, Valle M (2007) Muscle and tendon. In: Bianchi S, Martinoli C (ed.) Ultrasound of the musculoskeletal system. Springer, Berlin
15. Ahmed R, Nazarian LN (2010) Overview of musculoskeletal sonography. Ultrasound Q. 26: 27–35
16. Fanucci E, Masala S, Fabiano S, Perugia D, Squillaci E, Varrucciu V, Simonetti G (2004) Treatment of intermetatarsal Morton's neuroma with alcohol injection under US guide: 10 month follow-up. Eur Radiol 14(3):514–518
17. D'Agostino MA, Said-Nahal R, Hacquard-Bouder C, Brasseur JL, Dougados M, Breban M (2003) Assessment of peripheral enthesitis in the spondylarthropathies by ultrasonography combined with power Doppler: a cross-sectional study. Arthritis Rheum 48:523–533
18. Hirschmüller A, Frey V, Konstantinidis L, Baur H, Dickhuth HH, Südkamp NP, Helwig P (2012)

Prognostic value of achilles tendon doppler sonography in asymptomatic runners. Med Sci Sports Exerc. 44(2):199–205

19. Tok F, Demirkaya E, Özçakar L (2011) Musculoskeletal ultrasound in pediatric rheumatology. PediatrRheumatol Online J 9:25

20. Rist HJ, Mauch M (2012) Quantified TDI elastography of the patellar tendon in athletes. Sportverletz Sportschaden 26(1):27–32

21. Naredo E, Möller I, Acebes C, Batlle-Gualda E, Brito E, de Agustín JJ, de Miguel E, Martínez A, Mayordomo L, Moragues C, Rejón E, Rodríguez A, Uson J, Garrido J (2010) Three-dimensional volumetric ultrasonography, does it improve reliability of musculoskeletal ultrasound? Clin Exp Rheumatol. 28(1):79–82

22. Reimann AJ, Davison C, Bjarnason T, Yogesh T, Kryzmyk K, Mayo J, Nicolaou S (2012) Organ-based computed tomographic (CT) radiation dose reduction to the lenses: impact on image quality for CT of the head. J Comput Assist Tomogr 36(3):334–338

23. Incidental findings on computed tomography scans in children with mild head trauma (2012) Ortega HW, Vander Velden H, Reid S. ClinPediatr (Phila)

24. Buckwalter KA (2009) Current concepts and advances: computerized tomography in sports medicine. Sports Med Arthrosc 17(1):13–20

25. Calisir C, Fayad LM, Carrino JA, Fishman EK (2012) Recognition, assessment, and treatment of non-union after surgical fixation of fractures: emphasis on 3D CT. Jpn J Radiol 30(1):1–9

26. Perlowski AA, Jaff MR (2010) Vascular disorders in athletes. Vasc Med 15(6):469–479

27. Haake EM, Brown BW, Thompson MR, Venkatesan R (1999) Magnetic resonance imaging: physical principles and sequence design. J Wiley-Liss

28. Dwek JR, Cardoso F, Chung CB (2009) MR imaging of overuse injuries in the skeletally immature gymnast: spectrum of soft-tissue endosseous lesions in the hand and wrist. PediatrRadiol. 39(12):1310–6. Epub 2009 Oct 22

29. Megliola A, Eutropi F, Scorzelli A et al (2006) Ultrasound and magnetic resonance imaging in sports-related muscle injuries. Musculoskelet Radiol 111:836–845

30. Ho-Fung VM, Jaimes C, Jaramillo D (2011) MR imaging of ACL injuries in pediatric and adolescent patients. Clin Sports Med 30(4):707–726

31. Jans LB, Jaremko JL, Ditchfield M, Verstraete KL (2011) MR imaging findings of lesions involving cartilage and bone in the paediatric knee: a pictorial review. JBR-BTR 94(5):247–253

32. Chauvin NA, Jaimes C, Laor T, Jaramillo D (2012) Magnetic resonance imaging of the pediatric shoulder. Magn Reson Imaging Clin N Am 20(2):327–347

33. Hunter JV, Wilde EA, Tong KA, Holshouser BA (2012) Emerging imaging tools for use with traumatic brain injury research. J Neurotrauma 29(4):654–671

34. Zhang L, Heier LA, Zimmerman RD, Jordan B, Ulug AM (2006) Diffusion anisotropy changes in the brains of professional boxers. AJNR Am J Neuroradiol 27(9):2000–2004

Index

Printing and Binding: Stürtz GmbH, Würzburg